Practical Radiation Oncology for Surgeons

Editor

CHRISTOPHER G. WILLETT

SURGICAL ONCOLOGY CLINICS OF NORTH AMERICA

www.surgonc.theclinics.com

Consulting Editor
NICHOLAS J. PETRELLI

July 2013 • Volume 22 • Number 3

ELSEVIER

1600 John F. Kennedy Boulevard • Suite 1800 • Philadelphia, Pennsylvania, 19103-2899

http://www.theclinics.com

SURGICAL ONCOLOGY CLINICS OF NORTH AMERICA Volume 22, Number 3
July 2013 ISSN 1055-3207, ISBN-13: 978-1-4557-7614-6

Editor: Jessica McCool

Surgical Oncology Clinics of North America (ISSN 1055-3207) is published quarterly by Elsevier Inc., 360 Park Avenue South, New York, NY 10010-1710. Months of publication are January, April, July, and October. Business and Editorial Offices: 1600 John F. Kennedy Blvd., Ste. 1800, Philadelphia, PA 19103-2899. Customer Service Office: 3251 Riverport Lane, Maryland Heights, MO 63043. Periodicals postage paid at New York, NY and additional mailing offices. Subscription prices are $274.00 per year (US individuals), $401.00 (US institutions) $135.00 (US student/resident), $314.00 (Canadian individuals), $498.00 (Canadian institutions), $193.00 (Canadian student/resident), $392.00 (foreign individuals), $498.00 (foreign institutions), and $193.00 (foreign student/resident). Foreign air speed delivery is included in all *Clinics* subscription prices. All prices are subject to change without notice. **POSTMASTER**: Send address changes to *Surgical Oncology Clinics of North America*, Elsevier Health Science Division, Subscription Customer Service, 3251 Riverport Lane, Maryland Heights, MO 63043. **Customer Service: 1-800-654-2452 (US and Canada). 314-447-8871 (outside U.S. and Canada). Fax: 314-447-8029. E-mail: journalscustomerservice-usa@elsevier.com** (for print support); **journalsonline support-usa@elsevier.com** (for online support).

Reprints. For copies of 100 or more, of articles in this publication, please contact the Commercial Reprints Department, Elsevier Inc., 360 Park Avenue South, New York, New York 10010-1710. Tel. 212-633-3813; Fax: 212-462-1935; E-mail: reprints@elsevier.com.

Surgical Oncology Clinics of North America is covered in *MEDLINE/PubMed (Index Medicus)* and *EMBASE/ Excerpta Medica, Current Contents/Clinical Medicine,* and *ISI/BIOMED.*

Printed and bound by CPI Group (UK) Ltd, Croydon, CR0 4YY

Transferred to digital print 2012

Contributors

CONSULTING EDITOR

NICHOLAS J. PETRELLI, MD, FACS
Bank of America Endowed Medical Director, Helen F. Graham Cancer Center at Christiana Care, Newark, Delaware; Professor of Surgery, Thomas Jefferson University, Philadelphia, Pennsylvania

EDITOR

CHRISTOPHER G. WILLETT, MD
Professor and Chairman, Department of Radiation Oncology, Duke University Medical Center, Durham, North Carolina

AUTHORS

JONATHAN B. ASHMAN, MD, PhD
Department of Radiation Oncology, Mayo Clinic Arizona, Scottsdale, Arizona

CHRISTOPHER BEAUCHAMP, MD
Department of Orthopedic Surgery, Mayo Clinic Arizona, Scottsdale, Arizona

RACHEL C. BLITZBLAU, MD, PhD
Assistant Professor, Department of Radiation Oncology, Duke University Medical Center, Durham, North Carolina

BRIAN E. BRIGMAN, MD, PhD
Associate Professor, Departments of Orthopaedic Surgery and Pediatrics, Duke University Medical Center, Durham, North Carolina

DAVID M. BRIZEL, MD
Professor, Department of Radiation Oncology; Division of Otolaryngology, Department of Surgery, Duke University Medical Center, Durham, North Carolina

ALVIN R. CABRERA, MD
Assistant Professor, Department of Radiation Oncology, Duke University Medical Center, Durham, North Carolina

JUNZO CHINO, MD
Associate Professor for Angeles Secord, Assistant Professor, Department of Radiation Oncology, Duke University Medical Center, Durham, North Carolina

BRIAN G. CZITO, MD
Associate Professor, Department of Radiation Oncology, Duke University Medical Center, Durham, North Carolina

MARK W. DEWHIRST, DVM, PhD, FASTRO, FAAAS
Gustavo S. Montana Professor, Department of Radiation Oncology; Department
of Pathology, Duke University Medical Center; Biomedical Engineering Department,
Duke University, Durham, North Carolina

WILLIAM C. EWARD, DVM, MD
Assistant Professor, Department of Orthopaedic Surgery, Duke University Medical
Center, Durham, North Carolina

RICHARD J. GRAY, MD
Division of Surgical Oncology, Department of Surgery, Mayo Clinic Arizona,
Scottsdale, Arizona

LEONARD L. GUNDERSON, MD, MS
Emeritus Professor and Consultant, Department of Radiation Oncology, Mayo Clinic
Arizona, Scottsdale, Arizona

MICHAEL G. HADDOCK, MD
Department of Radiation Oncology, Mayo Clinic, Rochester, Minnesota

JACQUES HEPPELL, MD
Division of Colorectal Surgery, Department of Surgery, Mayo Clinic Arizona,
Scottsdale, Arizona

CHRISTINA L. HOFMANN, MS
Department of Biomedical Engineering, Duke University, Durham, North Carolina

THEODORE S. HONG, MD
Department of Radiation Oncology, Massachusetts General Hospital, Harvard Medical
School, Boston, Massachusetts

JANET K. HORTON, MD
Assistant Professor, Department of Radiation Oncology, Duke University Medical Center,
Durham, North Carolina

LISA A. KACHNIC, MD
Department of Radiation Oncology, Boston Medical Center, Boston University
School of Medicine, Boston, Massachusetts

CHRIS R. KELSEY, MD
Associate Professor, Department of Radiation Oncology, Duke Cancer Institute,
Duke University Medical Center, Durham, North Carolina

JOHN P. KIRKPATRICK, MD, PhD
Associate Professor, Department of Radiation Oncology; Assistant Professor,
Department of Surgery, Duke Cancer Institute, Duke University Medical Center,
Durham, North Carolina

DAVID G. KIRSCH, MD, PhD
Associate Professor, Departments of Radiation Oncology and Pharmacology and Cancer
Biology, Duke University Medical Center, Durham, North Carolina

BRIDGET F. KOONTZ, MD
Butler-Harris Assistant Professor, Department of Radiation Oncology, Duke University
Medical Center, Durham, North Carolina

CHELSEA D. LANDON, MS
Department of Pathology, Duke University Medical Center, Durham, North Carolina

NICOLE A. LARRIER, MD, MSc
Assistant Professor, Department of Radiation Oncology, Duke University Medical Center, Durham, North Carolina

W. ROBERT LEE, MD, MEd, MS
Professor, Department of Radiation Oncology, Duke University Medical Center, Durham, North Carolina

HOWARD LEVINSON, MD, FACS
Assistant Professor, Division of Plastic and Reconstructive Surgery, Department of Surgery, Duke University Medical Center, Durham, North Carolina

HARVEY J. MAMON, MD, PhD
Department of Radiation Oncology, Brigham and Women's Hospital/Dana-Farber Cancer Institute, Harvard Medical School, Boston, Massachusetts

JEFFREY MEYER, MD
Assistant Professor, Department of Radiation Oncology, The University of Texas Southwestern Medical Center, Dallas, Texas

ADYR MOSS, MD
Division of Transplant Surgery, Department of Surgery, Mayo Clinic Arizona, Scottsdale, Arizona

HEIDI NELSON, MD
Division of Colorectal Surgery, Department of Surgery, Mayo Clinic, Rochester, Minnesota

IVY A. PETERSEN, MD
Department of Radiation Oncology, Mayo Clinic, Rochester, Minnesota

BARBARA A. POCKAJ, MD
Division of Surgical Oncology, Department of Surgery, Mayo Clinic Arizona, Scottsdale, Arizona

JENNIFER L. PRETZ, MD
Harvard Radiation Oncology Program, Harvard Medical School, Boston, Massachusetts

RICHARD F. RIEDEL, MD
Assistant Professor, Division of Medical Oncology, Department of Internal Medicine, Duke University Medical Center, Durham, North Carolina

LEWIS ROSENBERG, MD, PhD
Department of Radiation Oncology, University of North Carolina, Chapel Hill, North Carolina

JOSEPH K. SALAMA, MD
Associate Professor, Department of Radiation Oncology, Duke Cancer Institute, Duke University Medical Center, Durham, North Carolina

JOHN H. SAMPSON, MD, PhD
Associate Professor, Department of Radiation Oncology; Professor, Department of Surgery, Duke Cancer Institute, Duke University Medical Center, Durham, North Carolina

ANGELES ALVAREZ SECORD, MD
Division of Gynecologic Oncology, Department of Obstetrics and Gynecology,
Duke Cancer Institute, Duke University Medical Center, Durham, North Carolina

PAUL R. STAUFFER, MSEE, CCE
Professor, Department of Radiation Oncology, Duke University Medical Center, Durham,
North Carolina

JOEL TEPPER, MD
Department of Radiation Oncology, University of North Carolina, Chapel Hill,
North Carolina

JENNIFER Y. WO, MD
Department of Radiation Oncology, Massachusetts General Hospital, Harvard Medical
School, Boston, Massachusetts

FANG-FANG YIN, PhD
Professor, Department of Radiation Oncology, Duke Cancer Institute, Duke University
Medical Center, Durham, North Carolina

DAVID S. YOO, MD, PhD
Assistant Professor, Department of Radiation Oncology, Duke University Medical Center,
Durham, North Carolina

Contents

Foreword　　　　　　　　　　　　　　　　　　　　　　　　　　　　　**xiii**

Nicholas J. Petrelli

Preface: Practical Radiation Oncology for Surgeons　　　　　　　　**xv**

Christopher G. Willett

Integration of Radiation Oncology with Surgery as Combined-Modality Treatment　　**405**

Leonard L. Gunderson, Jonathan B. Ashman, Michael G. Haddock,
Ivy A. Petersen, Adyr Moss, Jacques Heppell, Richard J. Gray,
Barbara A. Pockaj, Heidi Nelson, and Christopher Beauchamp

> Integration of surgery and radiation (external beam, EBRT; intraoperative, IORT) has become more routine for patients with locally advanced primary cancers and those with local-regional relapse. This article discusses patient selection and treatment from a more general perspective, followed by a discussion of patient selection and treatment factors in select disease sites (pancreas cancer, colorectal cancer, retroperitoneal soft-tissue sarcomas). Outcomes with combined modality treatment (surgery, EBRT alone or with concurrent chemotherapy, IORT) are discussed. The ultimate in contemporary integration of radiation and surgery is found in patients who are candidates for surgery plus both EBRT and IORT.

Practical Radiation Oncology for Extremity Sarcomas　　　　　　　**433**

Nicole A. Larrier, David G. Kirsch, Richard F. Riedel, Howard Levinson,
William C. Eward, and Brian E. Brigman

> Soft tissue sarcomas are rare cancers. They should be managed by a multidisciplinary team with experience caring for these diverse malignancies. Local control is frequently achieved with a combination of radiation therapy and surgery. This article reviews the data supporting the role of adjuvant radiotherapy in the care of patients with soft tissue sarcoma and describes the side effects of surgery and radiation therapy. Preoperative radiation therapy increases the risk of wound complication from surgery, but has fewer long-term side effects than postoperative radiation therapy. The timing of radiation therapy can be tailored to each patient.

Radiotherapy and Radiosurgery for Tumors of the Central Nervous System　　**445**

John P. Kirkpatrick, Fang-Fang Yin, and John H. Sampson

> In this article, the application of radiotherapy, alone and in combination with surgery and chemotherapy, in the treatment of metastases to the brain (the most common malignant brain lesion), primary malignant gliomas (the most common malignant primary brain tumor), and metastases to the osseous spine is reviewed. Brain metastases may be treated with surgical resection, whole-brain radiotherapy, stereotactic radiosurgery, or some combination of these treatments. The optimum treatment of brain

metastases is a matter of controversy, and patient and disease factors favoring one approach over another are presented.

Stereotactic Body Radiation Therapy for Treatment of Primary and Metastatic Pulmonary Malignancies   463

Chris R. Kelsey and Joseph K. Salama

Stereotactic body radiation therapy (SBRT) has become the preferred treatment approach for patients with stage I non–small cell lung cancer who are medically inoperable or refuse surgery. SBRT consists of 3 to 5 radiation treatments delivered over a 10- to 14-day period. Local control is achieved in approximately 90% of patients, and the risk of toxicity is relatively low. Ongoing studies are examining whether SBRT can replace surgery for certain patients, the optimal dose-fractionation scheme, and how best to treat patients having central tumors near the primary tracheo-bronchial tree.

Radiation Therapy for Prostate Cancer   483

Bridget F. Koontz and W. Robert Lee

Radiation therapy is an effective treatment for newly diagnosed prostate cancer, salvage treatment, or for palliation of advanced disease. Herein we briefly discuss the indications, results, and complications associated with brachytherapy and external beam radiotherapy, when used as mono-therapy and in combination with each other or androgen deprivation.

Image-guided Brachytherapy for Gynecologic Surgeons   495

Junzo Chino and Angeles Alvarez Secord

Brachytherapy is a fundamental component of the definitive treatment of many advanced gynecologic malignancies, most notably cancers of the uterine corpus and cervix, and allows high radiation doses to be delivered to the target while minimizing the normal tissue dose. However, dose specification has been based primarily on points visible on plain radio-graphs, with limited correlation to a patient's anatomy and extent of dis-ease. Recent advances have allowed more customized volume-based specification of dose, which has allowed improvements in outcomes. This article reviews these advances using cervical cancer as a model, and looks to future directions with this promising treatment.

Chemoradiation Therapy: Localized Esophageal, Gastric, and Pancreatic Cancer   511

Jennifer L. Pretz, Jennifer Y. Wo, Harvey J. Mamon, Lisa A. Kachnic, and Theodore S. Hong

Chemoradiation plays an important role in management of locally advanced gastrointestinal tumors. This article reviews data regarding chemoradiation for tumors of the upper gastrointestinal tract. For esophageal and gastro-esophageal junction cancers, chemoradiation is standard of care in the preoperative setting. In gastric cancer, two standards have emerged: defin-itively treating with perioperative chemotherapy alone and using chemora-diation postoperatively. For pancreatic cancer, the benefit of radiation is less well-defined. The future of treatment sites lies in trials evaluating new chemotherapy regimens, alternative systemic therapies, and different radiation fractionation schema. Because care of these patients is complex, multimodality team evaluation before treatment is encouraged.

Radiation Therapy in Anal and Rectal Cancer   525

Brian G. Czito and Jeffrey Meyer

Historically, squamous cell carcinoma of the anal canal was treated with abdominoperineal resection. Nigro discovered that radiation therapy combined with 5-fluorouracil and mitomycin resulted in high rates of local control and colostomy-free and overall survival without surgical intervention. Recent advances include the integration of PET into staging, radiation treatment planning, disease monitoring, and the use of intensity-modulated radiation therapy. For rectal cancer, clinical trials have established the role for neoadjuvant therapy for T3-4 and/or node-positive tumor presentations. Chemotherapy and targeted agents are under study in both anal and rectal cancers to improve on the standard combinations of chemotherapy and radiation.

Novel Approaches to Treatment of Hepatocellular Carcinoma and Hepatic Metastases Using Thermal Ablation and Thermosensitive Liposomes   545

Mark W. Dewhirst, Chelsea D. Landon, Christina L. Hofmann, and Paul R. Stauffer

Because of the limitations of surgical resection, thermal ablation is commonly used for the treatment of hepatocellular carcinoma and liver metastases. Current methods of ablation can result in marginal recurrences of larger lesions and in tumors located near large vessels. This review presents a novel approach for extending treatment out to the margins where temperatures do not provide complete treatment with ablation alone, by combining thermal ablation with drug-loaded thermosensitive liposomes. A history of the development of thermosensitive liposomes is presented. Clinical trials have shown that the combination of radiofrequency ablation and doxorubicin-loaded thermosensitive liposomes is a promising treatment.

Radiotherapy After Mastectomy   563

Rachel C. Blitzblau and Janet K. Horton

Classic randomized trials documented the benefit of postmastectomy radiotherapy in women with node-positive or locally advanced breast cancer. Modern advances in surgical therapy, systemic therapy, and radiotherapy, however, along with an improved understanding of cancer biology, have called into question previously assumed recurrence risks and treatment benefits. This article explores the impact of tumor biology and genomic medicine on utilization of postmastectomy radiotherapy and how treatment decision-making is moving beyond TNM-based predictors.

Contemporary Radiotherapy in Head and Neck Cancer: Balancing Chance for Cure with Risk for Complication   579

Alvin R. Cabrera, David S. Yoo, and David M. Brizel

Radiotherapy plays an integral role in the management of most patients with cancers of the head and neck. Better understanding of radiobiology and radiation physics has allowed radiation oncologists to enhance the tumoricidal effects of radiation and reduce the severity of normal tissue toxicities. This article reviews the biologic foundation of head and neck radiotherapy, the physical principles and technological innovations that enable delivery of highly conformal radiation, the acute and late complications of radiation-based treatments, and the clinical evidence supporting contemporary practice.

Present and Future Innovations in Radiation Oncology   **599**

Lewis Rosenberg and Joel Tepper

The purpose of this article is to provide a review of innovations in radiation oncology that have been recently adopted as well as those that are likely to be adopted in the near future. Physics and engineering innovations, including image-guidance technologies and charged particle therapy, are discussed. Biologic innovations, including novel radiation sensitizers, functional imaging for use in treatment planning, and altered fractionation, are also discussed.

Index   **619**

SURGICAL ONCOLOGY
CLINICS OF NORTH AMERICA

FORTHCOMING ISSUES

October 2013
Translational Cancer Research for Surgeons
William G. Cance, MD, *Editor*

January 2014
Colorectal Cancer
Nancy N. Baxter, MD, PhD and
Marcus Burnstein, MD, *Editors*

April 2014
Biliary Tract and Primary Liver Tumors
Timothy M. Pawlik, MD, *Editor*

RECENT ISSUES

April 2013
Multidisciplinary Care of the Cancer Patient
Gregory A. Masters, MD, *Editor*

January 2013
Laparoscopic Approaches in Oncology
James Fleshman, MD, *Editor*

October 2012
**Treatment of Peritoneal Surface
Malignancies**
Jesus Esquivel, MD, *Editor*

NOW AVAILABLE FOR YOUR iPhone and iPad

FORTHCOMING ISSUES

RECENT ISSUES

Foreword

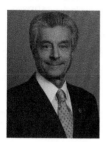

Nicholas J. Petrelli, MD, FACS
Consulting Editor

The editor for this edition of the *Surgical Oncology Clinics of North America* is Christopher G. Willett, MD, Professor and Chairman of Radiation Oncology at Duke University Medical Center. Dr Willett chairs one of the country's largest and most active academic radiation oncology programs.

This issue of the *Surgical Oncology Clinics of North America* is entitled, "Practical Radiation Oncology for Surgeons," and as Dr Willett highlights in his Preface, this issue emphasizes the role of radiation oncology in the management of patients with cancer that impacts the daily practice of surgeons. Radiation oncology is a key element in the multidisciplinary approach to cancer care. Surgeons work closely with radiation and medical oncologists along with subspecialities to deliver cutting-edge cancer treatment to patients.

In this issue of the *Surgical Oncology Clinics of North America*, Dr Willett has assembled an outstanding group of professionals emphasizing the complementary roles of radiation therapy and surgery in the management of patients with soft tissue sarcomas, brain metastases, lung cancer, prostate cancer, and gynecologic cancers.

Dr Willett has spent his career developing clinical trials for patients with gastrointestinal malignancies. His commitment to the care of patients with gastrointestinal malignancies has been at the bedside and in laboratory research. Hence, it is not surprising that there are outstanding articles in this issue highlighting the approaches to these malignancies and also a discussion of future treatment strategies.

Further excellent discussions center around breast cancer and head and neck cancers, where the involvement of the three major disciplines of surgery, radiation, and medical oncology are critical. As radiation technology continues to advance, surgeons need to understand the principles behind these advancements to communicate with their colleagues.

I would like to thank Dr Willett for the time and effort he and his colleagues have put into this issue of the *Surgical Oncology Clinics of North America*. This issue of the

Surg Oncol Clin N Am 22 (2013) xiii–xiv
http://dx.doi.org/10.1016/j.soc.2013.02.014
1055-3207/13/$ – see front matter © 2013 Published by Elsevier Inc.

surgonc.theclinics.com

Surgical Oncology Clinics of North America demonstrates the important relationship between radiation and surgical oncologists in the multidisciplinary approach to cancer care.

Nicholas J. Petrelli, MD, FACS
Helen F. Graham Cancer Center at Christiana Care
4701 Ogletown-Stanton Road, Suite 1213
Newark, DE 19713, USA

E-mail address:
npetrelli@christianacare.org

Preface

Practical Radiation Oncology for Surgeons

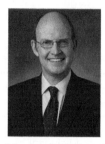

Christopher G. Willett, MD
Editor

This issue, devoted to "Practical Radiation Oncology for Surgeons" highlights the contemporary role of radiation oncology in the management of the cancer patient that impacts the daily practice of surgeons.

This issue is divided into 12 articles. Each article is written by expert radiation oncologists with extensive subspecialty experience and a record of effective collaboration with their surgical colleagues.

Dr Gunderson and colleagues first provide the context of the theme of this issue: the optimal integration of radiation therapy with surgery. This includes a thorough discussion of the principles, as well as illustrations of this integration, and a perspective of intraoperative radiation therapy, a therapy that truly forges the close collaboration of surgeons and radiation oncologists in the operating room.

In the second article, Dr Kirsch and associates thoroughly portray the complementary yet changing roles of radiation therapy and surgery in the management of patients with soft tissue sarcomas. There is a perspective of the important role of reconstructive surgery in the multimodality management of these challenging malignancies.

One of the more recent developments in radiation oncology is radiosurgery and stereotactic body radiation therapy (SBRT). Drs Kirkpatrick, Yin, and Sampson carefully examine the role of radiosurgery in the management of patients with cranial metastases. With increased experience and technological advances spurred by cranial radiosurgery, investigators have applied these principles and techniques to thoracic and abdominal malignancies. Drs Kelsey and Salama outline the techniques and the promising experience of SBRT in the treatment of patients with primary and metastatic lung malignancies. In selected patients, this technique provides potentially curative outcomes and is a viable alternative to surgery.

Facilitated by CT, MRI, and PET-CT imaging and impressive technical innovations in radiation therapy planning and administration, there has been substantive progress in brachytherapy for patients with prostate and gynecologic cancer. Brachytherapy

Surg Oncol Clin N Am 22 (2013) xv–xvi
http://dx.doi.org/10.1016/j.soc.2013.02.013
1055-3207/13/$ – see front matter © 2013 Published by Elsevier Inc.

has many clinical and practical advantages: an enhanced therapeutic ratio, lower cost, and enhanced convenience to patients and providers. Drs Koontz and Lee provide an excellent discussion of current clinical practices in prostate cancer as do Drs Chino and Secord in gynecologic cancers.

Over the past 20 years, there have been significant gains in the multimodality treatment of patients with localized gastrointestinal cancer. These gains have been achieved by technical advances in surgery, new cytotoxic and targeted systemic agents, and the effective integration of radiation therapy into these treatment plans. The articles by Drs Pretz, Wo, Mamon, Kachnic, and Hong in upper abdominal gastrointestinal cancers and Drs Meyer and Czito in lower gastrointestinal malignancies highlight these approaches and importantly emphasize the controversies in contemporary and future treatment strategies. In an interesting article, Dr Dewhirst and colleagues describe an innovative and cutting edge approach of thermal ablation and heat-sensitive liposomes in the treatment of patients with hepatic malignancies.

For decades, breast cancer and head and neck cancer have been managed jointly by surgeons and radiation oncologists. This collaboration is as relevant today as earlier and is increasingly based on enhanced understanding of the biology and natural history of these malignancies and facilitated by technical advances in imaging and treatment. In this setting, Drs Blitzblau and Horton describe the changing role of postoperative radiation therapy in the management of breast cancer. Drs Cabrera, Yoo, and Brizel outline the therapeutic gains in head and neck cancer patients by modern radiation therapy and imaging, and the important role of viral status on the outcome of patients with oral pharyngeal cancer.

Finally, Drs Rosenberg and Tepper conclude with an excellent overview of the innovations of radiation therapy and their relevance to surgeons. They look positively and critically to future approaches, as well as investigative opportunities.

I would like to thank the authors for their thoughtful contributions to this issue of *Surgical Oncology Clinics of North America*, as well as Dr Nicholas Petrelli for providing us with this unique opportunity.

Christopher G. Willett, MD
Department of Radiation Oncology
Duke University Medical Center, Box 3085
Durham, NC 27710, USA

E-mail address:
christopher.willett@duke.edu

Integration of Radiation Oncology with Surgery as Combined-Modality Treatment

Leonard L. Gunderson, MD, MS[a],*, Jonathan B. Ashman, MD, PhD[a],
Michael G. Haddock, MD[b], Ivy A. Petersen, MD[b], Adyr Moss, MD[c],
Jacques Heppell, MD[d], Richard J. Gray, MD[e],
Barbara A. Pockaj, MD[e], Heidi Nelson, MD[f],
Christopher Beauchamp, MD[g]

KEYWORDS

- Surgery and radiation integration • Combined modality treatment
- Patient selection criteria • Intraoperative radiation

KEY POINTS

- Patient selection criteria: For patients with locally advanced primary cancer (borderline resectable, locally unresectable) or local-regional cancer relapse, the decision to proceed with combined-modality treatment that includes both surgery and radiation (external beam [EBRT], intraoperative [IORT]) should be determined by the surgeon and radiation oncologist in the setting of a joint preoperative consultation, whenever feasible.
- Patient evaluation: The pretreatment patient workup should include a detailed evaluation of the extent of the locally advanced primary or locally recurrent lesion combined with studies to rule out hematogenous or peritoneal spread of disease.
- Sequencing of surgery, EBRT, and IORT: Optimal sequencing of surgery and EBRT for locally advanced primary or local-regionally recurrent cancers should be discussed and determined at the time of a joint multispecialty consultation involving a surgeon, radiation oncologist, and often a medical oncologist. This collaboration allows input from all specialists with regard to studies that would be helpful for IORT and EBRT treatment planning, as well as whether IORT may be appropriate.

Continued

[a] Department of Radiation Oncology, Mayo Clinic Arizona, 13400 East Shea Boulevard, Scottsdale, AZ 85259, USA; [b] Department of Radiation Oncology, Mayo Clinic, 200 First Street South West, Rochester, MN 55905, USA; [c] Division of Transplant Surgery, Department of Surgery, Mayo Clinic Arizona, 13400 East Shea Boulevard, Scottsdale, AZ 85259, USA; [d] Division of Colorectal Surgery, Department of Surgery, Mayo Clinic Arizona, 13400 East Shea Boulevard, Scottsdale, AZ 85259, USA; [e] Division of Surgical Oncology, Department of Surgery, Mayo Clinic Arizona, 13400 East Shea Boulevard, Scottsdale, AZ 85259, USA; [f] Division of Colorectal Surgery, Department of Surgery, Mayo Clinic, 200 First Street South West, Rochester, MN 55905, USA; [g] Department of Orthopedic Surgery, Mayo Clinic Arizona, 13400 East Shea Boulevard, Scottsdale, AZ 85259, USA
* Corresponding author.
E-mail address: llg.scottsdale@cox.net

Surg Oncol Clin N Am 22 (2013) 405–432
http://dx.doi.org/10.1016/j.soc.2013.02.003
1055-3207/13/$ – see front matter © 2013 Elsevier Inc. All rights reserved.

surgonc.theclinics.com

Continued

- Combined modality treatment–related morbidity: In patients with locally advanced primary or locally recurrent malignancies, the issue of morbidity following aggressive treatment is placed into clearer perspective by a comparison with tumor-related morbidity. For instance, when EBRT is used as the only radiation modality for patients with residual disease following surgical resection of locally advanced rectal cancer or those with locally recurrent colorectal cancers, more than 90% of patients have local persistence or relapse of disease, and most are dead within 2 to 3 years (end result is nearly 100% tumor-related morbidity and/or mortality).

INTRODUCTION

Integration of surgery and radiation has become more routine for patients with locally advanced cancers at many disease sites. The intent of this article is to discuss general patient selection, patient evaluation, and treatment factors with regard to issues that cross a variety of disease sites. This discussion is followed by presentation of patient selection and treatment factors for select disease sites (pancreas cancer, colorectal cancer, and retroperitoneal soft-tissue sarcomas) and a discussion of combined-modality treatment outcomes that include surgery, external-beam radiation (EBRT) alone, EBRT plus concurrent chemotherapy (chemoRT), and intraoperative radiation (IORT). The ultimate in contemporary integration of radiation oncology with surgery is found in patients who are candidates for surgery plus both EBRT and IORT.[1,2]

GENERAL PATIENT SELECTION, EVALUATION, AND TREATMENT FACTORS
Patient Selection Criteria

For patients with locally advanced (borderline resectable, locally unresectable) or locally recurrent cancers, the decision to proceed with combined-modality treatment that includes both surgery and radiation should be determined by the surgeon and radiation oncologist in the setting of a joint preoperative consultation, whenever feasible. Such a consultation allows input from both specialties with regard to studies that would be helpful for diagnosis and treatment planning, determination of optimal sequencing of surgery and external beam radiation (EBRT), as well as whether both EBRT and intraoperative radiation (IORT) are appropriate treatment modalities in addition to maximal surgical resection.

Patient Evaluation

The pretreatment patient workup should include a detailed evaluation of the extent of the locally advanced primary or locally recurrent lesion combined with studies to rule out hematogenous or peritoneal spread of disease. In addition to history and physical examination, the routine evaluation includes a complete blood count (CBC), liver and renal chemistries, chest film or computed tomography (CT), and tumor-specific serum tests (carcinoembryonic antigen [CEA], CA 19-9, CA-125, and so forth). When palpable pelvic primary tumors or relapses are immobile or fixed on rectal or bimanual examination, or symptoms suggest pelvic recurrence following primary resection, CT or magnetic resonance imaging (MRI) of the pelvis and abdomen can confirm lack of free space between the malignancy and a structure that may be surgically unresectable for cure (ie, presacrum, pelvic side wall). In such patients, preoperative chemoRT should be given before an attempt at resection. Distant metastatic spread should also be excluded with appropriate imaging (CT of chest/abdomen/thorax, positron emission tomography [PET or combined PET/CT], among others). If hematuria is present or findings on CT or MRI suggest bladder involvement, cystoscopy can be performed before or at the time of surgical exploration/resection.

Sequencing of Surgery, EBRT, and IORT

Optimal sequencing of surgery and EBRT for locally advanced or recurrent cancers should be discussed and determined at the time of a joint multispecialty consultation involving a surgeon, radiation oncologist, and, often, a medical oncologist.[2] Such collaboration allows input from all specialists with regard to studies that would be helpful for IORT and EBRT treatment planning as well as whether IORT may be appropriate. Specialized surgeons (vascular, plastics, and so forth) may also need to become involved in subsequent consultations.

For many patients with locally advanced primary or locally recurrent lesions, preoperative EBRT of 45 to 50 Gy in 1.8- to 2.0-Gy fractions (plus concurrent chemotherapy as indicated by disease site) followed by exploration and resection in 3 to 6 weeks offers theoretical advantages over a sequence of resection followed by EBRT. The potential advantages include the following: (1) deletion of patients with metastases detected at the restaging workup or laparotomy thus sparing the potential risks of aggressive surgical resection alone or plus IORT; (2) possible tumor shrinkage with an increased possibility of achieving a gross total R0 or R1 resection; (3) alteration of implantability of cells that may be disseminated at the time of an R1 or R2 surgical resection; (4) reduction of treatment interval between EBRT and IORT (when resection and IORT precede EBRT, if postoperative complications ensue, the delay to EBRT $\pm$ chemotherapy may be excessive); (5) intact vascular supply to tumor with better oxygenation; (6) better clinical tumor volume (CTV) definition when gross tumor is intact; (7) ability often to treat more conservative EBRT fields and exclude more dose-limiting organs and structures.

The following general criteria have guided the selection of appropriate patients for IORT at the authors' institution.[1,2] (1) By definition, there must be no medical contraindications for exploratory surgery and an attempt at gross total resection. (2) Surgery alone will not achieve acceptable local control because of the high probability of microscopic or gross residual disease after maximal resection, based on preoperative imaging. (3) EBRT doses needed for adequate local control following subtotal resection or unresectable disease would exceed normal tissue tolerance (60–70 Gy in 1.8–2.0 Gy for microscopic residual [R1 resection], 70–90 Gy for gross residual [R2 resection] or unresected disease). (4) IORT will be given at the time of a planned surgical procedure. (5) The IORT plus EBRT technique would likely result in a more suitable therapeutic ratio between cure and complications by permitting direct irradiation of unresected or marginally resected tumor while surgically displacing or shielding dose-limiting structures or organs. (6) There is no evidence of distant metastases or peritoneal seeding (rare exceptions: treatable single-organ metastasis, slow progression of systemic disease, or excellent systemic therapy options).

EBRT Doses and Technique

EBRT doses of 45 to 54 Gy are delivered in 1.8-Gy fractions, 5 days per week over 5 to 6 weeks in patients with no prior irradiation. For pelvic lesions, treatments are given with linear accelerators using at least 6 MV photons and 3-dimensional conformal radiation (3D-CRT) or intensity-modulated radiation (IMRT) techniques. With extrapelvic lesions, unresected or residual disease plus 3- to 5-cm margins of normal tissues are included to 40 to 45 Gy with 3D-CRT or IMRT. Reduced fields with margins of 2 to 3 cm are treated to 45 to 54 Gy. With a variety of disease sites (eg, gastrointestinal, gynecologic), concurrent chemotherapy is often given during EBRT with regimens based on 5-fluorouracil (5FU) or cisplatin.

For previously irradiated patients, an attempt is made to re-irradiate with low-dose preoperative EBRT (20–30 Gy in 1.8-Gy fractions or 1.5 Gy twice a day). This therapy is preferably delivered in combination with concurrent chemotherapy.

IORT Doses and Technique

In institutions that choose to have the availability of IORT as a component of treatment, a carefully constructed team needs to exist.[2] This team should include a surgeon, radiation oncologist, anesthesiologist, operating room nursing and radiation physicist (alone or plus a radiation therapist). IORT is delivered, after maximal surgical resection, with electron-beam radiation (IOERT), high-dose-rate brachytherapy (HDR-IORT), or electronic brachytherapy/low-kilovolt IORT, depending on institutional preference.[2,3]

IORT energy and dose are dependent on the amount of residual disease remaining after maximal resection, and on the EBRT component that has been given preoperatively or is feasible postoperatively.[2,3] For patients who have received standard preoperative EBRT doses of 45 to 54 Gy (1.8-Gy fractions, 5 days per week), the IORT dose usually varies from 10 to 20 Gy: narrow margins or microscopic residual, 10 to 12.5 Gy; gross residual, 15 to 20 Gy; unresectable disease, 20 Gy. In previously irradiated patients, the IORT dose is usually 15 to 20 Gy if EBRT doses of 20 to 30 Gy can be safely given preoperatively or postoperatively. IORT doses of 25 to 30 Gy have been given to patients in whom no or limited EBRT is planned, but such doses have higher risks of normal structure intolerance.

The biological effectiveness of single-dose IORT is considered equivalent to 1.5 to 2.5 times the same total dose of fractionated EBRT.[4] The effective dose in the IORT boost field, when added to the 45 to 50 Gy given with fractionated EBRT, is as follows: 60 to 70 Gy, IORT dose of 10 Gy; 75 to 87.5 Gy, 15-Gy IORT boost; 85 to 100 Gy, 20-Gy IORT boost.

Dose-Limiting Structures/Treatment-Related Morbidity

In patients with locally advanced primary or locally recurrent malignancies, the issue of morbidity following aggressive treatment is placed into clearer perspective by a comparison with tumor-related morbidity. For instance, when EBRT is used as the only radiation modality for patients with residual disease following surgical resection of locally advanced rectal cancer or those with locally recurrent colorectal cancers, more than 90% of patients have local persistence or relapse of disease, and most are dead within 2 to 3 years (the end result is nearly 100% tumor-related morbidity and/or mortality).

PATIENT SELECTION AND TREATMENT FACTORS BY DISEASE SITE
Pancreas Cancer

Patient evaluation and selection
The basic workup for a patient with pancreas cancer should consist of history, physical examination, basic laboratory studies (CBC, liver functions, renal function), and imaging studies. At present, most patients have a CT of the abdomen (with or without pelvis) followed by biopsy via CT or endoscopic ultrasonography (EUS) (**Table 1**). At Mayo Clinic Arizona (MCA), tissue diagnosis is preferably achieved at the time of EUS rather than with thin-needle biopsy at the time of an abdominal CT or ultrasound examination. Accurate clinical staging requires high-quality, multiphase, helical CT to accurately define the relationship of the pancreatic cancer to the celiac axis and superior mesenteric vessels in 3 dimensions, as well as the absence of extrapancreatic disease.

Table 1
Diagnostic algorithm for pancreas cancer, Mayo Clinic Arizona

Diagnostic Procedure	Diagnosis and Staging Capability	Recommend Routine Use
Primary tumor/regional nodes[a]		
Computed tomography (CT) of abdomen ± chest (pancreas protocol)	Most valuable modality to determine degree of extrapancreatic extension and distant metastases	Yes
Endoscopic ultrasonography (EUS) alone or with endoscopic retrograde cholangiopancreatography (ERCP)	More accurately defines involvement of pancreatic duct and inferior extent of biliary duct and lymph node involvement; predicts resectability	EUS: preferable, biopsy node(s), if feasible; ERCP: optional
Magnetic resonance imaging (MRI)	Clarify resectability if uncertain on CT	Optional
Metastatic workup		
Chest films	Screen for metastases (mets)	Yes
CT of chest	Will detect small mets better than chest film	Optional
Positron emission tomography (PET/CT)	Excellent for detecting unsuspected mets	Optional; encouraged with borderline or unresectable lesions before chemoradiation
Laparoscopy	May allow visualization of small surface liver metastases or peritoneal seeding	Optional; encouraged if plan preop. or primary chemoradiation and CA 19-9 markedly elevated (≥1000)

[a] Laboratory studies: complete blood count (CBC), creatinine, liver function studies (alkaline phosphatase [ALP], bilirubin, aspartate aminotransferase [AST], lactate dehydrogenase [LDH]), albumin. Tumor markers: CA 19-9 has high sensitivity (>90%) but low specificity (75%); carcinoembryonic antigen (CEA) (optional).

Objective, reproducible radiographic criteria are used to define disease extent and resectability. Potentially resectable disease is defined as: (1) the absence of extrapancreatic disease; (2) the absence of superior mesenteric or portal vein encasement, abutment or distortion, or associated thrombi, and presence of a patent superior mesenteric artery (SMA)–portal vein confluence; and (3) distinct fat planes around the SMA, celiac axis, and hepatic artery. The accuracy of CT in predicting unresectability and the inaccuracy of intraoperative assessment of resectability are both well established.[5,6] Borderline resectable tumors, which may benefit from neoadjuvant therapy, include tumors with (1) abutment or encasement of the SMV/portal vein without arterial involvement whereby sufficient vessel is present proximally and distally to permit resection and venous reconstruction; (2) gastroduodenal artery encasement without extension to the celiac axis and with or without abutment or minor encasement of the hepatic artery; and (3) abutment of less than 180° of the SMA.[7]

External-beam radiation

For patients with borderline resectable or unresectable cancers, preoperative chemoRT is preferably given before exploratory laparotomy and possible surgical resection alone or plus IOERT (**Table 2**).[8] At MCA, neoadjuvant gemcitabine plus

Table 2
Treatment algorithm for pancreas cancer, Mayo Clinic Arizona

Disease Extent	Surgery	Irradiation (Alone or with Chemotherapy)	Chemotherapy
TisN0M0	Pancreaticoduodenectomy and regional nodes	NR routinely; evaluate adjuvant concurrent chemo EBRT (CCRT)	NR routinely
Resectable	Pancreaticoduodenectomy (head lesion)[a] and regional nodes	Postop. CCRT, 45–54 Gy Evaluate preop. CCRT	CCRT: gemzar or 5FU based Systemic CT: gemzar based
Borderline resectable	Pancreaticoduodenectomy and regional nodes	Postop. CCRT, 45–54 Gy Evaluate preop. CCRT/ IOERT[b]	CCRT: gemzar or 5FU based Systemic CT: gemzar based Evaluate neoadjuvant gemzar-abraxane prior to CCRT and after resection
Locally unresectable	Evaluate for resection after preop. CCRT	Preop. CCRT,[b] 45–50 Gy Attempt resection and IOERT	CCRT: gemzar or 5FU based Systemic CT: gemzar based Evaluate neoadjuvant gemzar-abraxane Evaluate alternative CCRT, maintenance chemotherapy
Metastatic	Palliative bypass or stent may be indicated	Palliative CCRT if indicated	ICT phase I, II, or III; MACT

Abbreviations: CCRT, concurrent chemoradiation; EBRT, external-beam radiation; EBRT-CT, external-beam radiation + chemotherapy; ICT, investigational chemotherapy clinical trials; IOERT, intraoperative electron radiation; MACT, multiagent chemotherapy; NR, not recommended; postop., postoperative; preop., preoperative.

[a] If resectable body/tail lesion, distal pancreatectomy, and splenectomy plus regional nodes.

[b] Prefer preop. CCRT for borderline resectable and unresectable pancreas cancers, based on imaging.

abraxane is frequently given before preoperative chemoRT in view of the high risk of systemic relapse in these patient groups. For patients with resectable cancers, chemoradiation can be delivered either preoperatively or postoperatively (see **Table 2**). Some institutions prefer preoperative chemoradiation even for potentially resectable cancers.

EBRT is typically delivered through multiple fields (3D-CRT, IMRT) on a daily basis over a period of 5 to 6 weeks for a dose of 45.0 to 50.4 Gy in 1.8 daily fractions. Concurrent chemotherapy is given during EBRT 5 days per week (Monday to Friday) with infusional 5FU or capecitabine, or as weekly gemcitabine.

Nodal target volumes for tumors of the head of the pancreas include the pancreaticoduodenal, peripancreatic, porta hepatis, celiac, and suprapancreatic nodes. For lesions involving the body and tail of the pancreas, the suprapancreatic, celiac and splenic hilar nodes should be included; inclusion of more medially placed lymph nodes (pancreaticoduodenal and porta hepatis) can be optional, depending on the ability to spare normal organs and structures.

Normal tissue tolerances should be carefully respected with regard to kidneys, liver, stomach, small intestine, and spinal cord, and will influence the choice of beam direction and weighting. Use of non-coplanar beams can allow for greater sparing of normal liver and kidney parenchyma. When IORT is being considered as a component of treatment for patients with a medial lesion over the vertebral column (head of pancreas, medial body), the dose to the spinal cord should be limited to 35 to 40 Gy.

Intraoperative radiation

IORT for pancreatic cancer has predominantly been delivered with electrons.[9] The beam energy and dose of IOERT is determined by the resection status and geometry of the treated field. Unresectable tumors often require energies of 12 to 18 MeV to achieve adequate coverage of the depth of the target tumor volume. After marginal resection of initially borderline resectable or unresectable lesions, the tumor bed can be adequately treated with lower-energy electrons in the 9 to 12 MeV range. Intraoperatively, the radiation oncologist and surgeon consult regarding the unresectable tumor or retroperitoneal area at risk for residual tumor after maximal resection of the primary, and the volume at risk is encompassed within a field defined by an IOERT applicator with a margin of at least 1 cm (ie, 5 cm unresectable tumor or tumor bed = 7-cm applicator). For cancers resected with narrow margins or microscopic residual tumor, IOERT doses in the range of 10.0 to 12.5 Gy are given (preferably 12.5 Gy for microscopic residual). For gross residual or unresected cancers, IOERT doses of 15 to 20 Gy have been used. Preferably a library of predefined isodose curves for a range of IOERT applicator field shapes and electron energies should be available in the operating room for intraoperative consultation. An electron energy should be chosen to adequately encompass the target tissues within the 90% isodose curves while limiting the dose to the spinal cord.

Surgical technique: pancreaticoduodenectomy

Pancreaticoduodenectomy involves the excision of the pancreatic head, duodenum, gallbladder, and bile duct, with or without removal of the gastric antrum, after careful inspection of all intra-abdominal organs and peritoneal surfaces. Any suspicious lesions should be biopsied and sent for frozen-section examination, because presence of distant metastasis is a contraindication to proceeding with resection. Vascular resection of the superior mesenteric–portal vein confluence using either lateral venectomy or segmental venous resection and reconstruction should be performed when there is no tissue plane between the tumor and superior mesenteric and portal vein. Despite all efforts, a microscopically positive margin will occur in 10% to 20% of cases, owing to perineural invasion along the mesenteric plexus at the origin of the SMA and microscopic lymphatic spread beyond the extent of the palpable tumor.[10,11] Although there are numerous reports showing that a positive margin of resection is an independent predictor of poor long-term survival, this concept has been recently challenged.[12]

One of the most debated technical aspects of the pancreaticoduodenectomy is the extent of the associated lymphadenectomy (standard vs extended). To date there have been 3 prospective randomized controlled trials that compare standard lymphadenectomy with the extended lymphadenectomy in patients undergoing resection of the pancreatic head for malignant disease. The largest 2 series (Yeo and colleagues[13] from Johns Hopkins University, and Farnell and colleagues[14] from Mayo Clinic, Rochester [MCR]) have both failed to show any survival benefit of extended lymphadenectomy for pancreatic head carcinoma. The third study, by Pedrazzoli and colleagues,[15] also demonstrated no difference in the overall survival (OS), although patients with positive lymph nodes who underwent extended lymphadenectomy were noted to have improved survival. More recently, Iqbal and colleagues[16] published a meta-analysis comparing standard with extended pancreaticoduodenectomy. The investigators concluded that extended pancreaticoduodenectomy offers no survival benefit and is associated with increased morbidity.

Combined modality outcomes: borderline resectable and unresectable cancers

For unresectable cancer of the pancreas, EBRT with concurrent 5FU-based or gemzar-based chemotherapy results in a doubling of median OS when compared with surgical bypass or stents alone (3–6 vs 9–13 months) and a 2-year OS of 10% to 20%.[17–20] Five-year OS is rare, however, and local control is low. In a Thomas Jefferson University Hospital (TJUH) series, local control was achieved in 20% or fewer of patients treated with EBRT alone to doses of 60 to 70 Gy in 1.8- to 2.0-Gy fractions over 7 to 8 weeks.[17,18] With chemoRT, local control was achieved in approximately 30% of patients (**Table 3**).

Table 3
Pancreas: EBRT ± IOERT for unresectable/borderline resectable cancers

Series	Ref.	No. of Patients	Survival Overall (%)				Relapse (%)		
			Median (mo)	2-y	3-y	P	Local	P	Liver/PS
Thomas Jefferson									
EBRT ± CT	17	46	7.3	—	—		78		—
IOERT/5FU-Leuc/EBRT[a]	23	49	16	22	7		29		55
Massachusetts General									
EBRT ± 5FU/IOERT	24	22	16.5	33	20	>.05	31 (2 y)	>.05	—
EBRT ± 5FU/IOERT + Miso	24	63	12	20	—		45 (2 y)		—
EBRT ± 5FU/IOERT	25	150	13	15	7		—		—
Mayo Clinic Rochester									
EBRT ± CT	19	122	12.6	16.5	—		80 (2 y)		56
IOERT/Postop. EBRT ± 5FU	19	37	13.4	12	—	.25	34 (2 y)	.0005	54
IOERT/Postop. EBRT ± 5FU	22	56	10.5	6	0		35 (2 y)		—
Preop. EBRT + 5FU/IOERT	22	27	14.9	27	20	.001	32 (2 y)[b]		52
Mayo Clinic Arizona									
Preop. EBRT + 5FU or Gem/IOERT	26	31	19	31	16		16		71
R0/R1 resection after preop. CRT		16	23	48	35	.002	6	.1	69
R2 resection or Unresectable		15	10	13	0		27		73

Abbreviations: 5FU, 5-fluorouracil; CRT, chemoradiation; CT, chemotherapy; EBRT, external-beam radiation; Gem, gemcitabone; IOERT, intraoperative electron radiation; Leuc, leucovirin; PS, peritoneal seeding.
[a] Perioperative 5FU/leucovorin was given before, during, and after EBRT.
[b] 2-year local relapse of 19% in the 23 patients with tumor diameter ≤7 cm versus 75% in the 4 patients with tumors >7 cm.

The combination of EBRT and intraoperative electrons (IOERT) has appeared to improve local control in IOERT series from Massachusetts General Hospital (MGH), Mayo Clinic, and TJUH.[19–26] However, this has not translated into significant improvements in either median or 2-year OS (see **Table 3**).

In the latest update of MGH results, 150 patients with locally unresectable cancer of the pancreas received IOERT as a component of treatment from 1978 to 2001 in conjunction with EBRT and 5FU-based chemotherapy.[25] Long-term survival was seen in 8 patients, and 5 were alive at or beyond the 5-year interval. Actuarial 1-, 2-, 3-, and 5-year survival for the 150 patients was 54%, 15%, 7%, and 4%, respectively, and median survival was 13 months (see **Table 3**).

In the initial MCR series, IOERT usually preceded EBRT.[19] When results were compared with EBRT ± 5FU, local control at 1 year was 82% for EBRT plus IORT ± 5FU versus 48% for EBRT ± 5FU; at 2 years it was 66% versus 20%, respectively ($P = .0005$; see **Table 3**). This result did not translate into a difference in either median or 2-year OS (13.4 months median OS with IOERT vs 12.6 months without IOERT; 12% vs 16.5% 2-year OS) in view of a high incidence of abdominal relapse in both groups of patients (20 of 37 IOERT patients, or 54%, developed liver or peritoneal metastases vs 68 of 122, or 56%, in non-IOERT patients).

In an attempt to improve patient selection and survival, MCR investigators delivered the chemoRT preoperatively instead of postoperatively.[22] Median OS was 14.9 months with this sequence, and 2- and 5-year OS were respectively 27% and 7%. These findings were compared with results in 56 patients who had IOERT plus postoperative EBRT (median OS 10.5 months, 2-year OS 6%, $P = .001$; see **Table 3**). Although 2-year OS appeared to be better with the altered sequence of preoperative chemoRT followed by IOERT, this was likely due to altered patient selection, as the rate of liver plus peritoneal relapse did not change (14 of 27 at risk, 52%).

Investigators at MCA have used preoperative chemoradiation followed by restaging, and surgical exploration with resection/IOERT, as indicated, for select patients with borderline resectable or unresectable cancer of the pancreas.[26] A series of 31 patients with no prior treatment had subsequent surgical exploration after preoperative chemoRT. R0 or R1 resection was performed in 16 of 31 patients, and 28 of 31 received IOERT. As seen in **Table 3**, median OS for the total group of patients was 19 months, 2-year OS 31% and 3-year OS 16% (see **Table 3**). Survival outcomes appeared to be improved in the 16 patients with gross total resection (R0/R1) after preoperative chemoRT versus the 15 patients with R2 resection or unresectable disease (median OS 23 vs 10 months; 2-year OS 48% vs 13%; 3-year OS 35% vs 0%; $P = .002$, log rank). Liver or peritoneal relapse was documented in 22 of 31 patients (71%).

A pooled analysis of 270 patients from 5 European Institutions was presented at the 2008 meeting of the International Society of Intraoperative Radiation Therapy (ISIORT 2008) by Valentini and colleagues.[27] Radical surgery was performed in 247 cases (91.5%; R0 resection 53.4%, R1 resection 27.4%, R2 resection 19.2%) and exploratory laparotomy in 8.5%. Surgery was preceded by EBRT in 63 patients (concurrent chemotherapy, 38% of patients) and 106 received postoperative EBRT (concurrent chemotherapy, only 7.5% of patients). In the total group of patients, median OS was 19 months and 5-year OS was 17.7%. Survival and local control appeared to be better in patients treated with preoperative radiation or chemoRT before IORT (ie, preoperative EBRT or chemoRT/IORT) compared with either the postoperative sequence of treatment (IORT/postoperative EBRT or chemoRT) or IORT alone (median OS of 30 vs 22 and 13 months; local control: median not reached with preoperative EBRT/chemoRT group vs median 28 months with postoperative EBRT/chemoRT and median 8 months with IORT alone). On multivariate analysis, nodal status and timing of EBRT/chemoRT significantly affected survival.

Summary and future possibilities
Long-term survival and disease control are achievable in select patients with border-line resectable or locally unresectable cancer of the pancreas, and survival appears to be better in patients with resection after full-dose preoperative chemoRT. Accordingly, continued evaluation of curative-intent combined modality therapy is warranted in this high-risk population of patients. However, additional strategies are needed to improve both resectability rates after preoperative chemoRT and disease control (local, distant). The incidence of abdominal relapse must be decreased by using either more aggressive or new regimens of systemic or regional therapy (intrahepatic, intra-peritoneal). Targeted therapies (ie, epidermal growth factor receptor inhibitors, vascular endothelial growth factor inhibitors) and pancreas cancer vaccines are also being evaluated in an attempt to improve systemic disease control. As improvements are made in distant disease control, the benefit of improved local control with IORT-containing regimens may become even more apparent.

Colorectal Cancer

Patient selection and evaluation
For patients with locally unresectable or borderline resectable primary colorectal cancers (T4N0M0; tethered T3N0M0) or local or regional relapse, the indications for preoperative chemoRT alone or plus IORT should be determined by the surgeon and radiation oncologist in the setting of a joint preoperative consultation, whenever feasible. This collaboration allows input from both specialties with regard to studies that would be helpful in determining optimal sequencing of surgery and chemoRT, optimizing treatment planning for EBRT and deciding whether IORT is indicated (**Tables 4** and **5**). Patients with resectable but high-risk rectal cancers (T3N0, TanyN1–3M0) may also be candidates for combined-modality treatment that includes preoperative or postoperative chemoRT without IORT (see **Table 5**).

The pretreatment patient workup should include a detailed evaluation of the extent of the locally advanced primary or recurrent lesion plus studies to rule out hematoge-nous (liver/lung) or peritoneal spread of disease (see **Table 4**). In addition to history and physical examination, the routine evaluation includes CBC, liver and renal chem-istries, chest film, and CEA. If the rectum is still present, the local evaluation includes digital examination, and proctoscopy and/or colonoscopy. When low-rectal or mid-rectal lesions are immobile or fixed, or symptoms suggest pelvic recurrence following abdominoperineal resection, CT of the pelvis and abdomen can confirm lack of free space between the malignancy and a structure that may be surgically unresectable for cure (ie, presacrum, pelvic side wall). In these patients preoperative radiation plus 5FU-based chemotherapy should be given before an attempt at resection. MRI often provides greater anatomic detail regarding local extension of disease. Extrapel-vic spread to para-aortic nodes or liver and the pretreatment status of ureters with regard to presence or absence of obstruction can also be determined from a CT scan of the abdomen and pelvis. PET/CT is very useful in evaluating potential meta-static spread of disease (distant nodal, liver, lung, and so forth), but is used in the authors' institutions primarily in patients who present with recurrent disease. If hema-turia is present or findings on CT or MRI suggest bladder involvement, cystoscopy is done before or on the day of surgical confirmation.

General criteria for selection of IORT as a component of treatment for patients with locally unresectable, borderline resectable, or local-regionally recurrent colorectal

Table 4
Diagnostic algorithm for colorectal cancer, Mayo Clinic Arizona

Diagnostic Procedure	Diagnosis and Staging Capability	Recommend Routine Use
Primary tumor ± regional nodes[a]		
Colonoscopy	Very accurate modality for detecting and defining primary lesions in rectum, sigmoid (flexible sigmoidoscopy [flex sig]), or remaining colon (colonoscopy)	Yes
Endorectal ultrasonography (EUS)	Useful in defining depth of penetration of primary rectal cancers; may define suspicious lymph nodes	Yes, if preoperative chemoradiotherapy is considered; biopsy suspicious nodes
Computed tomography (CT) of abdomen + pelvis[b]	Most valuable of all modalities for determining extrarectal or extracolonic local invasion and nodal metastases	Yes
CT colonography with intravenous contrast	Highly accurate for detecting/ defining colon lesions before surgery, equal to CT of abdomen and pelvis for local and distal metastases	Optional. Recommend if need to localize and stage a known colon lesion. Can replace barium enema if incomplete colonoscopy
Barium enema	Double-contrast examination alone or single-contrast examination used in combination with flex sig to identify colon lesions. Less accurate than colonoscopy	Optional. Double- or single-contrast barium enema used in combination with flex sig for screening or for incomplete colonoscopy
Metastases		
Chest film; CT chest	Chest film used commonly for metastasis screening; CT chest is best for detecting metastases	Yes
CT of abdomen/pelvis or CT colonography with intravenous contrast	Useful in defining para-aortic node enlargement or liver metastases; CT colonography equal to CT of abdomen and pelvis for local and distant metastases	Yes regarding CT abdomen/ pelvis; Optional regarding CT colonography: recommend if need to localize and stage a known colon lesion
Positron emission tomography (PET)	Used to detect CT occult metastases or further evaluate indeterminate CT findings; preferable as a merged PET/CT study	Yes, with rising CEA and negative or indeterminate CT; before resection or radiofrequency ablation of liver metastases
Magnetic resonance imaging (MRI) of liver	Used primarily to evaluate indeterminate liver lesions on CT	Optional. Recommended for indeterminate liver lesion at CT or contraindication to CT (dye allergy, renal failure)

[a] Laboratory studies: CBC, creatinine, liver function studies (ALP, bilirubin, AST, LDH). Tumor markers: CEA is recommended; CA 19-9 is also being evaluated.
[b] Pelvic MRI is preferred in Europe and is an acceptable alternative to pelvic CT.

Table 5
Treatment algorithm for colorectal cancer, Mayo Clinic Arizona

Disease Extent, Stage Grouping	Surgery	Irradiation (Alone or with CT)	Chemotherapy
Primary Rectal			
T1–2N0M0 (I)	Low anterior or abdominoperineal resection (LAR, CAPR) and regional nodes; local excision of select lesions	Endocavitary irradiation, select lesions[a]; EBRT-CT before local excision or LAR of distal T2N0 lesions	NR as systemic treatment CCRT 5FU based with local excision of T2N0 lesions
T3N0M0 (IIA) T4N0M0 (IIB)	LAR or CAPR/regional nodes; Resect after preop. CCRT (or before for T3N0 lesions)	T4N0, preop. EBRT-CT 45–54 Gy; T3N0, Pre- or postop. EBRT-CT 45–54 Gy[b]	CCRT 5FU based, PVI 5FU 5–7 d/wk or capecitabine 825 g/m^2/bid 5–7 d/wk; Consider postop. MACT
T1–2N1M0 (IIIA) T1–2N2M0 (IIIC) T3N1–2M0 (IIIB/C)	LAR or CAPR/regional nodes; resect after CCRT (or before)	Preop. EBRT-CT 45–54 Gy, preferred if TN stage known[b]; postop. EBRT-CT, 45–54 Gy	CCRT 5FU based, PVI 5FU 5–7 d/wk or capecitabine 825 g/m^2/bid 5–7 d/wk; postop. MACT
Primary Colorectal			
T4N1M0 (IIIB) T4N2M0 (IIIC)	LAR or CAPR/regional nodes; resect after preop. CCRT; IOERT[c]	Preop. EBRT-CT, 45–54 Gy; IOERT[a]	CCRT 5FU based, PVI 5FU 5–7 d/wk or capecitabine 825 g/m^2/bid 5–7 d/wk; postop. MACT
Recurrent colorectal	Resect after preop. CCRT; IOERT[a]	Preop. EBRT-CT, 45–54 Gy if no prior EBRT; 20–40 Gy if prior EBRT; IOERT[a]	CCRT 5FU based, PVI 5FU 5–7 d/wk or capecitabine 825 g/m^2/bid 5–7 d/wk; postop. MACT

Abbreviations: CAPR, combined abdominoperineal resection; CCRT, concurrent chemoradiation; EBRT, external-beam radiation; EBRT-CT, external beam radiation + chemotherapy; ICT, investigational chemotherapy clinical trials; IOERT, intraoperative electron radiation; LAR, low anterior resection; MACT, multiagent chemotherapy; NR, not recommended; postop., postoperative; preop., preoperative; PVI, protracted venous infusion.

[a] 30 Gy × 3–4 surface dose; available at Mayo Clinic Cancer Center, Rochester.

[b] Prefer preop. CCRT for T4N0–2M0 cancers (based on physical examination and computed tomography) and for T3N0–2 or T1–2N1–2 cancers (based on endoscopic ultrasonography or pelvic MRI staging).

[c] IOERT dose dependent on amount of residual disease after maximal surgical resection: R0, 10–12.5 Gy; R1, 12.5–15 Gy; R2, 15–20 Gy.

cancers have been detailed previously in publications from both Mayo Clinic and MGH.[28–41] By definition, there must be no contraindications for exploratory surgery. Local control rates with surgery alone should be low, and EBRT doses needed for local control following subtotal resection or with EBRT alone should exceed normal tissue tolerance. An IORT approach should permit direct irradiation of unresected or marginally resected tumor with single or abutting IORT fields while allowing the ability to surgically displace or shield dose-limiting normal organs or tissue. Bowel should always be displaced out of the IORT field, and other critical tissues, such as ureter and bladder, can often be displaced if not at risk for harboring residual disease. Patients with documented distant metastases are not usually candidates because of their limited life span. However, with increasing survival observed with modern systemic therapies, many patients will outlive the palliative effects of local therapy, and aggressive locoregional therapy may be considered. In addition, patients with oligometastatic disease (limited liver or lung metastases) may be considered appropriate for curative-intent treatment.

Sequencing of treatment modalities

For most patients with locally unresectable, borderline resectable, or recurrent colorectal cancers, delivery of 45 to 55 Gy plus concomitant chemotherapy preoperatively, with reoperation in 3 to 6 weeks, offers the following theoretical advantages over the sequence of resection and IORT followed by postoperative chemoRT: (1) potential alteration of implantability of cells that may be disseminated intra-abdominally or systemically at the time of marginal or partial surgical resection; (2) deletion of patients with metastases detected at the restaging workup or laparotomy, thus sparing the potential risks of aggressive surgical resection ± IORT; (3) possible tumor shrinkage with an increased probability of achieving a gross total resection; and (4) reduction of treatment interval between the EBRT and IORT components of irradiation (if surgical resection and IORT are done initially and postoperative complications ensue, the delay to the EBRT-plus-chemotherapy component of treatment may be excessive).

There would seem to be no tumor-related advantages in having surgical resection and IORT precede the EBRT component of treatment in patients with locally unresectable, borderline resectable, or recurrent colorectal cancers. For patients with locally recurrent pelvic lesions, the altered sequencing may, however, provide an advantage for normal tissue tolerance. If fixed loops of small bowel were found at exploratory laparotomy, they could be mobilized out of the pelvis. Pelvic reconstruction could be performed with omentum or mesh to allow displacement of small bowel during subsequent chemoRT. However, performing 2 surgical procedures may be difficult to justify (exploration and reconstruction; exploration, resection, and IORT after preoperative chemoRT). An alternative approach would be to keep the planned preoperative dose at a level of 40 to 45 Gy, instead of a higher dose of 50.4 to 54 Gy, if fixed loops of small bowel were adjacent to the recurrent disease and could not be excluded after a dose of 40 to 45 Gy.

Chemotherapy should typically be instituted simultaneously with EBRT for locally recurrent colorectal cancers. The advantage of starting radiation and chemotherapy simultaneously is that effective local and systemic treatments are instituted simultaneously. There is less risk, therefore, that one component of disease will become uncontrollable owing to progression during single-modality treatment. The disadvantage of starting chemotherapy simultaneously with EBRT is that full-intensity chemotherapy may never be feasible. For tolerance reasons, the intensity of chemotherapy during EBRT is usually less than if chemotherapy precedes EBRT. If further cycles of chemotherapy are given after pelvic EBRT, full-intensity chemotherapy may not be feasible because of alterations in bone marrow reserve.

A potential advantage of altered sequencing of chemotherapy and EBRT (ie, deliver 2 or more cycles of multiple drug chemotherapy before starting combined radiation/chemotherapy) would be the ability to give full-intensity chemotherapy for at least 2 cycles. This approach may have an increased impact on occult systemic disease and thereby improve the ultimate rates of systemic disease control. The risk of starting chemotherapy before EBRT, however, is that the local component of disease may continue to progress and subsequent resection may never be feasible. However, for patients with limited metastatic disease in whom resection with IORT is being considered, this may be the preferred approach.

EBRT

Patients with locally unresectable or borderline resectable primary rectal cancer or local-regional relapse of colorectal cancer have been evaluated in aggressive local strategies including EBRT, IOERT, and maximal resection at MGH since 1978, at MCR since 1981, and at MCA since 2001.[28–41] Such patients currently receive full-dose preoperative EBRT with infusional 5FU (225 mg/m^2/d 5 days per week throughout irradiation) or capecitabine (825 mg/m^2 twice daily, Monday to Friday) if they have not received prior EBRT within their planned treatment field. Multiple-field techniques using 3D-CRT or IMRT techniques are used to carry extended fields to 45 Gy in 25 fractions over 5 weeks, and boost fields to tumor plus 2 to 2.5 cm are carried to 50.4 to 54 Gy. If external iliac nodes are at risk because of tumor adherence or fixation to anterior pelvic structures (bladder, prostate, cervix, uterus), IMRT can be useful in decreasing small-bowel volumes in the EBRT field and, thereby, improving acute tolerance.

If patients present with local or regional relapse of colorectal cancer after prior adjuvant treatment that included 45 to 50 Gy of EBRT, full doses of preoperative EBRT may not be feasible at the time of retreatment. In such instances, delivery of 20 to 30 Gy in 1.8- to 2.0-Gy fractions to conformal fields exclusive of small bowel may be followed immediately (1 day to 1 week) with surgical exploration and attempted resection plus IORT.

Surgery: primary and recurrent cancers

Following a course of preoperative chemoRT, surgical exploration is undertaken 3 to 6 weeks later, if IORT is thought to be a pertinent component of treatment. The delay allows ongoing tumor shrinkage after the cessation of preoperative treatment as well as resolution of treatment-induced acute inflammation. For non-IORT patients, an interval of 8 or more weeks is preferred by some surgeons and radiation oncologists to allow a potentially higher rate of pathologic complete response.

Surgery is usually best performed via a midline incision, which allows extension as necessary and permits multiple stomas. Adhesions are completely taken down, and the abdomen is carefully evaluated for liver and peritoneal metastases. If metastases are found that are not able to be treated with curative intent, IORT is not performed; palliative resection or diversion is followed by systemic therapy.

If no metastases are evident, or are limited and can be resected for cure, the patient undergoes abdominoperineal resection, low anterior resection, or pelvic exenteration, depending on the extent and location of the primary or recurrent cancer. En bloc wide resection is the goal; at least a grossly complete resection of the tumor is desirable, but if this cannot be done, as much of the cancer as possible is removed. For resection of locally unresectable primary rectal or sigmoid cancer or pelvic relapse of colorectal cancer, mobilization of the tumor off the sacrum and pelvic side wall can be difficult. Sometimes a large periosteal elevator (eg, Cobb elevator) functions well for this part of the resection; for recurrent cancers with sacral involvement, a distal sacrectomy may be necessary. Hemostasis after resection is important because pooled blood over the tumor bed could decrease the IOERT dose at depth.

If an anastomosis is to be done, it is completed after the delivery of IOERT. Following moderate doses of preoperative EBRT (45–50 Gy) ± 5FU-based chemotherapy, anterior resection and primary anastomosis may be safely accomplished if an unirradiated loop of large bowel can be used for the proximal limb of the anastomosis. Temporary diverting colostomies are preferable in patients who receive preoperative EBRT or chemoRT.

Surgical considerations for recurrent cancers

Pelvic recurrences are typically amenable to re-resection if they are strictly posterior or anterior. Evidence of lateral pelvic side-wall involvement diminishes the chance of complete resection; however, operative assessment and at least an opportunity for resection and IOERT are warranted, providing no other contraindications are identified. Although locoregional recurrences that occur above or below S2 of the sacrum are amenable to resection using anterior-table sacral resection or distal sacrectomy, respectively, the presence of tumor both above and below S2 precludes curative surgery. Similarly, although vascular tumor involvement of either the arterial or venous structures at or distal to the aorta may be resectable, involvement of both structures contraindicates curative surgery in most, if not all, cases.

At the time of surgery, careful assessment for extrapelvic disease is essential. If possible it is preferable to determine resectability before critical structures are sacrificed or injured. Adjacent involved organs should be removed en bloc with the specimen if the associated morbidity is acceptable to the patient and physician. When the recurrent tumor is locally adherent to the prostate or base of the bladder, because the side effects of pelvic exenteration are excessive it may be preferable to deliver preoperative EBRT with chemotherapy followed by gross total resection, with organ preservation, and supplemental IOERT to the site of adherence (thus sparing the organ involved by adherence). However, in view of severe adhesions caused by prior surgery and/or adjuvant EBRT, organ preservation is often not technically feasible in the setting of recurrent lesions, and exenterative procedures may be necessary to accomplish a gross total resection. The option to spare the bladder should be reserved for those cases whereby present function is good and there is minimal adherence, such that local-regional control could be accomplished with exenteration equally as well as with organ-preserving resection plus IOERT.

In the setting of pelvic recurrence of rectal cancer, it is rarely possible or reasonable to restore intestinal continuity. Most often a previous low anterior resection is being converted to an abdominal perineal resection (APR), or a previous APR to a sacrectomy or exenteration. In the face of local relapse, it is usually ill advised to place another anastomosis in this heavily treated field that is at risk for subsequent local relapse. Rarely, in a highly motivated patient with good sphincter function and a very proximal anastomotic recurrence, it may be reasonable to perform a coloanal anastomosis.

If at the end of resection it is decided that postoperative EBRT is indicated, small titanium or vascular clips should be placed around areas of adherence or residual disease for the purpose of defining postoperative EBRT fields. The pelvic floor should be reconstructed after resection to minimize the amount of small bowel within the true pelvis, and primary closure of the perineum should be performed after APR to hasten healing (2–6 weeks vs 2–3 months) and decrease the interval to postoperative EBRT and chemotherapy, if indicated.

In patients who have been heavily pretreated or those with large defects, vascularized myocutaneous flap closure or placement of a pedicled omentum should be strongly considered. The reconstructive procedure may decrease the risk of a leak from an anastomosis, minimize the risk of malignant small-bowel obstruction if pelvic recurrence occurs after abdominoperineal resection of a primary rectal cancer, keep small bowel out of the pelvis in case postoperative EBRT is necessary, and help prevent pelvic sepsis by eliminating dead space (a substantial risk especially after pelvic exenteration). The muscle closes the dead space of the pelvis, which is typically fibrotic and prone to small-bowel adhesion formation, and the fresh nonirradiated skin ensures perineal healing. For posterior sacrectomy wounds, myocutaneous flap closure has become the standard at Mayo Clinic.

If patients develop locally recurrent disease following prior adjuvant EBRT, preoperative and postoperative EBRT options are limited at the time of retreatment unless pelvic reconstruction can be accomplished to displace small bowel (eg, omentum, myocutaneous flap). In previously irradiated patients, IOERT as salvage is usually feasible only in the setting of gross total resection of disease, and extended organ resection (anterior exenteration, distal sacrectomy, and so forth) may be necessary to achieve total resection.

IORT

The decision to treat with IORT is based on the operative findings, status of pathologic margin, and pretreatment physical examination and imaging studies, and is an intraoperative collaborative judgment made by the surgeon and the radiation oncologist.[28–41] It is critical to define the area at highest risk for subsequent local relapse to determine the optimal position of the IORT field. Margins of resection are determined by frozen-section pathologic analysis of the surgical specimen and, sometimes, the tumor bed. The tumor bed is marked with sutures to facilitate later positioning of the IORT applicator.

If no tumor adherence existed after preoperative chemoradiation and adequate soft-tissue radial margins were present (>1 cm), IORT was not always delivered at MGH until an analysis suggested a high risk for relapse in patients with pretreatment adherence who had T3 or N(+) disease after preoperative treatment and who did not receive an IORT boost. Patients with gross residual cancer, with microscopically positive margins, or with close (≤5 mm) radial soft-tissue margins after preoperative chemoradiation, have always been candidates for IORT.

IOERT An IOERT applicator is selected according to the location and size of the area to be irradiated. The internal diameters of circular applicators range from 4 to 9 cm at MGH, and from 4 to 9.5 cm at MCR and MCA. Applicator size is selected to allow full coverage of the high-risk area, which is generally on the presacrum or pelvic side wall for primary or recurrent rectal cancers. Usually the largest applicator that will fit into the area is best. The applicator's shape is chosen so that the geometry fits the specific situation of tumor versus normal tissue. The applicator must abut the site being treated, which can be difficult if the high-risk area is located in an anatomically confined region such as the pelvis. Some applicators have beveled ends of 15° or 30°, enabling good apposition of the applicator to sloping surfaces in the pelvis so as to maximize dose homogeneity. It is important that the applicator be placed so that the tumor or tumor bed is fully covered, that sensitive normal tissues are not included in the beam, and that there is no fluid buildup in the treatment area. The applicator not only directs the electron beam accurately to the high-risk area but also serves to retract sensitive normal tissues out of the way, especially small bowel and ureter. Visceral retraction and packing are usually necessary also. If a distal rectal stump remains for later anastomosis, it should also be excluded from the IOERT field by retraction outside the applicator, with the IOERT applicator and packing, or with the use of lead sheets, which can be cut out to block sensitive normal tissues that cannot be removed from the path of the beam. During treatment, suction catheters are positioned to minimize fluid buildup within the applicator.

Most IOERT treatments in patients with cancer are given via a transabdominal approach because the area of concern is usually posterior presacrum or posterolateral pelvic side wall. A perineal approach is occasionally used after abdominoperineal resection to treat a very low-lying tumor involving the coccyx or distal presacrum, distal pelvic side wall, or portions of the prostate and base of the bladder when an exenteration is not performed. The perineal approach is technically more difficult. For institutions where IOERT is delivered with the x-band Mobetron accelerator (MCA and other North American, European, and Asian institutions), the perineal approach is especially challenging if the tumor was adherent to or invading anterior structures. In such instances, the patient has to be rotated from supine to prone position following resection and before IOERT delivery. On rare occasions it may be impossible to abut the applicator to the tumor bed if the lesion is located very low in the pelvic side wall in an obese male with a narrow pelvis, and HDR-IORT would be a preferable option for IORT delivery, if available.

After positioning the IOERT applicator it is docked to the linear accelerator, and IOERT is delivered. Typical doses of radiation delivered intraoperatively are in the range of 10 to 20 Gy, with the lower doses being given for minimal residual disease (narrow or microscopically positive margins) and the higher doses for gross residual disease after maximal resection. For patients undergoing complete resection with negative but narrow margins (R0), the IOERT dose is usually 10 to 12.5 Gy, whereas for patients undergoing subtotal resection with microscopically positive margins (R1) the dose is 12.5 to 15 Gy. For patients with macroscopic or gross residual after resection (R2), the dose is 17.5 Gy to 20 Gy. Typical electron energies used are 6 to 15 MeV, depending on the thickness of residual tumor. The dose is quoted at the 90% isodose.

Electron energies are chosen on the basis of maximum thickness of disease after maximal resection and the ability to achieve complete hemostasis after surgical resection. The lower energies of 6, 9, and 12 MeV are used after gross total resection or with minimal residual disease. If the 6-MeV energy is chosen, 0.5 to 1.0 cm of bolus material may need to be used to improve the surface dose. If surgical hemostasis is incomplete and suction drainage is not functioning properly, choice of either 6 or 9 MeV electrons could result in underdosage at depth. The 15- to 18-MeV energies and doses of 20 Gy are used more commonly in patients in whom gross residual or unresectable disease exists after attempts at resection.

The size and shape of the IOERT applicators used are dependent on tumor location. For pelvic tumors, circular applicators with 30° bevels are often needed to conform to the anatomy of the presacrum, pelvic side wall, or anterior pelvis. With the 30° bevel, the depth of isodose curves is shallower at the heel end than the toe end of the applicator, and should be considered when placing the treatment applicator relative to the tumor bed or residual tumor. For extrapelvic lesions, rectangular and elliptical applicators with flat or 20° bevel ends are occasionally used in institutions where they are available, in addition to circular applicators.

HDR-IORT As with IOERT, the decision to treat with HDR-IORT is based on operative findings, margin status, physical examination and imaging studies, and collaborative judgment between surgeon and radiation oncologist.[31] A primary limitation of IOERT that could favor use of HDR-IORT for a given patient is the nonflexible IOERT applicator, which makes treatment difficult or sometimes impossible in narrow cavities, steeply sloping surfaces, or regions requiring treatment delivery to bend around a corner. The deep pelvis can sometimes present such a challenge. Relative advantages must be weighed against HDR-IORT's lower dose homogeneity, longer treatment time, greater shielding requirement, lower dose at depth, and inability to treat areas at risk with a depth greater than 0.5 cm from the surface of the applicator.

Combined-modality outcomes: primary colorectal cancers

MGH results: EBRT + resection + IOERT Sixty-four patients with locally unresectable T4 rectal cancer had full-dose preoperative EBRT (alone or plus 5FU) followed by resection and IOERT at MGH.[28,29,31] The 5-year actuarial local control and disease-specific survival for 40 patients undergoing complete resection plus IOERT was 91% and 63%, respectively. For 24 patients undergoing partial resection, local control and disease-specific survival correlated with the extent of residual cancer: 65% and 47%, respectively, for microscopic residual disease, and 57% and 14%, respectively, for gross residual disease.

Mayo Clinic results: EBRT ± 5FU, resection, IOERT In an MCR comparison of 17 non-IOERT and 56 IOERT + EBRT patients with locally advanced primary rectal or colon cancers, local control was 24% versus 84%, median OS was 18 versus 40 months, and the 3-year OS was 24% versus 55% (**Table 6**).[30] The impact of degree of resection and amount of residual disease on disease control and survival was evaluated. The 5-year OS for the entire group of 56 colorectal IOERT + EBRT patients was 46%. Patients with R0 or R1 resection did better than those with R2 resection, with a 5-year OS of 59% versus 21% ($P = .0005$). Relapse within an irradiation field occurred in 4 of 16 patients (25%) with R2 resection versus 2 of 39 (5%) with R0 or R1 resection ($P = .01$).

A separate MCR analysis was done regarding the use of EBRT (alone or plus chemotherapy) alone or plus IOERT as a supplement to maximal resection for 103 patients with locally advanced colon cancers.[32] The local relapse rate at 5 years was 10% for patients with R0 resection, 54% for patients with R1 resection, and 79% for patients with R2 resection ($P<.0001$). For patients with residual disease, local relapse occurred in only 11% of patients receiving IOERT plus EBRT, compared with 82% of patients receiving only EBRT ($P = .02$). The 5-year OS was 66% for patients with R0 resection, 47% for patients with R1 resection, and 23% for those with R2 resection ($P = .0009$). The 5-year OS for patients with residual disease was 76% for patients receiving IOERT plus EBRT, and 26% for patients with EBRT alone ($P = .04$).

In the most recent MCR analysis, 146 patients with locally unresectable primary colorectal cancer had IOERT in addition to preoperative or postoperative chemoRT and resection.[33] Median and OS were slightly better than in the earlier series of patients with rectal cancer (see **Table 6**). The sequence of preoperative chemoRT before resection/IOERT appeared to have a survival advantage over postoperative chemoRT (median 76 vs 26 months, 5-year OS 55% vs 38%; $P = .02$).

European pooled analysis A pooled analysis of 651 IOERT patients from 4 major European centers was presented at ISIORT 2008 by Rutten and colleagues[42]; 5-year OS was 67% and 5-year local control was 88%. Positive margins of circumferential resection were a strong predictor for both OS ($P<.0001$) and local relapse ($P<.01$). Preoperative chemoradiation before resection and IOERT seemed to improve OS in comparison with resection/IOERT plus postoperative chemoRT (5-year OS 70% vs 64%, $P<.05$).

IOERT ± EBRT: locally recurrent colorectal cancers

MGH results In an MGH IOERT analysis of 41 patients with locally recurrent rectal cancer, 5-year disease-free survival (DFS) was 16% and 5-year OS was 30%,[34,35] which exceeds expected long-term survival of 5% or less when treated with non-IORT approaches. Patients with R2 resection had 5-year local control and DFS of 21% and 7%, versus 47% and 21% with R0 or R1 resection. Patients with R1 resection had better in-field disease control than those with R2 resection or unresected disease.

Table 6
Locally advanced primary and recurrent colorectal cancer: EBRT ± IOERT, Mayo Clinic Rochester

Disease Presentation/ Treatment/Reference	Ref.	No. of Patients	Survival Median (mo)	Overall Survival (%) 2-y	3-y	5-y	P	Relapse (3-y) (%) Local	Distant
Primary Disease, Colorectal									
EBRT alone[a]	30	17	18	35	24	24		76	59
EBRT + IOERT	30	56	40	70	55	46		16	49
EBRT + IOERT	33	146	44	74	61	52		10	43
P reop. EBRT/CT		124	76	—	65	55	.02	—	—
Postop. EBRT/CT		20	26	—	43	38		—	—
Localized Recurrence									
a. Suzuki et al, rectal	36	106							
No IOERT		64	17	26	18	7		93	54
IOERT		42	30	62	43	19	.0006	40	60
b. IOERT ± EBRT, colorectal									
Prior EBRT:									
None	37	123	28	62	39	20		25	64
Yes	38	51	23	48	28	12		49	71
c. IOERT ± EBRT, rectal	39	304	34	66	48	24		40	63
Prior EBRT:									
None		157	38	71	50	27	.001[b]	—	—
Yes		147	31	61	37	18		—	—
d. IOERT ± EBRT, colorectal	40	607[c]	36	70	50	30		27	54
Prior EBRT:									
None		359	37	71	51	34	.07	20	57
Yes		248	35	67	49	26		49	49
Systemic Chemotherapy:									
Yes		107	50	82	—	40	.03	—	—
No		500	34	67	—	28		(2-y)	(2-y)
Resection:									
R0		227	51	80	—	46	<.001	15	31
R1		224	35	69	—	27		22	51
R2		156	27	56	—	16		24	53

[a] All deaths within 30 months. Local failure range 3–15 months. Distant failure range 3–17 months.
[b] $P = .06$ univariate, .001 multivariate.
[c] Multivariate analysis: prior EBRT, $P = .897$; systemic chemotherapy, $P = .075$; R0 vs R1 vs R2, $P<.0001$; treated after 3 March 1997, $P = .012$.

Mayo Clinic results: IOERT ± EBRT MCR data supporting the use of IOERT for patients with locally recurrent cancer were initially found in an analysis of 106 patients with palliative resection of locally recurrent rectal cancers (see **Table 6**).[36] None had evidence of extrapelvic disease and 42 received IOERT as a component of treatment (R1 resection, 8 patients; R2 resection, 34 patients). The IOERT dose was 15 to 20 Gy in 40 of 42 patients, and EBRT was given in 41 of the 42 ($\geq$45 Gy in 38). Significant factors with regard to 3- and 5-year OS included amount of residual disease after maximal resection (R1 vs R2 resection: 3-year OS 44% vs 26%; 5-year OS 33% vs 9%; $P = .032$), IOERT versus none (3-year OS 43% vs 18%; 5-year OS 19% vs 7%; $P = .0006$), type of symptoms (asymptomatic vs symptomatic without or with pain: 3-year OS 49%, 28%, 7% $P = .0075$), and type of fixation (none or 1 vs 2, or $\geq$3 sites: 3-year OS 45%, 29%, 0%; $P<.0001$). For IOERT patients, 3-year OS with R2 resection or presentation with pain was 44% and 43%, respectively.

Subsequent Mayo Clinic analyses on patients with locally recurrent colorectal cancer without prior EBRT (n = 123)[34,37] or with prior EBRT (n = 51)[34,38] are shown in **Table 6**. Local relapse rates at 3 years appear higher in patients with prior EBRT.

A series of 304 patients with locally recurrent rectal cancer receiving IOERT as a component of treatment was presented at ISIORT 2002.[39] In the 159 patients without prior EBRT, 5-year OS was 27%, and in the 145 with prior EBRT 5-year OS was 20%. Improvements in long-term OS appeared to be related to more intensive treatment in recent years (patients usually receive protracted venous infusion [PVI] 5FU during EBRT in both groups; prior EBRT patients often receive reirradiation EBRT doses of 25.2–30.6 Gy plus PVI 5FU), including the use of maintenance systemic chemotherapy.

The most recent MCR analysis presented at ISIORT 2008 included 607 patients with recurrent colorectal cancer receiving IOERT as a component of treatment.[40] Five-year OS was 30% and, on multivariate analysis, complete resection, no prior chemotherapy, and treatment after 1997 were associated with improved OS (see **Table 6**). In patients with R0 resection, 5-year OS was 46%. Prior in-field radiation was associated with increased risk of local relapse (49% vs 20% at 3 years; $P<.0001$) but not with decreased survival.

European results: IORT ± EBRT The current philosophy in Europe is closely related to the United States concept, which uses IORT as a segment of a multidisciplinary approach in cancer management.[34,43–46] A component of EBRT ± 5FU-based chemotherapy is always attempted, either before or after surgery, if no previous EBRT has been delivered.

The most impressive European results have been achieved in consecutive series from Eindhoven.[45,46] Outcomes in a series of 147 consecutive IOERT patients were presented at ISIORT 2008.[46] Median OS was 28 months; 5-year OS, DFS, metastasis-free survival (MFS), and local control were 31.5%, 34.1%, 49.5%, and 54.1%, respectively. R0 resections were achieved in 84 patients (57.2%), R1 resections in 34 (23.1%), and R2 resections in 29 (19.7%). After R0 resections, 5-year OS, DFS, MFS, and local control were 48.4%, 52.3%, 65.5%, and 68.9%, respectively ($P<.001$ for OS, DFS, and local control when compared with outcomes of R1 or R2 resection). Patients treated with IOERT alone had worse outcomes than those who were reirradiated or treated with full-dose preoperative EBRT with regard to 5-year OS ($P = .043$), local control ($P = .038$), or MFS ($P<.001$).

IOERT for nodal presentation or relapse

An MCR analysis evaluated IOERT as a component of treatment in a series of 48 patients with colorectal cancer who had bulky mesenteric or para-aortic nodal disease at time of presentation, or nodal relapse.[41]

5-year OS was approximately 35% for all patients at risk and approximately 40% for those with colon cancer. These results strongly support the use of CT of the abdomen as a component of follow-up in resected high-risk patients with colon cancer.

Summary and future possibilities

Although encouraging trends exist with regard to improved local control and OS when IOERT or HDR-IORT is combined with standard treatment for locally advanced primary and recurrent colorectal cancers, the incidence of systemic failure is at least 50%, and relapses within IOERT and EBRT fields are significant if gross resection is not feasible. In attempts to improve local control, bolus 5FU plus leucovorin, infusion 5FU, or other enhancing or additive agents should be given during EBRT, and studies should be performed to evaluate the use of dose modifiers with IORT (eg, sensitizers, hyperthermia). In view of high rates of systemic failure, maintenance chemotherapy should become standard and more modern chemotherapy regimens including biologics (eg, Avastin) need to be evaluated both after and during EBRT (systemic FOLFOX/Avastin). Most published data were accumulated before the availability of more effective multi-agent systemic regimens and targeted agents. The benefits of IORT as a component of aggressive local-regional salvage attempts for local or nodal relapse may become more apparent in future analyses with more contemporary multi-modality treatment regimens, as suggested in sequential Mayo Clinic analyses.

Although it would be of scientific interest to randomly compare standard treatment ± IORT, such trials did not accrue well in the United States or Europe, and were closed. Trials that are feasible will standardize the aggressive local treatment of EBRT, resection, and IORT with IOERT or HDR-IORT, and randomize optimal chemo-therapy/targeted agents during as well as after EBRT, and the presence or absence of dose modifiers during IORT.

Retroperitoneal Sarcomas

EBRT and IORT factors

A current treatment approach at Duke University, MGH, and Mayo Clinic for patients with nonmetastatic retroperitoneal sarcoma is to use moderate-dose preoperative EBRT (usually 45–50 Gy in 1.8-Gy fractions over 4.5–5 weeks), surgical resection, and IORT (if technically feasible).[47–54] As with other cancers, the IORT dose (usually 10–20 Gy) is based on both the EBRT dose that can be delivered preoperatively and the amount of residual disease after maximal surgical resection.

When planning preoperative EBRT, the gross tumor volume with 3- to 5-cm margins is carried to 40 to 45 Gy, preferably with 3D-CRT or IMRT, and boost fields with 2- to 3-cm margins are treated to a total dose of 45 to 50.4 Gy. Dose-limiting organs/struc-tures include the liver, kidneys, spinal cord, stomach, and small intestine. In some instances, oblique or non-coplanar beams are helpful in minimizing the dose to normal structures such as the spinal cord and kidney, and the use of such is facilitated by the use of 3D treatment planning. Use of IMRT techniques to selectively escalate high-risk margins to a dose as high as 62.5 Gy in 25 fractions is under evaluation, if the high-risk region is not adjacent to small bowel or stomach. If irradiation of the tumor or tumor bed requires the inclusion of one kidney to doses beyond tolerance, function of the remaining kidney should be assessed with serum creatinine ± blood urea nitrogen levels and a contrast renal study (CT scan with intravenous contrast, renal scan).

Surgical factors

Surgical resection remains the cornerstone of the treatment of retroperitoneal sarcomas. Despite technical and supportive advances, the surgical management of patients with retroperitoneal sarcoma remains a therapeutic challenge. Published series of surgical resection alone for retroperitoneal sarcoma have shown poor local control and survival rates, even in the setting of margin-negative, radical excision. Because of the infiltrative nature of these tumors, their large size, and their anatomic origin, it is often difficult to obtain microscopically clear and not infrequently macroscopically clear resection margins. Contemporary series have suggested that locoregional relapse is a predominant mode of failure and cause of death, occurring in a high percentage of patients, even following complete resection.[47–54] Therefore, optimization of local control is an important outcome.

Surgical techniques
Four to 6 weeks following completion of EBRT, exploratory laparotomy is performed in the dedicated IORT suite in the authors' institutions. At laparotomy, the abdomen and pelvis are carefully examined for metastases to the liver and/or peritoneal surfaces. If no metastases are found the patient undergoes resection of the tumor, leaving as little residual sarcoma as possible. Every effort is made to resect the tumor and involved normal structures en bloc without violation or exposure of the tumor surface. Lateral mobilization of the tumor is generally easier because most vascularity arises from the medial aspect of the tumor. Every effort should be made to perform the dissection through normal tissue planes away from the tumor pseudocapsule, but anatomic restraints may preclude this relative to some portions of the tumor, thus increasing the risk of microscopic residual disease or tumor seeding.

For sarcomas of the iliac fossa and central retroperitoneum, major vascular resections are more often necessary for achieving gross total resection. Vascular reconstruction is generally required, usually with prosthetic graft material. If the anastomosis is not within a high-risk area for local relapse, it can be excluded from the IORT field. The vascular anastomoses and large irradiated vessels should be shielded from adjacent bowel, particularly bowel anastomoses, using the greater omentum, peritoneal flaps, or other normal tissues, to reduce the risk of fistula formation.

IORT factors: IOERT, HDR-IORT
To direct IOERT, applicators (circular, elliptical, or rectangular) are used.[47–54] Applicator geometry and size are carefully selected to fully cover the high-risk area. For large sarcomas, abutting fields may be needed to ensure that all high-risk areas are included. The IOERT dose and energy are dependent on amount of residual disease after maximal resection and the volume treated (ie, length of peripheral nerve in IOERT field, amount of bowel circumference, and so forth). For patients with completely resected tumors and negative margins, an IOERT dose of 10 Gy is usually selected, whereas a grossly resected tumor bed with positive microscopic margins will receive 12.5 to 15 Gy (depending on volume treated). For gross residual disease, doses will range from 15 to 20 Gy depending on the extent of residual tumor and volume treated. The electron energy is selected according to the desired depth of penetration, and ranges typically between 9 and 15 MeV. For HDR-IORT guidelines see the article elsewhere in this issue, and prior publications.[47,55,56]

Combined-modality outcomes: retroperitoneal sarcomas
EBRT ± chemotherapy/resection When surgery is the sole treatment modality for retroperitoneal sarcomas, subsequent local relapse rates are as high as 70% to 90%.[47,48,55] If EBRT is combined with resection, the dose of EBRT that can be delivered safely (45–50 Gy in 1.8–2-Gy fractions) is much lower than with extremity sarcomas in view of dose-limiting structures (small intestine, stomach, liver, kidney, spinal cord). In a randomized National Cancer Institute trial (NCI), patients with primary sarcomas randomized to EBRT alone after marginal resection had a local relapse rate of 80% and excessive acute and chronic small-bowel morbidity (see details below).[57] The use of IORT supplements is therefore reasonable and practical.[47–61]

NCI randomized trial: EBRT and resection ± IOERT NCI conducted a randomized trial in which 35 patients with retroperitoneal sarcomas were randomized to receive postoperative EBRT ± IOERT.[57] All had primary lesions; none had prior EBRT or chemotherapy. All had gross total resection; most had microscopic residual disease. Patients randomized to EBRT alone received 35 to 40 Gy to an extended field over 4 to 5 weeks and an additional 15 Gy over 2 weeks to a reduced field. The IOERT group received 35–40 Gy EBRT in 4 to 5 weeks to an extended field, and an IOERT dose of 20 Gy to abutting fields.

Some apparent advantages for IOERT patients were seen in outcomes analyses. Treatment-related small-bowel complications were substantially lower in the IOERT group. Severe acute enteritis occurred in 12 of 20 versus 1 of 15 patients (P<.01), chronic enteritis in 10 of 20 versus 2 of 15 (P<.05), and fistulae in 5 of 20 versus 0 of 15 (P = .06). Local failure in the irradiation fields occurred in 3 of 15 IOERT (20%) versus 16 of 20 non-IOERT patients (80%) (P<.01).

IOERT ± EBRT, resection

Mayo Clinic Rochester The initial MCR analysis involved 87 patients with retroperitoneal or pelvic sarcomas who had resection plus IOERT between March 1981 and September 1995 and a follow-up of 1 year or more (median >3 years).[47,48,50,52] EBRT was given in 77 patients (43 of 43 patients who presented with primary disease and 34 of 44 who presented with locally recurrent cancers). The majority of patients (69%) underwent preoperative EBRT and the remainder underwent postoperative EBRT. Subsequent local or central failure occurred in only 3 of 43 patients who presented with primary lesions (7%) versus 17 of 44 (39%) who presented with recurrent disease. With median follow-up of greater than 3.5 years, 5-year OS was 47%, which was not significantly different for primary versus recurrent status (52% vs 42%), and low-grade versus high-grade lesions (45% vs 47%). Patients with R0 or R1 resection had a trend toward improved survival in comparison with those with R2 resection (median OS 4.7 vs 3.2 years, 5-year OS 49% vs 36%; P = .08). Prognostic factor analyses for patients with primary disease are shown in **Table 7**.

The most recent analysis of MCR results was presented at ISIORT 2008 in a series of 231 patients treated from 1981 to 2008 who received IOERT as a component of treatment for retroperitoneal or pelvic sarcoma.[53] The series was almost equally divided between patients who presented with primary (52%) and recurrent (48%) disease. An R0 resection was achieved in 90 patients (40%) and R1 resection in 116 (51%). Five-year OS was 50% for the total group, and patients with R0 or R1 resection appeared to do better (5-year OS: R0 resection 52%, R1 resection 55%, R2 resection 28%; P = .08). Five-year local relapse rates also varied by degree of resection: R0 18%, R1 31%, and R2 61%. Central relapse in the IOERT field occurred in 10% of patients and distant metastases in 42%.

Massachusetts General Hospital Results were analyzed in a group of 37 MGH patients with retroperitoneal sarcoma (EBRT 17, EBRT + IOERT 20), all of whom received preoperative EBRT.[47,49,51] In patients with R0 or R1 resection, survival trends favored EBRT + IORT (16 patients) over EBRT alone (13 patients), with 5-year local control of 83% versus 61% and 5-year OS 74% versus 30%.

Mayo Clinic Arizona A series of 64 consecutive patients underwent surgical resection of primary or locally recurrent retroperitoneal sarcoma at MCA from 1996 to 2011; 24 had resection alone, 2 had preoperative EBRT plus resection, and 38 received both preoperative EBRT and IOERT.[54] In the IOERT group, 47% presented

Table 7
Primary retroperitoneal and pelvic sarcoma: IOERT + EBRT, Mayo Clinics

Prognostic Factor	n	Overall Survival (%)		Disease Control			
				Local (%)		Distant (%)	
		2 y	5 y	2 y	5 y	2 y	5 y
Residual at IOERT							
≤ Microscopic							
Margin (−)	11	91	62	100	100	71	53
Margin (+)	25	75	54	100	92	65	41
Gross	7	71	29	80	60	43	29
Grade							
Low (1, 2)	9	89	42	100	100	88	25
High (3, 4)	34	75	54	96	84	55	43
Tumor Size (cm)							
≤5	7	100	86	100	83	71	43
>5	35	76	45	96	92	62	46

Data from Refs.[47,48,52]

with locally recurrent disease. Local control at 5 years was 81% in IOERT patients versus 52% for non-IOERT patients (P = .002). IOERT was associated with a lower risk of local relapse on both univariate (P = .001) and multivariate analysis (P = .003). Five-year OS was 62% in the total group of 64 patients, with no significant difference in IOERT versus non-IOERT patients.

European pooled analysis Results of a pooled European analysis were presented at ISIORT 2008 by Krempien and colleagues[60] in a series of 122 patients with retroperitoneal sarcoma who received IOERT as a component of treatment from 1991 to 2007 (recurrent 81, primary 41). Postoperative EBRT was given in 75 patients; 40 patients were previously irradiated. The 5-year actuarial OS, DFS, local control, and freedom from distant metastasis of all patients was 64%, 28%, 40%, and 50%, respectively. Central relapse within the IOERT field was related to degree of resection: R0 5%, R1 23%, and R2 75%. Late complications of Grade 2 or higher occurred in 21% of patients, but only 5% of patients required surgical intervention.

Conclusions and future possibilities IORT combined with resection and preoperative EBRT offers an effective means of improving local control with retroperitoneal sarcomas. Based on the NCI randomized trial, use of adjuvant postoperative EBRT without IORT after marginal resection could be questioned, because the rate of tumor-bed relapse with adjuvant EBRT in that trial was 80%, which is equivalent to results with surgery alone. A more practical approach is to give preoperative EBRT (±concomitant or neoadjuvant chemotherapy) after fine-needle biopsy and perform the resection at an institution that has the capability of giving an IORT supplement with IOERT or HDR-IORT. Local, regional, and distant failures are still common, however, emphasizing the need for further improvement in local therapy and an effective systemic treatment. Increased use of IMRT to deliver the EBRT component of treatment may be useful in improving tolerance to the aggressive combined-modality treatment approaches that include EBRT/IOERT and maximal resection, and may allow some dose escalation of the EBRT component of treatment and the safe addition of concurrent chemotherapy during EBRT. A phase II Radiation Therapy Oncology Group study was performed to evaluate neoadjuvant adriamycin and ifosfamide plus preoperative EBRT, resection, and IORT for moderate and high-grade retroperitoneal sarcomas, but the study was closed prematurely because of inadequate accrual.[61]

REFERENCES

1. Gunderson LL, Tepper JE, Biggs DJ, et al. Intraoperative +/- external beam irradiation. Curr Probl Cancer 1983;7:1–69.
2. Gunderson LL, Willett CG, Harrison LB, et al. Intraoperative irradiation: techniques and results. 2nd edition. New York: Humana Press/Springer; 2011. p. 1–529.
3. Nag S, Gunderson LL, Willett CG, et al. IORT with electron-beam, high- dose-rate brachytherapy, or low-KV/electronic brachytherapy: methodological comparisons. In: Gunderson LL, Willett CG, Calvo FA, et al, editors. Intraoperative irradiation: techniques and results. 2nd edition. New York: Humana Press/Springer; 2011. p. 99–118.
4. Okunieff P, Sundararaman S, Metcalf S, et al. Biology of large dose per fraction irradiation. In: Gunderson LL, Willett CG, Calvo FA, et al, editors. Intraoperative irradiation: techniques and results. 2nd edition. New York: Humana Press/Springer; 2011. p. 27–50.
5. Fuhrman GM, Charnsangavej C, Abbruzzese JL, et al. Thin-section contrast-enhanced computed tomography accurately predicts the resectability of malignant pancreatic neoplasms. Am J Surg 1994;167(1):104–13.
6. Evans DB, Abbruzzese JL, Rich TA. Cancer of the pancreas. In: DeVita VT, Hellman S, Rosenberg SA, editors. Cancer, principles and practice of oncology. Philadelphia: J.B. Lippincott Co; 1997. p. 1054–87.
7. Callery M, Chang K, Fishman E, et al. Pretreatment assessment of resectable and borderline resectable pancreatic cancer: Expert consensus statement. Ann Surg Oncol 2009;16(7):1727–33.
8. Spitz FR, Abbruzzese JL, Lee JE, et al. Preoperative and postoperative chemoradiation strategies in patients treated with pancreaticoduodenectomy for adenocarcinoma of the pancreas. J Clin Oncol 1997;15(3):928–37.
9. Miller RC, Valentini V, Moss A, et al. Pancreas cancer. In: Gunderson LL, Willett CG, Calvo FA, et al, editors. Intraoperative irradiation: techniques and results. 2nd edition. New York: Humana Press/Springer; 2011. p. 249–72.
10. Nagakawa T, Kayahara M, Ohta T, et al. Patterns of neural and plexus invasion of human pancreatic cancer and experimental cancer. Int J Pancreatol 1991;10:113–9.
11. Nagakawa T, Mori K, Nakano T, et al. Perineural invasion of carcinoma of the pancreas and biliary tract. Br J Surg 1993;80:619–21.
12. Raut CP, Tseng JF, Sun CCP, et al. Impact of resection status on pattern of failure and survival after pancreaticoduodenectomy for pancreatic adenocarcinoma. Ann Surg 2007;246:52–60.
13. Yeo CJ, Cameron JL, Lillemoe KD, et al. Pancreaticoduodenectomy with or without distal gastrectomy and extended retroperitoneal lymphadenectomy for periampullary adenocarcinoma, Part 2: Randomized controlled trial evaluating survival, morbidity, and mortality. Ann Surg 2002;236:355–68.
14. Farnell MB, Pearson RK, Sarr MG, et al. A prospective randomized trial comparing standard pancreatoduodenectomy with pancreatoduodenectomy with extended lymphadenectomy in resectable pancreatic head adenocarcinoma. Surgery 2005;138:618–30.
15. Pedrazzoli SM, DiCarlo VM, Dionigi RM, et al. Standard versus extended lymphadenectomy associated with pancreatoduodenectomy in the surgical treatment of

adenocarcinoma of the head of the pancreas: a multicenter, prospective, randomized study. Ann Surg 1998;228:508–17.

16. Iqbal N, Lovegrove RE, Tilney HS, et al. A comparison of pancreaticoduodenectomy with extended pancreaticoduodenectomy: a meta-analysis of 1909 patients. Eur J Surg Oncol 2009;35:79–86.

17. Whittington R, Solin L, Mohiuddin M, et al. Multimodality therapy of unresectable pancreatic adenocarcinoma. Cancer 1984;54:1991–8.

18. Mohiuddin M, Cantor RJ, Bierman W, et al. Combined modality treatment of localized unresectable adenocarcinoma of the pancreas. Int J Radiat Oncol Biol Phys 1988;14:79–84.

19. Roldan GE, Gunderson LL, Nagorney DM, et al. External beam vs external beam and intraoperative irradiation for locally advanced pancreatic cancer. Cancer 1988;61:1110–6.

20. Foo ML, Gunderson LL, Urrutia R. Pancreatic cancer. In: Gunderson LL, Tepper JE, editors. Clinical radiation oncology. New York: Churchill Livingstone/ Harcourt Health Sciences Co; 2000. p. 686–706.

21. Shipley WU, Wood WC, Tepper JE, et al. Intraoperative electron beam irradiation for patients with unresectable pancreatic carcinoma. Ann Surg 1984;200:25–32.

22. Garton GR, Gunderson LL, Nagorney DM, et al. High dose preoperative external beam and intraoperative irradiation for locally advanced pancreatic cancer. Int J Radiat Oncol Biol Phys 1993;27:1153–7.

23. Mohiuddin M, Regine WF, Stevens J, et al. Combined intraoperative radiation in perioperative chemotherapy for unresectable cancers of the pancreas. J Clin Oncol 1995;13:2764–8.

24. Tepper JE, Shipley WU, Warshaw AL, et al. The role of misonidazole combined with intraoperative radiation therapy in the treatment of pancreatic carcinoma. J Clin Oncol 1987;5:579–84.

25. Willett CG, Del Castillo CF, Shih HA, et al. Long-term results of intraoperative electron beam irradiation (IOERT) for patients with unresectable pancreatic cancer. Ann Surg 2005;241:295–9.

26. Ashman JB, Moss A, Callister MG, et al. Neoadjuvant chemoradiation and intraoperative electron irradiation for locally unresectable or borderline resectable pancreas adenocarcinoma. Gastrointestinal Cancer Symposium. J Clin Oncol 2012;20(Suppl 4) [abstract 327].

27. Valentini V, D'Agostino G, Mattiucci GC, et al. IORT in pancreatic cancer: a joint analysis on 270 patients. ISIORT 2008 Proceedings. Rev Cancer 2008;22:34–5.

28. Gunderson LL, Cohen AM, Dosoretz DE, et al. Residual, unresectable or recurrent colorectal cancer: external beam irradiation and intraoperative electron beam boost +/- resection. Int J Radiat Oncol Biol Phys 1983;9:1597–606.

29. Willett CG, Shellito PC, Tepper JE, et al. Intraoperative electron beam radiation therapy for primary locally advanced rectal and rectosigmoid carcinoma. J Clin Oncol 1991;9:843–9.

30. Gunderson LL, Nelson H, Martenson J, et al. Locally advanced primary colorectal cancer: Intraoperative electron and external beam irradiation + 5-FU. Int J Radiat Oncol Biol Phys 1997;37:601–14.

31. Arvold ND, Hong TS, Willett CG, et al. Primary colorectal cancer. In: Gunderson LL, Willett CG, Calvo FA, et al, editors. Intraoperative irradiation: techniques and results. 2nd edition. New York: Humana Press/Springer; 2011. p. 297–322.

32. Schild SE, Gunderson LL, Haddock MG, et al. Radiotherapy as a component of treatment for locally advanced colon cancer. Int J Radiat Oncol Biol Phys 1997; 37:51–8.

33. Mathis KL, Nelson H, Pemberton JH, et al. Unresectable colorectal cancer can be cured with multi-modality therapy. Ann Surg 2008;248:592–8.
34. Haddock MG, Nelson H, Valentini V, et al. Recurrent colorectal cancer. In: Gunderson LL, Willett CG, Calvo FA, et al, editors. Intraoperative irradiation: techniques and results. 2nd edition. New York: Humana Press/Springer; 2011. p. 323–52.
35. Wallace HJ, Willett CG, Shellito PC, et al. Intraoperative radiation therapy for locally advanced recurrent rectal or rectosigmoid cancer. J Surg Oncol 1995; 60:122–7.
36. Suzuki K, Gunderson LL, Devine RM, et al. Intraoperative irradiation after palliative surgery for locally recurrent rectal cancer. Cancer 1995;75:939–52.
37. Gunderson LL, Nelson H, Martenson J, et al. Intraoperative electron and external beam irradiation with or without 5-fluorouracil and maximum surgical resection for previously unirradiated, locally recurrent colorectal cancer. Dis Colon Rectum 1996;39:1379–95.
38. Haddock M, Gunderson L, Nelson H, et al. Intraoperative irradiation for locally recurrent colorectal cancer in previously irradiated patients. Int J Radiat Oncol Biol Phys 2001;49:1267–74.
39. Haddock MG, Miller RC, Nelson H, et al. Intraoperative electron irradiation for locally recurrent rectal cancer. ISIORT 2002 Proceedings, Abstract 8.3. Aachen (Germany).
40. Haddock MG, Miller RC, Nelson H, et al. Intraoperative electron irradiation for locally recurrent colorectal cancer. Int J Radiat Oncol Biol Phys 2011;79: 143–50.
41. Haddock MG, Nelson H, Donahue J, et al. IORT as a component of salvage therapy for colo-rectal cancer patients with advanced nodal metastases. Int J Radiat Oncol Biol Phys 2003;56:966–73.
42. Rutten H, Valentini V, Krempien R. Calvo FA for European Working Party of ISIORT. ISIORT 2008 Proceedings. Rev Cancer 2008;22:45–6.
43. Abuchaibe O, Calvo FA, Tangeo E, et al. Intraoperative irradiation in locally advanced recurrent colorectal cancer. Int J Radiat Oncol Biol Phys 1993;26: 859–67.
44. Bussieres E, Gilly FN, Rouanet P, et al. Recurrences of rectal cancers: results of a multimodal approach with intraoperative radiation therapy. Int J Radiat Oncol Biol Phys 1996;34:49–56.
45. Mannaerts GH, Martijn H, Crommelin MA, et al. Intraoperative electron beam radiation therapy for locally recurrent rectal carcinoma. Int J Radiat Oncol Biol Phys 1999;45:297–308.
46. Dresen RC, Gosens MJ, Martijn H, et al. Radical resection after IORT containing multimodality treatment is important determinant for outcome in patients treated for locally recurrent rectal cancer. ISIORT 2008 Proceedings. Rev Cancer 2008; 22:45–6.
47. Czito B, Donohue J, Willett CG, et al. Retroperitoneal sarcomas. In: Gunderson LL, Willett CG, Calvo FA, et al, editors. Intraoperative irradiation: techniques and results. 2nd edition. New York: Humana Press/Springer; 2011. p. 353–86.
48. Gunderson LL, Peterson I, Pritchard D, et al. Role and methods of irradiation as a component of treatment for extremity and retroperitoneal soft tissue sarcomas. Probl Gen Surg 1999;16:43–61.
49. Willett CG, Suit HD, Tepper JE, et al. Intraoperative electron beam radiation therapy for retroperitoneal soft tissue sarcoma. Cancer 1991;68:278–83.

50. Gunderson LL, Nagorney DM, McIlrath DC, et al. External beam and intraoperative electron irradiation for locally advanced soft tissue sarcomas. Int J Radiat Oncol Biol Phys 1993;25:647–56.

51. Gieschen HL, Spiro IJ, Suit HD, et al. Long-term results of intraoperative electron beam radiotherapy for primary and recurrent retroperitoneal soft tissue sarcoma. Int J Radiat Oncol Biol Phys 2001;50:127–31.

52. Petersen I, Haddock M, Donohue J, et al. Use of intraoperative electron beam radiotherapy in the management of retroperitoneal soft tissue sarcomas. Int J Radiat Oncol Biol Phys 2002;52:469–75.

53. Petersen I, Haddock M, Stafford SL, et al. Use of intraoperative radiation therapy in retroperitoneal sarcomas: update of the Mayo Clinic Rochester Experience. ISIORT 2008 Proceedings. Rev Cancer 2008;22:57.

54. Chee-Chee HS, Wasif N, Ashman JB, et al. The combination of preoperative radiation therapy, surgical resection and intraoperative electron radiation therapy improves local control of retroperitoneal sarcoma, in press.

55. Harrison LB, Anderson L, White C, et al. HDR-IORT for retroperitoneal sarcomas. In: Gunderson LL, Willett CG, Harrison LB, et al, editors. Intraoperative irradiation: techniques and results. Totowa (NJ): Humana Press; 1999. p. 351–8.

56. Alektiar KM, Hu K, Anderson L, et al. High-dose-rate intraoperative radiation therapy (HDR-IORT) for retroperitoneal sarcomas. Int J Radiat Oncol Biol Phys 2000;47:157–63.

57. Sindelar WF, Kinsella TJ, Chen PW, et al. Intraoperative radiotherapy and retroperitoneal sarcomas: Final results of a prospective, randomized, clinical trial. Arch Surg 1993;128:402–10.

58. Calvo FA, Azinovic I, Martinez R, et al. Intraoperative radiotherapy for the treatment of soft tissue sarcomas of central anatomic sites. 5th International IORT Symposium [abstracts]. Hepato Gastroenterol 1994;41:4.

59. Dubois JB, Hay MH, Gely S, et al. Intraoperative radiation therapy (IORT) in soft tissue sarcomas. 5th International IORT Symposium [abstracts]. Hepato Gastroenterol 1994;41:3.

60. Krempien R, Roeder F, Buchler MW, et al. for European Working Party of ISIORT. Intraoperative radiation therapy (IORT) for primary and recurrent retroperitoneal soft tissue sarcoma: first results of a pooled analysis. ISIORT 2008 Proceedings. Rev Cancer 2008;22:56–7.

61. Pisters PW, Ballo MT, Fenstermacher MJ, et al. Phase I trial of preoperative concurrent doxorubicin and radiation therapy, surgical resection and intraoperative electron-beam radiation therapy for patients with localized retroperitoneal sarcoma. J Clin Oncol 2003;21:3092–7.

Practical Radiation Oncology for Extremity Sarcomas

Nicole A. Larrier, MD, MSc[a], David G. Kirsch, MD, PhD[a,b,]*,
Richard F. Riedel, MD[c], Howard Levinson, MD[d],
William C. Eward, DVM, MD[e], Brian E. Brigman, MD[e,f]

KEYWORDS

- Soft tissue sarcoma • Radiation therapy • Surgery • Side effects

KEY POINTS

- Sarcomas should be managed by a multidisciplinary team with experience in caring for patients with sarcoma.
- Surgery is the cornerstone for management, but many patients with sarcoma are treated with adjuvant radiation therapy to improve local control.
- Preoperative and postoperative radiation therapy have similar rates of local control, but different side effect profiles. Therefore, combining radiation therapy with surgery should be tailored to each patient.

INTRODUCTION

Sarcomas encompass a diverse array of malignancies that originate in the musculoskeletal system. The cell of origin is most often muscle, fat, or bone. Overall, there are approximately 10,000 of these malignancies diagnosed in the United States annually.[1] Most occur in an extremity (50%). Other major sites are the retroperitoneum, trunk, and head and neck regions.

This article focuses on the use of radiation therapy for adult-type soft tissue sarcomas. Special mention is made of other sarcomas (eg, the management of retroperitoneal sarcoma) where appropriate. Although this article focuses on the use of

[a] Department of Radiation Oncology, Duke University Medical Center, 450 Research Drive, Durham, NC 27708, USA; [b] Department of Pharmacology & Cancer Biology, Duke University Medical Center, 450 Research Drive, Durham, NC 27708, USA; [c] Division of Medical Oncology, Department of Internal Medicine, Duke University Medical Center, 450 Research Drive, Durham, NC 27708, USA; [d] Division of Plastic and Reconstructive Surgery, Department of Surgery, Duke University Medical Center, 450 Research Drive, Durham, NC 27708, USA; [e] Department of Orthopaedic Surgery, Duke University Medical Center, 450 Research Drive, Durham, NC 27708, USA; [f] Department of Pediatrics, Duke University Medical Center, 450 Research Drive, Durham, NC 27708, USA
* Corresponding author. Department of Radiation Oncology, Duke University Medical Center, 450 Research Drive, Durham, NC 27708.
E-mail address: david.kirsch@duke.edu

Surg Oncol Clin N Am 22 (2013) 433–443
http://dx.doi.org/10.1016/j.soc.2013.02.004
1055-3207/13/$ – see front matter © 2013 Elsevier Inc. All rights reserved.
surgonc.theclinics.com

radiotherapy, emphasis is placed on the multidisciplinary management of these malignancies.

IMPORTANCE OF MULTIDISCIPLINARY EVALUATION

Because of the rarity and marked heterogeneity of soft tissue sarcomas, it is crucial that patients be evaluated in centers with clinical expertise.[2] The heterogeneity of histologic subtypes and varied clinical presentations observed require treatment plans that are ideally discussed and formulated in the context of a multidisciplinary setting. Pathologic expertise is essential in making an initial diagnosis. Radiologic evaluation is appropriate for adequate and complete staging. Discussion between the radiologist and surgeon additionally provides for a carefully planned surgical approach, allowing a determination of the proximity of disease to vital neurovascular and visceral structures. In addition, an open dialogue among the treating surgeons and medical and radiation oncologists allows timely consensus regarding the need, timing, and sequence of respective therapies in an effort to limit treatment-related morbidity while maintaining functional outcomes and performance status. Plastic and reconstructive and vascular surgical specialties may be used in specific scenarios. In addition, the evaluation and management of patients in a center with expertise may provide a sense of patient comfort and reduced anxiety in knowing that providers have experience and a working knowledge of an otherwise rare disease.

STAGING WORK-UP

The American Joint Committee on Cancer (AJCC) 7th Edition (2010) staging for sarcoma is now used.[3] For soft tissue sarcoma, not only are tumor size, lymph node status, and distant metastatic status integral to staging but tumor grade is also incorporated in the system. All grade 1 tumors are considered stage I given their low risk of malignancy-related death. All metastatic tumors are stage IV. Stage III tumors are considered to be those greater than 5 cm and grade 3, or those with involved lymph nodes. The remainder are considered stage II.

The staging of individuals diagnosed with sarcoma requires adequate imaging not only of the primary site but also as an assessment for disseminated disease. A determination of tumor size, relationship to fascial planes, proximity to vital structures, and presence or absence of metastasis all aid in determining an optimal treatment plan for patients. Magnetic resonance imaging (MRI) is the preferred imaging for sarcomas of the extremity, whereas computed tomography (CT) may be appropriate for retroperitoneal and truncal sarcomas. Adequate imaging of the chest is essential because the lungs are the most common site for distant spread. Staging should be individualized based on histologic subtype because some histologic subtypes show varying patterns of metastasis. Cross-axial imaging of the abdomen and pelvis should additionally be considered for histologies prone to abdominal spread, including leiomyosarcoma, epithelioid sarcoma, angiosarcoma, and myxoid round cell liposarcoma.[2–5] Myxoid round cell liposarcoma has additionally been associated with spinal metastasis,[5] whereas alveolar soft part sarcoma has been associated with the development of brain metastasis.[6] Positron emission tomography/CT may additionally be considered and has both prognostic[7] and predictive abilities.[8,9]

Individuals with localized or locally advanced disease (stage I–III) are often treated with multimodality therapies, primarily surgery with additional consideration for radiation and/or chemotherapy as part of a neoadjuvant or adjuvant approach. Individuals with disseminated disease (stage IV) are traditionally treated with palliative systemic therapies, although the degree of disease burden, particularly in the setting of oligometastatic disease, may warrant aggressive treatment approaches, including metastasectomy.

SURGICAL CONSIDERATIONS
Role of Biopsy

The primary focus of the orthopedic oncologist is the execution of an operative plan that resects the tumor and a surrounding margin of normal tissue while preserving or reconstructing as much functional tissue as possible. Before the widespread use of adjuvant radiation therapy, radical resections and amputations were common. The recognition that a limb-sparing resection plus adjuvant radiation therapy offered an equivalent outcome to amputation represented a landmark shift in the management of patients with soft tissue sarcoma of the extremity.[10] Therefore, the importance of a multidisciplinary team approach to treating patients with soft tissue sarcoma cannot be overstated. The critical first step in planning this treatment is the biopsy. Because normal tissue encountered during biopsy potentially becomes contaminated by neoplastic cells, definitive resections are performed so that all tissue contacted by biopsy instruments is included in the resection and the radiation field, which means that a biopsy tract or incision that passes outside the planned surgical field requires a more extensive resection and a wider radiation field, and incurs additional morbidity to the patient. Although many types of biopsy are possible (typically either a core needle biopsy or an incisional biopsy), all biopsies should be planned with the definitive resection in mind. To that end, an important consideration for the diagnostician is whether or not an unknown soft tissue tumor may be a sarcoma. Referral to an orthopedic oncologist for a planned biopsy should be considered for any soft tissue tumor that has one or more of the following: (1) size greater than 5 cm, (2) location deep to fascia, and (3) heterogeneous signal intensity on MRI. By planning the radiation therapy, the biopsy, and the definitive resection together, radiation oncologists and orthopedic oncologists are able to optimize the treatment plan for the greatest chance of successful limb preservation.

Surgical Margins

Because sarcomas often grow along fascial planes, the battle for local control seems to begin and end with a wide resection. However, such resections, where a surrounding margin of normal tissue is removed along with the tumor, are not definitive without adjuvant therapy. Patients treated with a negative-margin excision and no adjuvant radiation therapy might be expected to have local control of their disease. In reality, they experience rates of local recurrence of up to 40%.[11] It is now accepted that cancer cells are commonly found beyond the boundaries of the sarcoma pseudocapsule, but no one has been able to show a correct amount of normal tissue that should be resected to remove all cancer present,[12] in part because of the difficulty of determining where these satellite cells are found relative to the tumor. One author has shown cancer cells in the supposedly normal tissue peripheral to the tumor in two-thirds of cases.[12] In this study, cells were found up to 4 cm beyond the pseudocapsule of the tumor. There was no correlation between the presence of cancer beyond the pseudocapsule and signal changes on the MR imaging.[12] It is this uncertainty about when and where cancer is located beyond the pseudocapsule and even beyond the surgical margins that may explain the benefit of adjuvant radiation therapy in obtaining local control. The presence of residual sarcoma cells in the tumor bed is associated not only with local recurrence but also with decreased disease-specific survival.[13] With adjuvant radiation therapy, whether administered preoperatively or postoperatively, rates of local recurrence decrease from nearly 40% to approximately 10%.[14] Even when adjuvant radiation therapy is not part of the initial treatment plan, it should be elected to treat patients with unplanned positive margins identified on histopathology after resection.

The concept of the planned positive margin has been made possible by the use of adjuvant radiation therapy. A planned positive margin describes a situation in which the surgeon anticipates and executes a margin-positive resection to spare a critical structure (typically a nerve, vessel, or bone) adjacent to a tumor. Provided that the structure is not fixed to the tumor and that adjuvant radiation therapy is used, this carefully planned and anticipated margin-positive situation provides similar outcomes to margin-negative controls.[15]

EVIDENCE FOR THE USE OF RADIOTHERAPY IN SARCOMA MANAGEMENT

Classic studies from the 1970s and 1980s established the role of radiotherapy in the management of extremity sarcomas.[16] A randomized trial at the National Cancer Institute comparing amputation versus limb-sparing surgery followed by radiotherapy showed similar overall survival rates with an acceptable local recurrence rate in the surgery and radiotherapy arm (15%). The benefit of radiation therapy in addition to limb-sparing surgery was evaluated in a second National Cancer Institute study that randomized patients with extremity sarcoma to a compartmental resection versus tumor resection followed by radiotherapy.[17] The surgery alone arm had a lower local control rate (80% vs 100%) and again overall survival was not affected. Another prospective, randomized trial at Memorial Sloan Kettering Cancer Center compared limb-sparing surgery alone versus surgery plus brachytherapy.[11] The addition of brachytherapy increased the rate of local control from 69% to 82%.

The seminal contemporary contribution to this area is the randomized study of preoperative versus postoperative radiotherapy conducted by the National Cancer Institute of Canada (NCIC).[18] The radiotherapy techniques consisted of 50 Gy in the preoperative setting and 66 Gy given postoperatively. Longitudinal expansions around the tumor were 5 cm and radial expansions were 2 cm. The local control rate (90%) and overall survival were similar. There was a doubling (35% vs 17%) of the wound complications within 120 days after surgery in preoperative versus postoperative radiotherapy arms. However, these wound complications were predominantly in the lower extremity. Moreover, long-term complications such as fibrosis, edema, and joint stiffness seemed to be decreased in the preoperative radiotherapy arm.[19]

Therefore, the body of randomized data suggests that radiotherapy in combination with tumor resection provides excellent local control at the primary site. The optimal timing of radiotherapy (preoperative or postoperative) can be influenced by individual factors such as overall life expectancy of the patient and therefore the concern regarding long-term complications, and the underlying risk and potential complications from a wound infection (eg, vascular disease or uncontrolled diabetes).

RADIATION THERAPY FOR UNRESECTED SARCOMAS

As described in detail earlier, surgery is the foundation of local therapy for sarcomas. However, there are clinical scenarios in which surgery is not an option. In some cases, patient comorbidities may make certain surgeries too risky. In other cases, en bloc surgical resection may cause such significant morbidity that patients decline surgery. In these cases, the multidisciplinary team needs to consider creative options to try to achieve local control. In these situations, radiation therapy alone can be considered. In contrast with the radiation doses used in preoperative (50 Gy) or postoperative (60 Gy) radiation therapy, to achieve local control with radiation therapy alone, a higher dose of radiation is generally required for most soft tissue sarcomas.

The sarcoma group at the Massachusetts General Hospital reported the outcome of 112 patients whose unresected soft tissue sarcomas were treated with radiation therapy.[20] At the time of the analysis, median follow-up was 139 months. Tumor size at the time of radiation therapy and radiation therapy dose influenced local control. Local control at 5 years for sarcomas less than 5 cm, 5 cm to 10 cm, and greater than 10 cm was 51%, 45%, and 9%, respectively. Five-year local control for tumors treated with less than 63 Gy was 22%, whereas 5-year local control was 60% for tumors treated to doses of 63 Gy or greater. Use of chemotherapy, histologic grade, and tumor location did not influence the results of this retrospective study. Fourteen percent of all patients had a major complication from radiation therapy. The complication rate from radiotherapy increased to 27% for patients treated with at least 68 Gy. Although these results of radiotherapy for the treatment of unresected soft tissue sarcomas are inferior to the combination of surgery and adjuvant radiation therapy, they show that radiation therapy alone with a dose of at least 63 Gy can achieve local control in approximately half of all soft tissue sarcomas up to 10 cm in size. Therefore, for select patients who are unable or unwilling to undergo surgery, radiation therapy alone or with concurrent ifosfamide chemotherapy[21,22] should be considered.

SURGERY AS SOLE TREATMENT

Patients who are at low risk for local recurrence may not need any adjuvant therapy. These may include patients with superficial tumors and small tumors (<5 cm). In addition, low-grade sarcomas that have a very low propensity to metastasize may also be considered for resection alone. Pisters and colleagues[23] prospectively analyzed extremity and truncal T1 sarcomas (<5 cm) treated with oncologic resection alone. The long-term local recurrence rate was 7.9% at 5 years, which is comparable with the use of surgery and radiotherapy for higher risk tumors.[23]

TECHNICAL DETAILS OF RADIATION THERAPY PLANNING FOR SOFT TISSUE SARCOMAS
External Beam Radiotherapy

As with other types of cancer, the goal of radiation therapy for soft tissue sarcomas is to deliver radiation dose to the tumor (gross tumor volume) and the adjacent area at risk (clinical tumor volume) while sparing critical normal tissues from a radiation dose that has a high chance of causing a clinically meaningful complication. With the routine use of MRI to assess the extent of the primary tumor and adjacent peritumoral edema, which can harbor sarcoma cells,[12] and the availability of CT for treatment planning, investigators are currently seeking to define the appropriate clinical target volume to treat sarcomas in prospective clinical studies.

Kim and colleagues[24] reported a retrospective study of 56 patients with stage I to III extremity soft tissue sarcomas treated with preoperative radiation therapy. The clinical target volume was defined as the T1 postgadolinium-defined gross disease with 3.5 cm longitudinal margins and a 1-cm to 1.5-cm radial margin. With a median follow-up of 41 months after starting preoperative radiation therapy, the 5-year local control rate was 88.5%. At the time of the analysis, only 3 patients had developed a local recurrence at the site of first failure. All of these patients had a positive surgical margin. Two other patients developed distant disease first and then developed a late local recurrence. Three of the local failures occurred within the clinical target volume and 2 local recurrences occurred within, and also extending beyond, the clinical target volume. To evaluate similar treatment of preoperative radiation therapy in the multiinstitutional setting, the Radiation Therapy Oncology Group (RTOG) performed a prospective phase II clinical trial of patients with extremity soft tissue sarcomas (RTOG 0630). In this trial, the clinical target volume was defined as a 3-cm longitudinal and 1.5-cm radial margin for intermediate to high grade sarcomas larger than 8 cm, but other sarcomas were treated with a 2-cm longitudinal margin and a 1-cm radial margin. This trial met its accrual target of approximately 100 patients treated with pre-operative radiation therapy and follow-up is now in progress.

A prospective radiation field–size clinical trial is also underway in the United Kingdom for postoperative radiation therapy. In the VORTEX: Randomised trial of volume of post-operative radiotherapy given to adult patients with extremity soft tissue sarcoma trial, patients with extremity soft tissue sarcomas are treated with 66 Gy in 33 treatments for postoperative radiation therapy. Patients are randomized to 1 of 2 regions. Half of the patients are initially treated with a large field to 50 Gy: clinical target volume extends 2 cm radially beyond the location of the excised tumor and at least 5 cm in the longitudinal direction, but must include the scar by 1 cm. Then, the final 16 Gy boost is delivered using a clinical target volume that extends 2 cm in all directions beyond the resected tumor volume. The remaining patients are randomized to the smaller boost field for the entire 66 Gy. The VORTEX trial continues to accrue patients with a goal of 200 patients in each arm.

In addition to covering the clinical target volume with radiation, treatment planning should also try to minimize radiation dose to normal tissues to prevent long-term side effects. For example, in extremity sarcomas, a strip of normal tissue that is usually in the compartment opposite to the tumor is spared from radiation exposure to preserve lymphatic channels, and thus limit the risk and severity of lymphedema. In addition, for lower extremity sarcomas, the radiation dose to the femur should be limited when possible. A mean dose of 45 Gy is associated with fracture, but a mean dose of 37 Gy is not.[25]

Treatment immobilization is accomplished with the use of a custom mold and/or mesh to prevent motion and rotation of the extremity. Special measures of shielding may need to be taken if irradiation of the male genitals is of concern.

Verification of the setup of individual radiation beams or the center of the radiation field (called the isocenter) is critical to ensuring accurate treatment delivery. Traditional setup verification (port film) is done using the megavoltage image of the treatment field before or after the treatment is delivered. The image quality of these megavoltage port films may vary significantly depending on the anatomic location and the patient's body habitus. Current techniques for setup verification now include the use of kilovoltage orthogonal images and/or cone beam CT using devices mounted on the treatment machine, which allows the acquisition of a high-quality image just before or after the delivery of a treatment dose. This technique is often referred to as image-guided radiation therapy (IGRT). Depending on the location of the tumor and the criticality of adjacent normal structures, daily verification images may be acquired to verify an accurate setup.

With the advances in treatment verification discussed earlier, the use of advanced treatment planning techniques such as intensity modulated radiotherapy for sarcomas can be considered. In extremity lesions, this technique has been investigated primarily to decrease risk of bone fracture, which can lead to severe morbidity. Alektiar and colleagues[26] published a series suggesting excellent local control rates with this technique, although the follow-up is too short to assess for decrease in long-term complications. In the retroperitoneum, intensity-modulated radiotherapy may be considered as a dose painting technique to allow a higher radiation dose to be given to areas at high risk for local recurrence while sparing critical normal structures such as kidney and liver.[27]

X-rays, Electrons, and Particle Therapy for Sarcomas

To achieve coverage of the clinical target volume and minimize radiation dose to the normal strip of uninvolved tissue and the bone, different types of radiation therapy can be used. These include x-rays (often referred to as photons), electrons, protons, and radioactive sources for brachytherapy. Each type of radiation has different properties that may have advantages or disadvantages in different clinical situations. High energy x-rays are used most frequently because they are widely available and provide excellent coverage of the clinical target volume. One potential disadvantage of x-rays is that they enter one side of the patient and exit the other side after depositing energy in the tumor, which means that normal tissue in the entrance and exit path of the x-rays is exposed to radiation. For superficial sarcomas (<5 cm depth), electrons can be considered. Because of their negative charge, electrons deposit most of their energy over a narrow range and only a small fraction of the energy exits the patient. Because of its positive charge and large size, proton radiation therapy has no exit radiation dose beyond the tumor. For some sarcomas, such as retroperitoneal sarcomas, the radiation exposure to normal organs can be decreased compared with the most sophisticated treatment plans with x-rays.

Brachytherapy

In some cases, brachytherapy may provide the best coverage of the clinical target volume while sparing normal tissue. For brachytherapy, catheters are placed in the tumor bed at the time of surgery. Then, 5 or 6 days, later the catheters are loaded with a radioactive source to deliver the radiation treatment. Because the radiation dose decreases with the square of the distance from the source, for anatomic locations where the geometry is favorable for placing brachytherapy catheters, this approach can successfully cover the clinical tumor volume while sparing normal structure.[11] Pisters and colleagues[11] showed that the use of adjuvant low-dose-rate brachytherapy for high-grade sarcomas provided excellent local control compared in a randomized fashion with surgery alone. As an alternative, brachytherapy may be used as an adjuvant or boost to external beam radiotherapy when positive surgical margins are anticipated. Either low-dose-rate brachytherapy (in which the radioactive implant is left in place for a few days) or high-dose-rate brachytherapy (in which the radioactive source is administered in several sessions each lasting several minutes over the course of a few days) can be used.

Intraoperative Radiotherapy

An additional technique for delivering radiotherapy to areas adjacent to critical normal tissues is the use of intraoperative radiotherapy. The radiation is delivered directly to the operative bed at the time of surgery using either electrons or a high-dose-rate brachytherapy applicator. This technique may improve local control when delivered in conjunction with external beam radiotherapy in retroperitoneal sarcomas. However, caution must be exercised because this approach uses a single dose of 10 to 20 Gy, which can cause peripheral neuropathy and other late effects.[28]

COMPLICATIONS OF RADIOTHERAPY
Wound Complications

The rate of wound complications in patients who receive surgery and radiotherapy ranges from 17% to 35% during the first 6 months after surgery.[19] Access to the expertise of a reconstructive surgeon may be required at the time of initial surgery or after a wound complication has occurred.

Wound Reconstruction

From a reconstructive microsurgeon's perspective, sarcoma defects should be reconstructed as quickly as possible to expedite healing so that adjuvant chemotherapy and/or radiation therapy (typically initiated 6 weeks after reconstruction) can begin expeditiously. Reconstruction reduces patient morbidity and controls expenditures. There are many reconstructive options for sarcoma defects. Primary closure (tension free) is almost always the best option when possible. When wounds cannot be closed primarily, such as in large wounds or irradiated tissue beds, grafts and flaps should be used. There are 4 key concepts that guide decision making in reconstruction of sarcoma defects: (1) characterize the defect and replace like with like to restore form and function, (2) analyze the recipient bed niche, (3) understand the reconstructive ladder and choose the simplest approach that will optimize outcomes, and (4) think of defects in terms of regional anatomy to facilitate flap selection. A well-planned reconstruction optimizes aesthetic appearances, maximizes function, and provides stable tissue coverage with minimal morbidity.

The first thing to consider when planning reconstruction is to define the defect. How large is the defect, where is the defect, what tissues have been resected, and how are the form (aesthetic) and function being affected? By defining the defect, clinicians can decide which reconstructive approach best restores the missing tissue. Missing tissue can be categorized as skin, tendon, nerve, blood vessels, fascia, teeth, and bone. For example, for a patient who has a thigh extremity sarcoma that is treated by resection of skin, fat, and a small portion of the rectus femoris muscle without affecting leg function, the defect may only require skin coverage. However, more than skin is needed for a patient with an upper extremity sarcoma in which the forearm extensors are resected along with skin, fat, and tendon. Reconstruction of an area crucial to limb function may include a functioning muscle transfer along with skin and free-tendon grafts such as an innervated myocutaneous gracilis flap with palmaris grafts.[29–31] In the unusual circumstance in which like tissue cannot be used (eg, replacing a femur with a femur), then an allograft or prosthetic may be used.[32–34] Allografts and prosthetics can provide a good reconstruction, but autologous tissue (sometimes with allografts) is a common first choice.[33,35]

Bone Fracture

Fracture of the adjacent bone can impart severe morbidity to the patient, especially if it is a weight-bearing bone. The risk of bone fracture is related to the volume included in the radiotherapy fields and the preexisting conditions such as osteoporosis. The dose-volume relationship between risk of fracture and dose delivered has not been well studied. Current treatment planning techniques are allowing investigation into the radiotherapy factors that affect fracture risk.[36] Standard treatment consists of placement of an intramedullary nail for weight-bearing bones and maintenance of good bone health. There are no data on the use of bisphosphonates in this population, either prophylactically or after a fracture has occurred.

Edema

Edema of the involved extremity can occur and peaks during the first year after combined modality therapy.[17] In the randomized trial of preoperative versus postoperative radiotherapy, fewer patients experienced edema in the preoperative radiotherapy arm.[20] Treatment consists of symptomatic management of the edema using compressive stockings and physical therapy.

Other

Joint stiffness and muscle fibrosis are also reported after treatment of extremity sarcoma. However, the tools to evaluate these complications are not standard. In addition, in younger patients, there is a small risk of a second malignancy associated with radiotherapy.

SUMMARY

Radiotherapy is an integral part of the management of many patients with extremity soft tissue sarcoma. Individualized treatment planning can optimize local control and minimize morbidity. Because sarcomas are rare, multidisciplinary evaluation and management by a team of physicians with experience in caring for patients with sarcomas is recommended.

REFERENCES

1. American Cancer Society. Cancer facts and figures 2012. Atlanta (GA): American Cancer Society; 2012.
2. Demetri GD, Antonia S, Benjamin RS, et al. Soft tissue sarcoma. J Natl Compr Canc Netw 2010;8(6):630.
3. Edge SB, Byrd DR, Compton CC, et al, editors. AJCC Cancer staging manual. 7th edition. New York: Springer; 2010.
4. Behranwala KA, Roy P, Giblin V, et al. Intra-abdominal metastases from soft tissue sarcoma. J Surg Oncol 2004;87(3):116.
5. Moreau LC, Turcotte R, Ferguson P, et al. Myxoid\round cell liposarcoma (MRCLS) revisited: an analysis of 418 primarily managed cases. Ann Surg Oncol 2012;19(4):1081.
6. Portera CA Jr, Ho V, Patel SR, et al. Alveolar soft part sarcoma: clinical course and patterns of metastasis in 70 patients treated at a single institution. Cancer 2001; 91(3):585.
7. Fuglo HM, Jørgensen SM, Loft A, et al. The diagnostic and prognostic value of (18)F-FDG PET/CT in the initial assessment of high-grade bone and soft tissue sarcoma. A retrospective study of 89 patients. Eur J Nucl Med Mol Imaging 2012;39(9):1416.
8. Herrmann K, Benz MR, Czernin J, et al. 18F-FDG-PET/CT Imaging as an early survival predictor in patients with primary high-grade soft tissue sarcomas under-going neoadjuvant therapy. Clin Cancer Res 2012;18(7):2024.
9. Folpe AL, Lyles RH, Sprouse JT, et al. (F-18) Fluorodeoxyglucose positron emission tomography as a predictor of pathologic grade and other prognostic variables in bone and soft tissue sarcoma. Clin Cancer Res 2000;6(4):1279.
10. Rosenberg SA, Tepper J, Glatstein E, et al. The treatment of soft-tissue sarcomas of the extremities: prospective randomized evaluations of (1) limb-sparing surgery plus radiation therapy compared with amputation and (2) the role of adjuvant chemotherapy. Ann Surg 1982;196:305–15.
11. Pisters PW, Harrison LB, Leung DH, et al. Long-term results of a prospective randomized trial of adjuvant brachytherapy in soft tissue sarcoma. J Clin Oncol 1996;14(3):859–68.
12. White LM, Wunder JS, Bell RS, et al. Histologic assessment of peritumoral edema in soft tissue sarcoma. Int J Radiat Oncol Biol Phys 2005;61(5):1439–45.

13. Sabolch A, Feng M, Griffith K, et al. Risk factors for local recurrence and metastasis in soft tissue sarcomas of the extremity. Am J Clin Oncol 2012;35:151–7.

14. Lewis JJ, Leung D, Casper ES, et al. Multifactorial analysis of long-term follow-up (more than 5 years) of primary extremity sarcoma. Arch Surg 1999;134:190–4.

15. Gerrand CH, Wunder JS, Kandel RA, et al. Classification of positive margins after resection of soft-tissue sarcoma of the limb predicts the risk of local recurrence. J Bone Joint Surg Br 2001;83(8):1149–55.

16. Rosenberg SA, Kent H, Costa J, et al. Prospective randomized evaluation of the role of limb-sparing surgery, radiation therapy, and adjuvant chemoimmunotherapy in the treatment of adult soft-tissue sarcomas. Surgery 1978;84(1):62.

17. Yang JC, Chang AE, Baker AR, et al. Randomized prospective study of the benefit of adjuvant radiation therapy in the treatment of soft tissue sarcomas of the extremity. J Clin Oncol 1998;16(1):197–203.

18. O'Sullivan B, Davis AM, Turcotte R, et al. Preoperative versus postoperative radiotherapy in soft-tissue sarcoma of the limbs: a randomised trial. Lancet 2002;359(9325):2235–41.

19. Davis AM, O'Sullivan B, Turcotte R, et al. Late radiation morbidity following randomization to preoperative versus postoperative radiotherapy in extremity soft tissue sarcoma. Radiother Oncol 2005;75(1):48–53.

20. Kepka L, DeLaney TF, Suit HD, et al. Results of radiation therapy for unresected sarcomas. Int J Radiat Oncol Biol Phys 2005;63(3):852–9.

21. Eckert F, Matuschek C, Mueller AC, et al. Definitive radiotherapy and single-agent radiosensitizing ifosfamide in patients with localized, irresectable soft tissue sarcoma: a retrospective analysis. Radiat Oncol 2010;16(5):55.

22. Cuneo KC, Riedel RF, Dodd LG, et al. Pathologic complete response of a malignant peripheral nerve sheath tumor in the lung treated with neoadjuvant ifosfamide and radiation therapy. J Clin Oncol 2012;30(28):e291–3.

23. Pisters PW, Pollock RE, Lewis VO, et al. Long-term results of prospective trial of surgery alone with selective use of radiation for patients with T1 extremity and trunk soft tissue sarcomas. Ann Surg 2007;246(4):675–81.

24. Kim B, Chen YL, Kirsch DG, et al. An effective preoperative three-dimensional radiotherapy target volume for extremity soft tissue sarcoma and the effect of margin width on local control. Int J Radiat Oncol Biol Phys 2010;77(3):843–50.

25. Dickie CI, Parent AL, Griffin AM, et al. Bone fractures following external beam radiotherapy and limb-preservation surgery for lower extremity soft tissue sarcoma: relationship to irradiated bone length, volume, tumor location and dose. Int J Radiat Oncol Biol Phys 2009;75(4):1119–24.

26. Alektiar KM, Brennan MF, Healey JH, et al. Impact of intensity-modulated radiation therapy on local control in primary soft-tissue sarcoma of the extremity. J Clin Oncol 2008;26(20):3440–4.

27. Bossi A, De Wever I, Van Limbergen E, et al. Intensity modulated radiation-therapy for preoperative posterior abdominal wall irradiation of retroperitoneal liposarcomas. Int J Radiat Oncol Biol Phys 2007;67(1):164–70.

28. Sindelar WF, Kinsella TJ, Chen PW, et al. Intraoperative radiotherapy in retroperitoneal sarcomas. Final results of a prospective, randomized, clinical trial. Arch Surg 1993;128(4):402–10.

29. Koshima I, Nanba Y, Tsutsui T, et al. Vascularized femoral nerve graft with anterolateral thigh true perforator flap for massive defects after cancer ablation in the upper arm. J Reconstr Microsurg 2003;19:299–302.

30. Nelson AA, Frassica FJ, Gordon TA, et al. Cost analysis of functional restoration surgery for extremity soft-tissue sarcoma. Plast Reconstr Surg 2006;117:277–83.

31. Pritsch T, Malawer MM, Wu CC, et al. Functional reconstruction of the extensor mechanism following massive tumor resections from the anterior compartment of the thigh. Plast Reconstr Surg 2007;120:960–9.
32. Aponte-Tinao L, Farfalli GL, Ritacco LE, et al. Intercalary femur allografts are an acceptable alternative after tumor resection. Clin Orthop Relat Res 2012;470: 728–34.
33. Brigman BE, Hornicek FJ, Gebhardt MC, et al. Allografts about the knee in young patients with high-grade sarcoma. Clin Orthop Relat Res 2004;(421):232–9.
34. Donati D, Giacomini S, Gozzi E, et al. Proximal femur reconstruction by an allograft prosthesis composite. Clin Orthop Relat Res 2002;(394):192–200.
35. Ozger H, Akgul T, Yildiz F, et al. Biological reconstruction of the femur using double free vascularized fibular autografts in a vertical array because of a large defect following wide resection of an osteosarcoma: a case report with 7 years of follow-up. J Pediatr Orthop B 2013;22(1):52–8.
36. Pak D, Vineberg KA, Griffith KA, et al. Dose–effect relationships for femoral fractures after multimodality limb-sparing therapy of soft-tissue sarcomas of the proximal lower extremity. Int J Radiat Oncol Biol Phys 2012;83(4):1257–63.

Radiotherapy and Radiosurgery for Tumors of the Central Nervous System

John P. Kirkpatrick, MD, PhD[a,b,*], Fang-Fang Yin, PhD[a],
John H. Sampson, MD, PhD[a,b]

KEYWORDS

- Central nervous system • Brain tumors • Brain metastases • Spine tumors
- Stereotactic radiosurgery • Malignant gliomas • Intensity-modulated radiotherapy

KEY POINTS

- Options for the treatment of brain metastases include stereotactic radiosurgery, whole-brain radiotherapy, surgical resection, or some combination of these techniques, with the optimum therapy dependent on the size, number, and location of the brain lesions, the type and extent of primary tumor, and the patient's performance status and preferences.
- The standard of care for malignant gliomas remains maximal safe resection followed by concurrent conformal radiotherapy and temozolomide.
- Metastatic lesions to the osseous spine compressing the spinal cord are optimally treated with decompressive surgery followed by radiotherapy—nonsurgical candidates should be considered for stereotactic radiosurgery or conventional external beam radiotherapy.

INTRODUCTION

Radiation therapy is an integral component of the management of primary and metastatic tumors of the central nervous system (CNS).[1] In this article, the application of radiotherapy, alone and in combination with surgery and chemotherapy, in the treatment of metastases to the brain (the most common malignant brain lesion), malignant gliomas (the most common malignant primary brain tumor), and metastases to the osseous spine is reviewed. Minimizing radiation-induced damage to normal tissues is a fundamental objective in radiotherapy and it is a particular concern in the treatment of CNS lesions.

[a] Department of Radiation Oncology, Duke Cancer Institute, Duke University Medical Center, Durham, NC 27710, USA; [b] Department of Surgery, Duke Cancer Institute, Duke University Medical Center, Durham, NC 27710, USA
* Corresponding author. Duke University Medical Center, DUMC Box 3085, Durham, NC 27710.
E-mail address: john.kirkpatrick@dm.duke.edu

Surg Oncol Clin N Am 22 (2013) 445–461
http://dx.doi.org/10.1016/j.soc.2013.02.008
1055-3207/13/$ – see front matter © 2013 Elsevier Inc. All rights reserved.
surgonc.theclinics.com

BRAIN TUMORS
Radiotherapy Techniques

Whole-brain radiotherapy

Radiation therapy to the entire brain (whole-brain radiotherapy [WBRT]) uses a relatively simple technique, typically using 2 parallel opposed lateral fields with the patient in the supine position. In preparation for planning and treatment, the patient is positioned on a head rest and immobilized using either a custom-molded thermoplastic mask or simply tape (**Fig. 1**A). Before treatment, radiographic or computed tomographic (CT) images are acquired and a treatment plan is developed using opposed megavoltage radiographic beams (see **Fig. 1**B). The central axis of the beam is typically placed near the canthus to minimize the divergence of radiation beams into the eyes. In addition, the face and anterior eyes/lenses are blocked and the beam is shaped, using lead blocks or a multileaf collimator. At the time of treatment, the correct position of the treatment field is verified by either kilovoltage or megavoltage imaging of the treatment fields with the patient appropriately positioned on the radiation treatment table.

Intracranial stereotactic radiosurgery

In stereotactic radiosurgery (SRS) of brain lesions, a high dose of radiation is delivered in a single fraction or a few fractions with rapid dose falloff from the periphery of the target lesion into the surrounding normal brain tissue. Although a variety of disparate radiotherapy systems (eg, GammaKnife [Elekta, Stockholm, Sweden], CyberKnife [AccuRay, Sunnyvale, California], Novalis Tx [Varian Medical Systems, Palo Alto, California and BrainLAB, Munich, Germany]) are used in intracranial SRS, all share common features, as described in the attached consensus definition for radiosurgery (**Box 1**).[2] Radiosurgery systems demand and demonstrate exquisite accuracy (<1-mm deviation) for patient immobilization, target localization, and dose delivery. Typically, a patient is immobilized with either a semirigid, custom-molded, removable head mask (**Fig. 2**A) or a stereotactic head ring fixed to the patient's skull. Target delineation is performed using fine-cut CT scans (~1-mm slice thickness) fused with magnetic resonance imaging (MRI) images and occasionally functional imaging modalities, such as positron emission tomography. Intravenous contrast agents are often used to better define the target lesion.

In a collimator-based linear-accelerator system, such as the Novalis Tx, a typical treatment plan for an ellipsoid lesion, such as a small brain metastasis, consists of 3 to 5 non-coplanar conformal arcs (as illustrated in **Fig. 2**B), yielding the conformal dose distribution shown in **Fig. 2**C. Multiple intensity-modulated beams are often

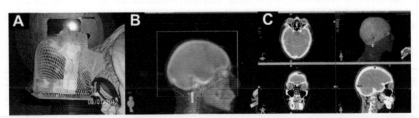

Fig. 1. Sample patient immobilization and field setup for whole-brain radiotherapy (WBRT) via opposed lateral fields. (*A*) Custom headholder with field shape outlined on mask. (*B*) Multileaf collimator outline (*dark blue lines*) and (*C*) radiation dose distribution—starting from upper righthand corner and moving clockwise: 3D rendering of dose distribution and isodose lines for sagittal, coronal, and axial cross-sections.

Box 1
Abridged consensus definition of stereotactic radiosurgery

- Stereotactic radiosurgery (SRS) uses externally generated ionizing radiation to inactivate/eradicate defined target(s) in the head or spine without the need to make an incision.
- The target is defined by high-resolution imaging.
- To assure quality care, the procedure involves a multidisciplinary team consisting of a neurosurgeon, radiation oncologist, and medical physicist.
- Although SRS typically is carried out in a single session, it can be administered in up to 5 sessions.
- SRS is performed using a rigidly attached stereotactic guiding device, other immobilization technology, and/or an image-guidance system.
- Technologies used to perform SRS include linear accelerators, particle beam accelerators, and multisource Cobalt 60 units.
- To enhance precision, these devices may incorporate robotics and real-time imaging.

Data from Barnett GH, Linskey ME, Adler JR, et al. Stereotactic radiosurgery—an organized neurosurgery-sanctioned definition. J Neurosurg 2007;106:1–5.

---

used for treating irregularly shaped targets and/or those that are intimately associated with critical organs. The correlation between the patient geometry (and/or immobilization device geometry) and the treatment machine geometry is achieved through 2 different approaches: (1) matching the geometry of the immobilization device with the machine isocenter through dedicated measurement devices with the assistance of room lasers; (2) matching planning/simulation images with treatment images (either 2D orthogonal images or 3D cone-beam CT images) acquired using an imaging device mounted in the treatment room (or machine) while patient is in the treatment position. Both approaches are able to achieve localization accuracy of about 1 mm. Radiation delivery consists of multiple beams intersecting at a single point (isocenter), shaped by fixed geometry cones and delivered in multiple arcs, dynamically conformal arcs continuously shaped by a multileaf collimator, or multiple intensity-modulated static beams or dynamic arcs. In the CyberKnife system, multiple collimated small-diameter beams are delivered to an intracranial lesion using a linear accelerator attached to a highly mobile robotic arm.

In contrast, the GammaKnife system uses hundreds of γ-ray sources (Co-60) precisely collimated to intersect at a single isocenter, yielding a small spherical or

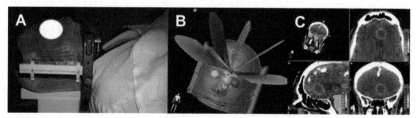

Fig. 2. Sample patient immobilization and field setup for stereotactic radiosurgery (SRS) via dynamic conformal arcs to a medial a medial left frontal brain metastasis. (*A*) Custom U-frame mask; (*B*) multiple arc paths; and (*C*) radiation dose distribution—starting from upper lefthand corner and moving clockwise: 3D rendering of dose distribution and isodose lines for axial, coronal, and sagittal cross-sections.

ellipsoid high-dose "cloud," the diameter of which is determined by the size of the collimator opening. Dose falloff from the cloud into the surrounding tissue is extremely rapid. Treatment of irregular and/or large targets is achieved by "packing" together multiple dose clouds, positioned in the target by precisely repositioning the stereotactic headframe with respect to the machine isocenter.

Brain Metastases

Primary cancer metastatic to the brain (brain metastases) is the most common malignant lesion in the brain, developing in greater than 200,000 patients with cancer in the United States each year.[3] Although brain metastases from lung, breast, kidney, and skin (melanoma) are most frequently encountered, virtually any histology from any anatomic site can metastasize to the brain. The optimal management of brain metastases is controversial, given the improved control of extracranial disease and increased longevity after the diagnosis of cancer; multiple tumor and patient factors influence prognosis, evolving patient expectations for treatment and a large number of treatment options. Treatment typically consists of WBRT, radiosurgery, surgical resection, or some combination of these modalities, as described in later discussion. Chemotherapy does not yet play a significant role in the management of brain metastases.[4]

WBRT with and without surgery

WBRT is widely used for the treatment of patients with brain metastases. WBRT can temporarily halt the growth of brain metastases, gradually reducing mass effect and neurologic deficits and extending life. However, there is a substantial risk of recurrence and neurologic death, and WBRT is typically delivered with palliative intent. Survival following WBRT is quite variable and an analysis of Radiation Therapy Oncology Group (RTOG) trials involving 1200 patients with brain metastases suggested the important factors influencing survival.[5] A technique termed Recursive Partitioning Analysis (RPA) was used to identify 3 RPA classes that predicted median overall survival (OS). The most favorable outcome (median OS 7.1 months) was observed in patients less than 65 years of age with well-controlled extracranial disease and a Karnofsky performance status $\geq$70 (RPA class 1). Patients with a Karnofsky performance status less than 70 were classified as RPA class 3 and demonstrated a median OS of 2.3 months. Patients who did not meet criteria in one of the above classes (RPA class 2) had a median OS of 4.2 months.

Acute side effects of WBRT include complete hair loss and mild scalp erythema and pruritus in nearly all patients, occasional sensation of fullness in the ears and parotid swelling, and mild anorexia and moderate fatigue, which can be severe in the debilitated and/or elderly patient.[6] Steroids (primarily dexamethasone) should be given judiciously, using the lowest dose to control symptoms while carefully managing the many potential side effects. Prophylactic antiepileptic drugs should not be routinely administered.[7] The long-term impact of WBRT on neurocognition and quality of life is a common concern of patients and their families. A frequently cited study of patients from Memorial Sloan-Kettering with single brain metastases treated with WBRT reported that "radiation-induced dementia" was observed in 5 of 47 patients at 1 year (11% crude rate). Four of the 5 patients who developed dementia were treated with a high dose per fraction (three 5- to 6-Gy fractions) and that the other received a concurrent radiosensitizer. In contrast, none of the 15 patients treated in ten 300-cGy fractions developed dementia. Typically, patients with brain metastases receive ten 300-cGy, fourteen to fifteen 250-cGy, or twenty 200-cGy fractions, although shorter and more protracted courses can be used. Although there are data from low-grade primary tumors suggesting that a more protracted course affords better preservation of neurocognition,[8,9] the optimal dose/fractionation regimen for brain metastases has not been determined.[10]

Studies of single brain metastases treated with WBRT with and without surgery have yielded conflicting results.[11-13] For example, Patchell and colleagues'[13] randomized trial of WBRT alone versus surgery plus WBRT in 48 patients suggests that surgery be considered in all surgical candidates with a single resectable lesion. The rate of recurrence at the original site of metastasis was significantly lower in patients who were resected and irradiated (20 vs 52%, P<.02); overall survival was higher (40 vs 15 weeks, P<.01) and functional independence was longer (38 vs 8 weeks, P<.005) compared with those who received WBRT alone. In contrast, Mintz and colleagues'[11] randomized study of WBRT with and without surgery in 84 patients with single brain metastases showed no significant difference with the addition of surgery (5.6 vs 6.3 months).

Surgery with and without WBRT
Although surgical resection can alleviate the mass effect associated with a brain metastasis and substantially reduce the tumor burden, recurrence of disease at the resection cavity and in other areas of the brain occurs frequently. In a randomized trial by Patchell and colleagues[14] of 95 patients with a solitary brain metastasis randomized to surgery with or without WBRT, recurrence of tumor anywhere in the brain was less frequent in the group receiving WBRT (18% vs 70%; P<.001). The addition of WBRT prevented brain recurrence at both the site of the original metastasis (10 vs 46%, P<.001) and other sites in the brain (14% vs 37%, P<.01). Patients in the group receiving WBRT were also less likely to die of neurologic causes (14% vs 44%, P = .003). However, the study showed no significant difference in overall survival with or without WBRT.

A subsequent study from the European Organization for Research and Treatment of Cancer (EORTC) randomized 359 patients with 1 to 3 brain metastases status either after surgery or after SRS observation versus WBRT.[15] Of the 160 surgically resected patients, 79 were randomized to observation alone versus 81 to WBRT. The primary endpoint was deterioration in performance status. Similar to the Patchell study, recurrence at the resection site was significantly higher when WBRT was omitted (27 vs 59% at 2 years, P<.001, for the surgical resection group), as was distant recurrence in the brain (23 vs 42%, P<.008). Patients in the group receiving WBRT were less likely to die of intracranial progression (28 vs 44%, P<.002, for the overall group). However, the study found no difference in time to deterioration of performance status (10.0 months for observation alone vs 9.5 months with WBRT, P = .71) or in overall survival (10.7 months for observation alone vs 10.9 months with WBRT, P = .87).

WBRT with and without SRS
The RTOG randomized 333 adult patients with 1 to 3 brain metastases treated with WBRT to SRS within 1 week of completing WBRT versus observation (RTOG 9508[16]). Of the 164 patients assigned to the SRS arm, 31 did not complete SRS with the principal reasons being refusal (9 patients) or disease progression/death (12 patients). Although local control was significantly improved in the group undergoing SRS (82 vs 71% at 1 year, P = .01), recurrent disease anywhere in the brain was not significantly better. Nonetheless, median overall survival was significantly higher with the addition of SRS in patients with a single brain metastasis (median overall survival time 6.5 vs 4.9 months, P = .039), patients less than 65 years old with controlled extracranial disease and Karnofsky performance status ≥70 (median overall survival time 11.6 vs 9.6 months, P = .045), and patients with brain metastasis ≥2 cm

in greatest diameter (P = .045 vs WBRT alone). In addition, patients treated with SRS exhibited significantly reduced steroid use and less deterioration in Karnofsky performance status than those who did not. Rates of acute and late toxicities were quite similar between the 2 groups, although SRS carried an approximate 0.5% monthly rate of radionecrosis.

SRS with or without WBRT
SRS alone with close follow-up to detect and treat recurrent disease has been suggested as an alternative to WBRT, as it potentially avoids neurocognitive and systemic sequelae encountered with treatment of the entire brain. On the other hand, omitting WBRT carries a significantly higher risk of recurrence, which in turn may result in increased neurocognitive deficits. Sneed and colleagues[17] performed a retrospective analysis of 569 patients from 10 institutions treated with SRS alone versus SRS with up-front WBRT. There was no significant difference in the median overall survival time for patients receiving SRS alone versus SRS and WBRT for any RPA class, with the hazard ratio for overall survival of 1.09 (P = .033) when adjusted for RPA class.

Aoyama and colleagues[18] randomized 132 adult patients with 1 to 3 brain metastases to SRS alone versus SRS and WBRT. The addition of WBRT improved control both at the site of the original metastases (89 vs 73% at 1 year, P = .002) and at distant sites in the brain (58 vs 36% at 1 year, P = .003). However, overall survival was not significantly different in either arm, 7.5 months with SRS alone vs 8.0 months with SRS and WBRT, P = .42). As measured by mini-mental status examination, neurocognition did not differ between these arms,[19] although mini-mental status examination is not a sensitive instrument for detecting changes in cognition.

Chang and colleagues[20] conducted a trial of 58 patients with brain metastases randomized to SRS alone versus SRS and WBRT. The primary endpoint of the trial was neurocognitive decline measured by a comprehensive battery of tests. Four months after SRS, neurocognitive decline was substantially higher in the group receiving WBRT, 52% versus 24%. However, in contrast to most other studies, survival was substantially poorer in patients treated with WBRT alone, with median and 1-year overall survivals of 5.7 versus 15.2 months and 63% versus 21%, respectively (P = .003). Similar to other studies, the 1-year freedom from recurrence anywhere in the brain was 27% for SRS alone versus 73% for SRS plus WBRT (P = .0003). As the neurocognitive decline was measured at a time when many of the patients in the WBRT group were close to death, the results of this study are somewhat difficult to interpret.

SRS with surgery
Following resection of a single brain metastasis, the surgical cavity alone can be treated with radiosurgery, omitting whole-brain radiotherapy, with the objective of decreasing the high rates of local recurrence observed with surgery alone[14] and avoiding the side effects of WBRT.[21] For example, Choi and colleagues[22] irradiated 120 resection cavities in 112 patients with brain metastases. At 1 year, the rate of recurrence at the cavity was 9.5%, whereas the rate of distant failure in the brain was 54%. They also examined the effect of irradiating only the resection cavity versus the resection cavity expanded by 2 mm and found that the rate of local failure at 1 year was significantly lower in the 2-mm group (3 vs 16%, P = .042). No significant difference in toxicity was observed as a function of resection margin.

Decision-making
All patients with brain metastases should be treated with some form of radiation therapy. In determining which patients should be treated with surgery before or after

radiation, there are generally 6 features to consider, as follows: comorbidities, patient prognosis, size, location of metastasis, number of metastasis, and patient preference. In general, patients with comorbidities such that perioperative risk is extraordinary should be treated with radiation alone. In addition, patients with a poor prognosis because of fulminant metastatic disease or other comorbidities should also be treated with radiation only, as the time to recover from surgery is generally a minimum of 3 to 6 weeks and surgery imparts risks that may increase the recovery time. Given increasing tumor burden and decreasing maximum tolerated dose for radiosurgery as tumor diameter increases, many patients with tumors greater than 3 cm, and most patients with lesions less than 4 cm, should be considered for surgery. Similarly, the size and location of the mass also may suggest surgery. For example, a 3-cm mass in the frontal lobe can be safely treated with radiation alone, but a similarly sized lesion in the cerebellum may produce obstructive hydrocephalus; radiation without surgical decompression may worsen the hydrocephalus. It is also generally accepted that patients with a single metastasis or more than one metastasis that can all be accessed through a reasonably sized craniotomy should be considered for surgical resection. Finally, patient preference should always be taken into account given the lack of level I data to support specific recommendations, particularly with regard to the choice between surgery plus radiation versus radiation alone; this discussion must involve the neurosurgeon, radiation oncologist, and the patient.

Primary Brain Tumors

Malignant gliomas

Anaplastic astrocytomas and glioblastomas (World Health Organization grade III and IV malignant gliomas, respectively[23]) account for about two-thirds of primary malignant brain tumors in adults with an annual incidence in the United States of approximately 6 cases per 100,000 person-years.[24] Although meningiomas are more frequently encountered, these are overwhelmingly benign tumors[24] and the discussion in this section focuses on the management of the far more aggressive malignant gliomas. Malignant gliomas arise from neuroepithelial tissue with a peak incidence in the sixth decade of life. The cause of most cases of malignant gliomas is unknown in more than 90% of cases, although exposure to ionizing radiation and certain genetic syndromes are associated with an increased risk of this disease.[25]

Surgery

Maximum safe resection of malignant glioma is a key element in the management of malignant gliomas, as outcomes seem to be more favorable in patients undergoing a gross or near total resection compared with minimal debulking or biopsy alone.[26] However, there are no randomized control studies proving the superiority of a gross total resection and it is unlikely that such a trial would be performed. With surgery alone, median progression-free survival and overall survival are on the order of only a few months, as tumor cells are present well beyond the gross lesion. Thus, surgery and radiotherapy are typically both used, as described below.

Radiotherapy

Radiation therapy following surgical resection of malignant gliomas has been a recommended component of the management strategy since the 1970s, because it improves overall survival compared with surgery alone.[27–29] At that time, the present standard total dose of 60-Gy radiation delivered in 1.8- to 2-Gy daily fractions was established.[30,31] Trials to improve outcome by dose escalation using conventionally fractionated radiotherapy (RT),[32] hyperfractionation,[33] brachytherapy,[34,35] or a stereotactic radiosurgery[36] boost have not revealed a benefit to increasing dose beyond

60 Gy. For example, in RTOG 9305, 203 patients with glioblastoma were randomized to receive SRS versus no SRS before a course of conventional RT (a total of 60 Gy in 2-Gy daily fractions) and concurrent carmustine. No significant differences in survival (14.1 vs 13.7 months with or without SRS), neurocognition, quality of life, or patterns of failure were found, with 90% of failures occurring at the treatment field in both arms. Thus, standard RT typically consists of thirty or thirty-three 2.0- or 1.8-Gy daily fractions to a total dose of 59.4 to 60 Gy delivered over a 6-week to 7-week period. However, there is evidence in elderly patients that treatment at a slightly higher dose per day for a significantly shorter period (eg, 40 Gy delivered over 3 weeks) yields reasonable outcome.[37]

Although the entire brain was initially irradiated due to the concern about the widespread and insidious distribution of tumor cells throughout the brain, various trials showed no significant differences in outcome when the volume of brain irradiated was reduced.[38,39] Pattern-of-failure analyses show that most failures occur with 2 to 3 cm of the enhancing lesion visualized on CT are MRI scan and that a distant failure is almost always associated with a local failure.[38,40] Thus, to avoid toxicity associated with whole-brain irradiation to 60 Gy, the current standard practice is to irradiate only the involved portion of the brain. Typically, the initial target for irradiation is the volume of brain exhibiting T2 hyperintensity on MRI expanded by 2 cm, and this target volume is treated to 45 to 46 Gy, which is followed by a "boost" of an additional 14 to 14.4 Gy to the contrast-enhancing residual lesion and/or resection cavity on T1-weighted MRI imaging, bringing the total dose to 59.4 to 60 Gy. To minimize the volume of normal brain irradiated and keep the dose to critical structures within tolerance limits, multiple shaped, intersecting radiation beams are used and intensity-modulated RT is often necessary to satisfy dose constraints.

Surgery, RT, and chemotherapy

Meta-analyses of the outcome in patients with malignant glioma treated with or without nitrosureas suggested a small but significant benefit from the addition of these intravenous agents.[41,42] However, in 2005, Stupp and colleagues[43] reported the results an EORTC trial that randomized 573 patients with glioblastoma receiving RT (60 Gy in 2-Gy daily fractions) with or without the oral alkylating agent, temozolomide (TMZ). TMZ was administered once daily during RT and then for 5 days each month for the next 6 months. The addition of TMZ was associated with significantly improved overall survival ($P<.0001$), with median, 2-year overall survival, and 5-year overall survival of 15 versus 12 months, 27% versus 11%, and 10% versus 2%, respectively.[44] Patients expressing lower levels of the enzyme responsible for repair of DNA damage, MGMT, exhibited a much more favorable response, although an improvement in survival was noted in the RT/TMZ arm even in those patients with unfavorable MGMT status. Likewise, although younger age, performance status, and increased extent of resection were associated with better outcome, the addition of TMZ conveyed improved survival in all prognostic groups. Consequently, the standard of care for adult patients with newly diagnosed glioblastomas includes maximum safe resection followed by conventionally fractionated RT with concurrent and adjuvant chemotherapy. This practice has been extended to cover all malignant gliomas, although data from randomized trials in anaplastic astrocytomas, for example, are absent.

Even with the optimum combination of surgery, RT, and chemotherapy, the typical prognosis in malignant gliomas remains poor with virtually all patients recurring and less than 10% surviving 5 years after diagnosis.[44] A variety of novel approaches are under trial to improve outcome in newly diagnosed glioblastoma, including vaccine therapies[45] and the use of anti-angiogenic agents.[46–48] Of particular importance, a large phase III randomized trial from the RTOG (RTOG 0825) is examining the impact of anti-angiogenic bevacizumab (BVZ) on survival in newly diagnosed glioblastoma, when added to conventional regimen of RT and concurrent TMZ. Accrual is complete and the results are expected in the next few years. Given the extremely high rates of recurrence in malignant gliomas, improved treatment of recurrent disease is also a matter of great interest. BVZ has been approved by the Food and Drug Administration for the treatment of recurrent disease based on the results of phase II trials[49–51] and SRS, alone[52] or, particularly, in combination with BVZ,[53–55] may offer benefits in this setting. However, randomized trials demonstrating the efficacy of SRS/BVZ have not been completed.

Normal tissue toxicity
The tolerance of normal CNS tissue to therapeutic radiation depends on a variety of factors, including the total radiation dose, dose/fraction, the size and location of the target lesion, and concomitant chemotherapy.[56,57] A joint task force sponsored by the American Society of Radiation Oncology and American Association of Physics in Medicine recently published a comprehensive review quantifying normal tissue toxicity in clinical radiation oncology to a variety of organ systems, including the brain,[58] brainstem,[59] optic nerves/chiasm,[60] hearing apparatus,[61] and spinal cord.[62]

SPINE AND SPINAL CORD TUMORS
Radiotherapy Techniques

External-beam radiotherapy
External-beam radiotherapy (EBRT) for spine tumors typically uses 1 of the 3 following techniques: (1) a single radiation beam entering posterior aspect of the patient (PA field, **Fig. 3**A); (2) 2 parallel-opposed radiation beams entering the patient from both anterior and posterior (AP-PA fields); or (3) 3 or more radiation beams, often shaped by multileaf collimators (conformal 3D beam arrangement; see **Fig. 3**B). All of these EBRT techniques result in irradiation of the full width of the vertebral body, with the spinal canal and its contents receiving essentially the full dose of radiation. Thus, if tumor control is the primary objective of treatment, it is necessary to treat the target using multiple modest doses of radiation (typically, ranging from five 4-Gy daily fractions up to twenty 2-Gy fractions). Alternatively, if palliation is the goal, it may be possible to treat with a single 8-Gy fraction, although this may limit durability of response, as described below. Both the PA and the AP-PA fields are relatively quick and straightforward to execute. The PA field may limit exit dose into the chest and abdomen, but is limited in the depth of treatment, particularly for lesions located in

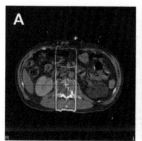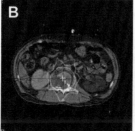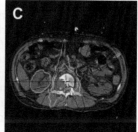

Fig. 3. Sample axial plane radiation dose distributions for (A) external-beam radiotherapy to the spine via posterior-anterior fields and (B) multiple beam 3D conformal beams. (C) Spinal single-fraction stereotactic radiosurgery via intensity-modulated radiotherapy.

the anterior aspect of lumbar vertebral bodies. AP-PA fields are capable of treating deep lesions but deliver higher radiation doses to the viscera. In contrast, 3D conformal EBRT plans are more complex to plan and execute but significantly reduce the maximum dose to adjacent organs by spreading out the dose (see **Fig. 3**B).

Spinal SRS

For metastatic disease involving one or a few contiguous vertebral bodies, SRS can be used to treat the osseous spine, while sparing the spinal cord with one or a few high-dose fractions. To do so, it is essential to use intensity-modulated radiation therapy or volumetric modulated arc therapy to treat the concave target while minimizing dose to the canal,[63–66] as shown in **Fig. 3**C. As in intracranial radiosurgery, this is a technically demanding procedure, requiring the appropriate commitment, effort, and expertise. Key elements of spinal SRS include high-resolution imaging (typically CT and MRI scans) for planning, immobilization, and imaging for position verification and, if necessary, adjustment immediately before and during treatment.[67,68] Treatment systems for spinal SRS include Novalis Tx, CyberKnife, and Synergy.

Primary Spine Tumors

Primary tumors of the spinal cord, nerves, and meninges are rare, comprising less than 5% of primary CNS tumors. In adults, the most common primary tumors are meningiomas, nerve sheath neoplasms, and ependymomas.[24] The incidence of metastases to the cord or intradural/extramedullary space is not well-characterized, although these so-called "drop metastases" are frequently encountered in late-stage disease. These tumors are characterized by substantial morbidity, including pain, parathesias, paralysis, and loss of bowel/bladder continence, with the severity of signs and symptoms related to the extent of tumor and the specific site of cord affected.

Tumors of the spinal canal and cord may be surgically resected to relieve mass effect and reduce the severity of symptoms, to obtain a tissue diagnosis, and/or, in the case of benign tumors such spinal myxopapillary ependymomas, to achieve a cure. Following surgery, radiation therapy is frequently recommended in the setting of residual and/or malignant disease, typically covering the entire circumference of the spine and canal at the involved levels. Irradiation of the entire craniospinal axis is appropriate in rare circumstances and carries significant morbidity. Alternatively, RT may be the sole treatment modality in patients who are not surgical candidates because of the extent of systemic disease, short life expectancy, potential morbidity, and/or refusal of surgery. Again, the radiation field typically includes the entire level of the involved cord/canal plus a margin of one vertebral body above and below this level. SRS is typically reserved for spinal nerve schwannomas with minimal intracanalicular extension.

The choice of radiation technique and dose depends on the objective of treatment. For definitive treatment of primary spinal cord tumors, doses in the range of 54 to 60 Gy, delivered at 1.8 to 2.0 Gy daily, are typically used. At these doses, there is a substantial risk of gastrointestinal toxicity if a simple AP-PA beam arrangement is used and, thus, highly conformal, multiple beam plans are often selected. In addition, the risk of radiation-induced myelopathy becomes substantial above 54 Gy[62] and it is important to treat the cord/canal with a relatively uniform dose, again favoring 3D planning and, often, an intensity-modulated technique. In contrast, effective palliation can be achieved at lower doses (eg, three 5-Gy, five 4-Gy, or ten 3-Gy daily fractions) and these treatments can be administered with minimal risk of long-term neurologic or gastrointestinal toxicity.

Metastatic Disease to the Osseous Spine

Although primary tumors of the bony spine are rare, metastases to the spine are quite common, with about 10% of all patients with cancer developing symptomatic spinal metastases and a far greater number having occult disease.[69–71] The most frequently presenting symptom of osseous spinal metastases is back pain,[71–73] although paralysis, parathesias, radicular pain, and bowel/bladder incontinence are seen in many cases, particularly when the spinal canal is compromised and the cord is compressed. Radiographically, lytic lesions and pathologic fracture are readily apparent on plain films and CT scans, although MRI is most sensitive for identifying more subtle lesions and defining the extent of cord/canal compromise and epidural disease. Time is of the essence in diagnosing and treating malignant spinal cord compression, necessitating the emergent initiation of steroids, concurrent consultation with radiation oncologist and spinal surgeon, and rapid intervention.[73–76]

In appropriate patients with neurologic compromise from metastatic disease to the bony spine, surgical decompression followed by radiation therapy is the treatment of choice. Patchell and colleagues[77] randomized 101 patients with malignant spinal cord compression diagnosed by MRI to surgical decompression, followed 2 weeks later by RT, versus RT alone. In both arms, RT consisted of ten 300-cGy daily fractions delivered as opposed AP-PA fields. The surgical arm exhibited superior outcome, including rate of ambulation following treatment (84 vs 57%, $P = .001$), duration of ambulation ability (median 122 vs 13 days, $P = .003$), return of ambulation after treatment in non-ambulatory patients (62 vs 19%, $P = .012$), urinary continence (74 vs 57%, $P = .005$), and overall survival (median 126 vs 100 days, $P = .033$). However, the selection criteria for this study were quite restrictive, excluding patients with radiosensitive tumors, short life expectancy, and multifocal disease, limiting the eligible patient population to only 10% to 15% of the patients with malignant spinal cord compression.[78] A retrospective matched pair analysis of patients with malignant spinal cord compression (without these strict exclusion criteria) treated with decompressive surgery and RT versus RT alone showed no significant difference in any functional outcome.[78]

In any case, many patients will not be surgical candidates because of medical comorbidities, short life expectancy, extent of disease, lack of neurologic deficits and impending fracture, and/or a desire to forego surgery. Radiation therapy delivered with palliative intent is appropriate in these patients, assuming that a diagnosis of malignancy has been established. However, patients frequently present with a symptomatic spinal lesion as the first manifestation of malignant disease and then the issue of proceeding with treatment of the spine without confirmation of malignancy arises. In such cases, it may be necessary to begin RT to the spine without a definitive diagnosis, but this must be performed with the full understanding of the patient (and other members of the care team) that a diagnosis has not been established and that RT may preclude making a diagnosis, particularly in the setting of a radiosensitive tumor (eg, lymphoma or germinoma). In such cases, it is often worthwhile to obtain a biopsy specimen of the lesion before RT and initiate RT while awaiting the results.

Treatment of spinal metastases may consist of conventional EBRT or SRS. Treatment of spinal metastases with EBRT has a long history and treatment may be set up and initiated rapidly, often within a few hours of the decision to treat. A variety of dosing schemes have been evaluated, ranging from a single 8-Gy fraction to twenty 2-Gy fractions. For bone metastases in general, there does not seem to be a significant difference in pain relief between the various regimens, with about one-third of patients exhibiting complete pain relief and the majority experiencing a substantial decrease in pain following RT.[79] However, a prospective study of short-course (one 8-Gy or five

4-Gy fractions) versus long-course (ten 3-Gy or twenty 2-Gy fractions) spinal RT showed that the more protracted regimens were associated with a significantly reduced rate of recurrence, 19 versus 39% 1-year after RT.[80] This study showed no significant difference in functional outcome between the regimens. Many patients with spinal metastases have been previously treated with RT for thoracic or abdominal malignancies and have received some dose of radiation to the spine. Potentially, this places the patient at greater risk of radiation-induced myelopathy and it is essential to obtain and consider the history of prior RT before making a decision on the treatment modality and radiation dose.

In treatment of a metastasis to the osseous spine with SRS, the target is the portion of the vertebral body at risk with delivery of a purposely low dose of radiation to the spinal cord. Thus, it seems particularly useful in treatment in the setting of previous irradiation to the involved level of the spinal cord. In comparison to conventional RT, this is a much more technically demanding and time-consuming procedure, requiring specialized expertise, equipment, and procedures.[68] Although very high rates of palliation and freedom from recurrence,[67,69,70] along with low rates of radiation-induced myelopathy,[62,81,82] have been reported, no randomized trial of SRS versus conventional RT in spinal metastases has been completed. The RTOG is currently conducting a randomized trial (RTOG 0618) comparing SRS versus conventional RT, delivered as a single 16- to 18-Gy versus 8-Gy fraction, respectively.

Normal tissue toxicity

Although uncommon, RT-induced damage of the spinal cord (ie, myelopathy) can be severe, resulting in pain, paresthesias, sensory deficits, paralysis, Brown-Sequard syndrome, and bowel/bladder incontinence. Based on published reports of radiation myelopathy in 335 and 1946 patients receiving RT to their cervical and thoracic spines, respectively, Kirkpatrick et al and Schultheiss[62,83] predicted a 0.2, 5%, and 50% risk of radiation-induced myelopathy at a total cord dose of 50, 59, and 69 Gy delivered in 2-Gy daily fractions, respectively. In 1400 cases of spinal SRS, only 12 cases of radiation-induced myelopathy were reported and it seems that the rate of myelopathy in SRS is low (<1%) when the maximum point dose to the spinal cord is less than 13 Gy for single-fraction SRS.[62] However, myelopathy has been reported at much lower doses[81] and longer term follow-up with careful reporting of dose distribution and neurologic deficits is required to establish the risk of radiation myelopathy as a function of dose and volume.

REFERENCES

1. Black PM, Loeffler JS. Cancer of the nervous system. 2nd edition. Philadelphia: Lippincott Williams & Wilkins; 2005.
2. Barnett GH, Linskey ME, Adler JR, et al. Stereotactic radiosurgery–an organized neurosurgery-sanctioned definition. J Neurosurg 2007;106:1–5.
3. Sperduto PW, Chao ST, Sneed PK, et al. Diagnosis-specific prognostic factors, indexes, and treatment outcomes for patients with newly diagnosed brain metastases: a multi-institutional analysis of 4,259 patients. Int J Radiat Oncol Biol Phys 2010;77:655–61.
4. Mehta MP, Paleologos NA, Mikkelsen T, et al. The role of chemotherapy in the management of newly diagnosed brain metastases: a systematic review and evidence-based clinical practice guideline. J Neurooncol 2010;96:71–83.
5. Gaspar LE, Scott C, Murray K, et al. Validation of the RTOG recursive partitioning analysis (RPA) classification for brain metastases. Int J Radiat Oncol Biol Phys 2000;47:1001–6.

6. Mikkelsen T, Paleologos NA, Robinson PD, et al. The role of prophylactic anticonvulsants in the management of brain metastases: a systematic review and evidence-based clinical practice guideline. J Neurooncol 2010;96:97–102.

7. Ryken TC, McDermott M, Robinson PD, et al. The role of steroids in the management of brain metastases: a systematic review and evidence-based clinical practice guideline. J Neurooncol 2010;96:103–14.

8. Klein M, Heimans JJ, Aaronson NK, et al. Effect of radiotherapy and other treatment-related factors on mid-term to long-term cognitive sequelae in low-grade gliomas: a comparative study. Lancet 2002;360:1361–8.

9. Douw L, Klein M, Fagel SS, et al. Cognitive and radiological effects of radiotherapy in patients with low-grade glioma: long-term follow-up. Lancet Neurol 2009;8:810–8.

10. Tsao MN, Lloyd N, Wong RK, et al. Whole brain radiotherapy for the treatment of newly diagnosed multiple brain metastases. Cochrane Database Syst Rev 2012;(4):CD003869.

11. Mintz AH, Kestle J, Rathbone MP, et al. A randomized trial to assess the efficacy of surgery in addition to radiotherapy in patients with a single cerebral metastasis. Cancer 1996;78:1470–6.

12. Noordijk EM, Vecht CJ, Haaxma-Reiche H, et al. The choice of treatment of single brain metastasis should be based on extracranial tumor activity and age. Int J Radiat Oncol Biol Phys 1994;29:711–7.

13. Patchell RA, Tibbs PA, Walsh JW, et al. A randomized trial of surgery in the treatment of single metastases to the brain. N Engl J Med 1990;322:494–500.

14. Patchell RA, Tibbs PA, Regine WF, et al. Postoperative radiotherapy in the treatment of single metastases to the brain: a randomized trial. JAMA 1998;280:1485–9.

15. Kocher M, Soffietti R, Abacioglu U, et al. Adjuvant whole-brain radiotherapy versus observation after radiosurgery or surgical resection of one to three cerebral metastases: results of the EORTC 22952-26001 study. J Clin Oncol 2011; 29:134–41.

16. Andrews DW, Scott CB, Sperduto PW, et al. Whole brain radiation therapy with or without stereotactic radiosurgery boost for patients with one to three brain metastases: phase III results of the RTOG 9508 randomised trial. Lancet 2004;363: 1665–72.

17. Sneed PK, Suh JH, Goetsch SJ, et al. A multi-institutional review of radiosurgery alone vs. radiosurgery with whole brain radiotherapy as the initial management of brain metastases. Int J Radiat Oncol Biol Phys 2002;53:519–26.

18. Aoyama H, Shirato H, Tago M, et al. Stereotactic radiosurgery plus whole-brain radiation therapy vs stereotactic radiosurgery alone for treatment of brain metastases: a randomized controlled trial. JAMA 2006;295:2483–91.

19. Aoyama H, Tago M, Kato N, et al. Neurocognitive function of patients with brain metastasis who received either whole brain radiotherapy plus stereotactic radiosurgery or radiosurgery alone. Int J Radiat Oncol Biol Phys 2007;68:1388–95.

20. Chang EL, Wefel JS, Hess KR, et al. Neurocognition in patients with brain metastases treated with radiosurgery or radiosurgery plus whole-brain irradiation: a randomised controlled trial. Lancet Oncol 2009;10:1037–44.

21. Soltys SG, Adler JR, Lipani JD, et al. Stereotactic radiosurgery of the postoperative resection cavity for brain metastases. Int J Radiat Oncol Biol Phys 2008;70: 187–93.

22. Choi CY, Chang SD, Gibbs IC, et al. Stereotactic radiosurgery of the postoperative resection cavity for brain metastases: prospective evaluation of target margin on tumor control. Int J Radiat Oncol Biol Phys 2012;84(2):336–42.

23. Louis DN, Ohgaki H, Wiestler OD, et al. The 2007 WHO classification of tumours of the central nervous system. Acta Neuropathol 2007;114:97–109.
24. CBTRUS Statistical Report: Primary brain and central nervous system tumors diagnosed in the United States in 2004-2008 (March 23, 2012 Revision), 2012.
25. Ricard D, Idbaih A, Ducray F, et al. Primary brain tumours in adults. Lancet 2012; 379:1984–96.
26. Stummer W, van den Bent MJ, Westphal M. Cytoreductive surgery of glioblastoma as the key to successful adjuvant therapies: new arguments in an old discussion. Acta Neurochir (Wien) 2011;153:1211–8.
27. Laperriere N, Zuraw L, Cairncross G. Radiotherapy for newly diagnosed malignant glioma in adults: a systematic review. Radiother Oncol 2002;64:259–73.
28. Walker MD, Alexander E Jr, Hunt WE, et al. Evaluation of BCNU and/or radiotherapy in the treatment of anaplastic gliomas. A cooperative clinical trial. J Neurosurg 1978;49:333–43.
29. Walker MD, Green SB, Byar DP, et al. Randomized comparisons of radiotherapy and nitrosoureas for the treatment of malignant glioma after surgery. N Engl J Med 1980;303:1323–9.
30. Bleehen NM, Stenning SP. A Medical Research Council trial of two radiotherapy doses in the treatment of grades 3 and 4 astrocytoma. The Medical Research Council Brain Tumour Working Party. Br J Cancer 1991;64:769–74.
31. Walker MD, Strike TA, Sheline GE. An analysis of dose-effect relationship in the radiotherapy of malignant gliomas. Int J Radiat Oncol Biol Phys 1979;5:1725–31.
32. Chang CH, Horton J, Schoenfeld D, et al. Comparison of postoperative radiotherapy and combined postoperative radiotherapy and chemotherapy in the multidisciplinary management of malignant gliomas. A joint Radiation Therapy Oncology Group and Eastern Cooperative Oncology Group study. Cancer 1983;52:997–1007.
33. Nelson DF, Curran WJ Jr, Scott C, et al. Hyperfractionated radiation therapy and bis-chlorethyl nitrosourea in the treatment of malignant glioma–possible advantage observed at 72.0 Gy in 1.2 Gy B.I.D. fractions: report of the Radiation Therapy Oncology Group Protocol 8302. Int J Radiat Oncol Biol Phys 1993;25: 193–207.
34. Laperriere NJ, Leung PM, McKenzie S, et al. Randomized study of brachytherapy in the initial management of patients with malignant astrocytoma. Int J Radiat Oncol Biol Phys 1998;41:1005–11.
35. Selker RG, Shapiro WR, Burger P, et al. The Brain Tumor Cooperative Group NIH Trial 87-01: a randomized comparison of surgery, external radiotherapy, and carmustine versus surgery, interstitial radiotherapy boost, external radiation therapy, and carmustine. Neurosurgery 2002;51:343–55 [discussion: 355–7].
36. Souhami L, Seiferheld W, Brachman D, et al. Randomized comparison of stereotactic radiosurgery followed by conventional radiotherapy with carmustine to conventional radiotherapy with carmustine for patients with glioblastoma multiforme: report of Radiation Therapy Oncology Group 93-05 protocol. Int J Radiat Oncol Biol Phys 2004;60:853–60.
37. Minniti G, Lanzetta G, Scaringi C, et al. Phase II study of short-course radiotherapy plus concomitant and adjuvant temozolomide in elderly patients with glioblastoma. Int J Radiat Oncol Biol Phys 2012;83:93–9.
38. Hochberg FH, Pruitt A. Assumptions in the radiotherapy of glioblastoma. Neurology 1980;30:907–11.
39. Shapiro WR, Young DF. Treatment of malignant glioma. A controlled study of chemotherapy and irradiation. Arch Neurol 1976;33:494–50.

40. Wallner KE, Galicich JH, Krol G, et al. Patterns of failure following treatment for glioblastoma multiforme and anaplastic astrocytoma. Int J Radiat Oncol Biol Phys 1989;16:1405–9.
41. Fine HA, Dear KB, Loeffler JS, et al. Meta-analysis of radiation therapy with and without adjuvant chemotherapy for malignant gliomas in adults. Cancer 1993;71: 2585–97.
42. Stewart LA. Chemotherapy in adult high-grade glioma: a systematic review and meta-analysis of individual patient data from 12 randomised trials. Lancet 2002;359:1011–8.
43. Stupp R, Mason WP, van den Bent MJ, et al. Radiotherapy plus concomitant and adjuvant temozolomide for glioblastoma. N Engl J Med 2005;352:987–96.
44. Stupp R, Hegi ME, Mason WP, et al. Effects of radiotherapy with concomitant and adjuvant temozolomide versus radiotherapy alone on survival in glioblastoma in a randomised phase III study: 5-year analysis of the EORTC-NCIC trial. Lancet Oncol 2009;10:459–66.
45. Ajay D, Sanchez-Perez L, Choi BD, et al. Immunotherapy with tumor vaccines for the treatment of malignant gliomas. Curr Drug Discov Technol 2012;9(4):237–55.
46. Lai A, Tran A, Nghiemphu PL, et al. Phase II study of bevacizumab plus temozolomide during and after radiation therapy for patients with newly diagnosed glioblastoma multiforme. J Clin Oncol 2011;29:142–8.
47. Vredenburgh JJ, Desjardins A, Reardon DA, et al. The addition of bevacizumab to standard radiation therapy and temozolomide followed by bevacizumab, temozolomide, and irinotecan for newly diagnosed glioblastoma. Clin Cancer Res 2011;17:4119–24.
48. Narayana A, Gruber D, Kunnakkat S, et al. A clinical trial of bevacizumab, temozolomide, and radiation for newly diagnosed glioblastoma. J Neurosurg 2012; 116:341–5.
49. Cohen MH, Shen YL, Keegan P, et al. FDA drug approval summary: bevacizumab (Avastin) as treatment of recurrent glioblastoma multiforme. Oncologist 2009;14: 1131–8.
50. Kreisl TN, Kim L, Moore K, et al. Phase II trial of single-agent bevacizumab followed by bevacizumab plus irinotecan at tumor progression in recurrent glioblastoma. J Clin Oncol 2009;27:740–5.
51. Vredenburgh JJ, Desjardins A, Herndon JE 2nd, et al. Phase II trial of bevacizumab and irinotecan in recurrent malignant glioma. Clin Cancer Res 2007;13:1253–9.
52. Fogh SE, Andrews DW, Glass J, et al. Hypofractionated stereotactic radiation therapy: an effective therapy for recurrent high-grade gliomas. J Clin Oncol 2010;28:3048–53.
53. Cabrera HN, Almeida AN, Silva CC, et al. Use of intraoperative MRI for resection of gliomas. Arq Neuropsiquiatr 2011;69:949–53.
54. Cuneo KC, Vredenburgh JJ, Sampson JH, et al. Safety and efficacy of stereotactic radiosurgery and adjuvant bevacizumab in patients with recurrent malignant gliomas. Int J Radiat Oncol Biol Phys 2012;82:2018–24.
55. Gutin PH, Iwamoto FM, Beal K, et al. Safety and efficacy of bevacizumab with hypofractionated stereotactic irradiation for recurrent malignant gliomas. Int J Radiat Oncol Biol Phys 2009;75:156–63.
56. Bentzen SM, Constine LS, Deasy JO, et al. Quantitative Analyses of Normal Tissue Effects in the Clinic (QUANTEC): an introduction to the scientific issues. Int J Radiat Oncol Biol Phys 2010;76:S3–9.
57. Marks LB, Ten Haken RK, Martel MK. Guest editor's introduction to QUANTEC: a users guide. Int J Radiat Oncol Biol Phys 2010;76:S1–2.

58. Lawrence YR, Li XA, el Naqa I, et al. Radiation dose-volume effects in the brain. Int J Radiat Oncol Biol Phys 2010;76:S20–7.
59. Mayo C, Yorke E, Merchant TE. Radiation associated brainstem injury. Int J Radiat Oncol Biol Phys 2010;76:S36–41.
60. Mayo C, Martel MK, Marks LB, et al. Radiation dose-volume effects of optic nerves and chiasm. Int J Radiat Oncol Biol Phys 2010;76:S28–35.
61. Bhandare N, Jackson A, Eisbruch A, et al. Radiation therapy and hearing loss. Int J Radiat Oncol Biol Phys 2010;76:S50–7.
62. Kirkpatrick JP, van der Kogel AJ, Schultheiss TE. Radiation dose-volume effects in the spinal cord. Int J Radiat Oncol Biol Phys 2010;76:S42–9.
63. Ma L, Sahgal A, Cozzi L, et al. Apparatus-dependent dosimetric differences in spine stereotactic body radiotherapy. Technol Cancer Res Treat 2010;9:563–74.
64. Nelson JW, Yoo DS, Sampson JH, et al. Stereotactic body radiotherapy for lesions of the spine and paraspinal regions. Int J Radiat Oncol Biol Phys 2009;73:1369–75.
65. Wu QJ, Wang Z, Kirkpatrick JP, et al. Impact of collimator leaf width and treatment technique on stereotactic radiosurgery and radiotherapy plans for intra- and extracranial lesions. Radiat Oncol 2009;4:3.
66. Wu QJ, Yoo S, Kirkpatrick JP, et al. Volumetric arc intensity-modulated therapy for spine body radiotherapy: comparison with static intensity-modulated treatment. Int J Radiat Oncol Biol Phys 2009;75:1596–604.
67. Sahgal A, Bilsky M, Chang EL, et al. Stereotactic body radiotherapy for spinal metastases: current status, with a focus on its application in the postoperative patient. J Neurosurg Spine 2011;14:151–66.
68. Sahgal A, Larson DA, Chang EL. Stereotactic body radiosurgery for spinal metastases: a critical review. Int J Radiat Oncol Biol Phys 2008;71:652–65.
69. Ahmed KA, Stauder MC, Miller RC, et al. Stereotactic body radiation therapy in spinal metastases. Int J Radiat Oncol Biol Phys 2012;82:e803–9.
70. Hall WA, Stapleford LJ, Hadjipanayis CG, et al. Stereotactic body radiosurgery for spinal metastatic disease: an evidence-based review. Int J Surg Oncol 2011;979214:2011.
71. Sciubba DM, Petteys RJ, Dekutoski MB, et al. Diagnosis and management of metastatic spine disease. J Neurosurg Spine 2010;13:94–108.
72. Bach F, Larsen BH, Rohde K, et al. Metastatic spinal cord compression. Occurrence, symptoms, clinical presentations and prognosis in 398 patients with spinal cord compression. Acta Neurochir (Wien) 1990;107:37–43.
73. Helweg-Larsen S, Sorensen PS. Symptoms and signs in metastatic spinal cord compression: a study of progression from first symptom until diagnosis in 153 patients. Eur J Cancer 1994;30A:396–8.
74. Loblaw DA, Mitera G, Ford M, et al. A 2011 updated systematic review and clinical practice guideline for the management of malignant extradural spinal cord compression. Int J Radiat Oncol Biol Phys 2012;84:312–7.
75. Rades D, Blach M, Nerreter V, et al. Metastatic spinal cord compression. Influence of time between onset of motoric deficits and start of irradiation on therapeutic effect. Strahlenther Onkol 1999;175:378–81.
76. Rades D, Heidenreich F, Karstens JH. Final results of a prospective study of the prognostic value of the time to develop motor deficits before irradiation in metastatic spinal cord compression. Int J Radiat Oncol Biol Phys 2002;53:975–9.
77. Patchell RA, Tibbs PA, Regine WF, et al. Direct decompressive surgical resection in the treatment of spinal cord compression caused by metastatic cancer: a randomised trial. Lancet 2005;366:643–8.

78. Rades D, Huttenlocher S, Dunst J, et al. Matched pair analysis comparing surgery followed by radiotherapy and radiotherapy alone for metastatic spinal cord compression. J Clin Oncol 2010;28:3597–604.
79. Lutz S, Berk L, Chang E, et al. Palliative radiotherapy for bone metastases: an ASTRO evidence-based guideline. Int J Radiat Oncol Biol Phys 2011;79:965–76.
80. Rades D, Lange M, Veninga T, et al. Final results of a prospective study comparing the local control of short-course and long-course radiotherapy for metastatic spinal cord compression. Int J Radiat Oncol Biol Phys 2011;79: 524–30.
81. Sahgal A, Ma L, Gibbs I, et al. Spinal cord tolerance for stereotactic body radiotherapy. Int J Radiat Oncol Biol Phys 2010;77:548–53.
82. Sahgal A, Weinberg V, Ma L, et al. Probabilities of radiation myelopathy specific to stereotactic body radiation therapy to guide safe practice. Int J Radiat Oncol Biol Phys 2013;85(2):341–7.
83. Schultheiss TE. The radiation dose-response of the human spinal cord. Int J Radiat Oncol Biol Phys 2008;71:1455–9.

Stereotactic Body Radiation Therapy for Treatment of Primary and Metastatic Pulmonary Malignancies

Chris R. Kelsey, MD*, Joseph K. Salama, MD

KEYWORDS

- Stereotactic body radiation therapy • Stereotactic ablative radiotherapy
- Lung cancer • Pulmonary metastases • Surgery

KEY POINTS

- Stereotactic body radiation therapy (SBRT) is an effective treatment for medically inoperable stage I non–small cell lung cancer with local control achieved in approximately 90% of patients.
- Most patients tolerate treatment exceptionally well. As high doses of radiation therapy are used, care is necessary when treating tumors that are located near the brachial plexus, primary tracheobronchial tree, skin, or chest wall. SBRT is currently being compared with surgery in randomized trials.
- SBRT has also been used for limited pulmonary metastases and studies are ongoing to determine the optimal method of integrating SBRT with systemic therapy.

INTRODUCTION

A conventional course of radiation therapy for most epithelial malignancies consists of daily treatments over a period of approximately 6 to 8 weeks. Stereotactic radiosurgery (SRS) has been successfully used for many years to manage both benign and malignant intracranial tumors. SRS contrasts dramatically with conventional radiation therapy. Instead of small daily fractions over many weeks, a single large treatment is precisely administered to a target while minimizing the dose to surrounding tissues. This approach has been adapted for extracranial targets whereby either a single or small number of dose-intense treatments are given over a 1- to 2-week period.[1] This technique is commonly referred to as both stereotactic body radiation therapy (SBRT) and stereotactic ablative radiotherapy.

Department of Radiation Oncology, Duke Cancer Institute, Duke University Medical Center, Box 3085, Durham, NC 27710, USA
* Corresponding author.
E-mail address: christopher.kelsey@dm.duke.edu

Surg Oncol Clin N Am 22 (2013) 463–481
http://dx.doi.org/10.1016/j.soc.2013.02.011
1055-3207/13/$ – see front matter © 2013 Elsevier Inc. All rights reserved.

Because SBRT consists of large radiation doses, which are associated with a greater potential for local tumor control but also normal tissue complications, with the radiation dose highly conformal to the target (making precise delivery critical), 3 components are mandatory for the successful and safe implementation of SBRT. The first component is reproducible and comfortable patient immobilization to prevent movement during the radiation treatment. This immobilization is most commonly performed using a Styrofoam (The Dow Chemical Company, Midland, Michigan) mold, vacuum bag, or a body frame. The second component is the assessment of respiratory-induced motion. Liver and lung tumors, in particular, are not stationary during the respiratory cycle and their motion must be taken into account during both the planning and treatment phase. Numerous strategies have been implemented to minimize and/or account for this. The third component includes the ability to image the tumor immediately before the treatment to ensure that the target and radiation dose distribution are aligned properly. This process is termed image-guided radiation therapy and is typically performed with computed tomography (CT) imaging or with implanted fiducial markers.

SBRT has emerged as an attractive, and potentially more effective, alternative to conventional radiation therapy for a variety of malignancies. Numerous prospective studies have evaluated SBRT for medically inoperable stage I non–small cell lung cancer (NSCLC). For most other malignancies, the data remains preliminary, although numerous prospective studies are currently ongoing. SBRT is being formally investigated for prostate cancer, pancreatic cancer, breast cancer, painful bone metastases, and liver and lung oligometastases, to name just a few. This article aims to summarize the data on SBRT, with a particular focus on stage I lung cancer and pulmonary metastases.

SBRT: STAGE I NSCLC

Surgery remains the preferred treatment modality for stage I NSCLC. However, patients with lung cancer often present with serious medical comorbidities, often related to tobacco abuse, which make them high-risk operative candidates. Many such patients are observed and do not receive any cancer-directed treatment.[2,3] Despite their other comorbidities, most patients who are observed eventually die of lung cancer.[4] Many other patients have minimal pulmonary reserve and undergo sublobar resections (eg, wedge resection), which are associated with a higher risk of local disease recurrence.[5–10] Other patients, particularly the elderly, wish to avoid surgery and seek out less-invasive alternatives.

Historically, conventional radiation therapy was the treatment of choice for patients with inoperable stage I NSCLC. The typical treatment was 60 to 66 Gy in 1.8- to 2.0-Gy daily fractions. Although this was generally well tolerated, 5-year survival was poor (~15%), with approximately 25% to 50% of tumors recurring at the treated site.[11–15] The primary reason for such a high risk of treatment failure may have been an inadequate radiation dose. Therefore, beginning in the early 1990s, investigators from around the world began exploring SBRT as an alternative approach. Biologically, a few very large treatments are more potent than many small treatments, even when the total radiation dose is the same. Furthermore, multiple radiation fields from different directions are used in SBRT. This method helps create a dose distribution that is conformal to the target, limiting the high dose to surrounding tissues and allowing for the safer administration of larger radiation doses (**Figs. 1** and **2**).

The first phase I dose-escalation study was performed by Robert Timmerman and colleagues[16] at Indiana University. Eligible patients were required to have stage I

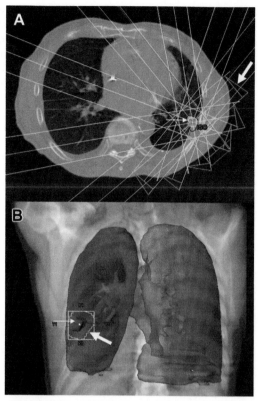

Fig. 1. Axial image (*A*) showing tumor (*thin arrow*) treated with 7 individual radiation fields. A left anterior oblique field is demarcated with a thick arrow. (*B*) The beam's eye view of the left anterior oblique field (*thin arrow*, tumor; *thick arrow*, radiation field edge).

NSCLC measuring 7 cm or less, with medical comorbidities precluding an operation. Patients were grouped into 3 cohorts (T1, T2 <5 cm, T2 >5–7 cm). SBRT consisted of 3 treatments over approximately 2 weeks, beginning with a total radiation dose of 24 Gy (8 Gy × 3), with the dose progressively escalated to 72 Gy (24 Gy × 3). The maximum tolerated dose was not reached for T1 and T2 tumors less than 5 cm and was 66 Gy in 3 fractions for T2 tumors larger than 5 cm.

A subsequent phase II study from Timmerman and colleagues[17] treated 70 patients with medically inoperable stage I NSCLC using the fractionation scheme established in the phase I study (20–22 Gy × 3). After a median follow-up of 50 months, 3-year actuarial local control, cancer-specific survival, and overall survival was 88%, 82%, and 43%, respectively. Local control with SBRT far exceeded results with conventional radiation techniques. However, as mentioned previously, larger radiation doses can potentially lead to toxicities not typically observed with more conventional fractionation schedules. It was observed that patients with central tumors and larger tumors were at higher risk of high-grade toxicity compared with patients with smaller and more peripheral lesions.[18]

A multicenter phase II study performed by the Radiation Therapy Oncology Group (RTOG; 0236) was the first North American multicenter, cooperative group study to evaluate SBRT in medially inoperable patients.[19] Given the complexity of SBRT, each center was required to pass central credentialing standards for protocol

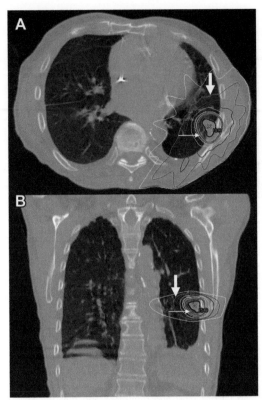

Fig. 2. Axial (*A*) and coronal (*B*) images showing SBRT dose distribution around a primary tumor (*dark blue*). The patient received three 18-Gy fractions (54 Gy) over an 8-day period. The 54-Gy (*red, thin arrow*) and 20-Gy (*pink, thick arrow*) isodose lines are demonstrated.

participation. Because of the findings from the Indiana University phase II study, only patients with smaller (<5 cm) and peripheral (greater than 2 cm from the proximal bronchial tree) tumors were eligible. Patients deemed medically operable were ineligible. All patients (n = 55) were treated with 3 fractions of 20 Gy without tissue density heterogeneity corrections (equivalent to approximately 18 Gy $\times$ 3 with corrections).[20] After a median follow-up of 34 months, the 3-year actuarial local tumor control was 98%. The most common site of failure was distant metastases, occurring in 22% of patients. The overall survival at 3 years was 56%. Grade 3 to 4 toxicity occurred in 15% of patients, which was primarily pulmonary toxicity, including decreased pulmonary function tests, pneumonitis, and hypoxia.

These excellent results have been corroborated by multiple prospective studies conducted in different countries (**Table 1**). Although a variety of dose fractionation schemes have been used, actuarial local control in most studies approaches or exceeds 90%, particularly when the biologic effective dose is more than 100 Gy_{10}.[21,22] In a population of patients who are medically inoperable, 3-year actuarial survival rates of 50% to 60% are also promising and seem to be greater than series in which conventional radiation therapy techniques were used.[23] Patterns of failure seem to have shifted with SBRT,[17,19,24–28] with distant metastases being the most common site of failure compared with conventional radiation therapy[13,15,29–31] where local failure is more prominent (**Fig. 3**).

Table 1 SBRT for stage I NSCLC (prospective trials)				
Study	n	Dose (Fractionation)	Survival (%) (Year)	Local Failure (%) (Year)
Nagata et al,[27] Japan	45	48 Gy (12 Gy × 4)	83: T1 (5) 72: T2 (5)	5: T1 (5) 0: T2 (5)
Baumann et al,[24] Sweden	57	45 Gy (15 Gy × 3)	60 (3)	8 (3)
Fakiris et al,[17] Indiana	70	60–66 Gy (20–22 Gy × 3)	43 (3)	12 (3)
Ricardi et al,[28] Italy	62	45 Gy (15 Gy × 3)	57 (3)	12 (3)
Bral et al,[25] Belgium	40	60 Gy (20 Gy × 3)[a] 60 Gy (15 Gy × 4)[b]	52 (2)	16 (2)
Hoyer et al,[26] Denmark	40	45 Gy (15 Gy × 3)	47 (2)	15 (2)
Timmerman et al,[19] RTOG	55	54 Gy (18 Gy × 3)[c]	56 (3)	2 (3)

[a] Peripheral tumors.
[b] Central tumors.
[c] With lung heterogeneity correction.

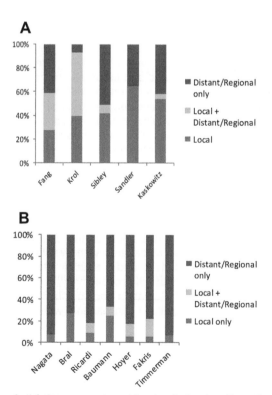

Fig. 3. Percentage of all failures occurring at local only, local + distant/regional, or distant/regional sites only with conventional radiation therapy (*A*) or SBRT (*B*) in published studies cited in references.

SBRT: COMPLICATIONS AND RISKS

Overall, most patients tolerate SBRT exceptionally well. It is an outpatient procedure that takes approximately 45 minutes to administer. The actual treatment only takes a few minutes, with most of the time dedicated to patient setup and tumor position verification. SBRT consists of large doses, which can be associated with complications even when carefully administered. Fortunately, high-grade toxicity occurs in only a minority of patients (~15%).[19]

Pulmonary Toxicity

Most patients develop increased tissue density on CT in the high-dose region after SBRT.[32,33] This increased density is typically asymptomatic but it can be difficult to differentiate from persistent or progressive tumor. Most studies have shown that pulmonary function tests are relatively preserved after SBRT,[34] permitting the use of SBRT even in patients with severely compromised pulmonary function.

Other pulmonary complications have been reported after SBRT, including radiation pneumonitis[16,26,27] and pneumonia.[18] High-grade toxicity has been reported to be higher in patients with central tumors and larger tumors after SBRT, particularly with high-dose 3-fraction regimens (20 Gy × 3).[18]

Chest Wall/Skin Toxicity

Many patients with inoperable stage I lung cancer have peripheral tumors in close proximity to the chest wall. In patients with breast cancer receiving conventionally fractionated radiation therapy, there is a small increased risk of rib fractures.[35] Rib fractures and chronic chest wall pain have also been observed after SBRT.[36–39] Defining the chest wall as the bone and soft tissues 3 cm from the lung/chest wall interface,[36] one study noted that grade 3 chest wall pain or rib fractures were observed when the volume of chest wall receiving 30 Gy or higher (in 3–5 fractions) exceeded 30 cm^3. The risk of chest wall toxicity increased to 30% when the volume receiving 30 Gy exceeded 35 cm^3. Similar findings were noted from MD Anderson.[39] In another study specifically evaluating rib fractures, the risk was related to the total dose delivered to 2 cm^3 of the rib.[37] These studies suggest that there is a dose response but further work is necessary to refine our understanding of chest wall toxicity after SBRT.

Skin reactions are very common after conventionally fractionated radiation therapy and are almost universally transient without long-term complications. However, with large radiation fractions used during SBRT, the risk of severe toxicity increases. In a large series of patients with peripheral lung tumors from MD Anderson, the risk of grade 0, 1, 2, and 3 toxicity after lung SBRT (12.5 Gy × 4–50 Gy) was 61%, 29%, 7%, and 3%, respectively.[39] A case of grade 4 skin necrosis has also been reported.[40] Radiation oncologists must be vigilant in evaluating the dose to the skin, especially in thin patients with posterior tumors near the chest wall.[39,40]

Brachial Plexopathy

In patients with apical lesions, the brachial plexus should be contoured on the treatment planning software and the amount of radiation administered to that structure assessed. It has been shown that the risk of brachial plexopathy is unacceptably high when the maximum dose exceeds 26 Gy.[41]

SBRT: FUTURE DIRECTIONS IN LUNG CANCER
Surgery Versus SBRT

Although there are theoretical reasons why lobectomy may be advantageous over SBRT for operable patients (surgical staging, chemotherapy use for incidental stage II disease, removal of interlobar lymphatics that may harbor cancer, and so forth), there are compelling reasons to think that SBRT may be equivalent to, or perhaps even preferred over, wedge resection. A recent single-institution analysis compared SBRT with wedge resection in patients with stage I lung cancer who were not eligible for lobectomy.[42] Patients undergoing SBRT were older, with more comorbidities, and generally medically inoperable. There was a trend for a lower risk of local failure with SBRT (4% vs 20%, $P = .07$), although ultimate cause-specific survival was equivalent. The overall survival was higher in patients undergoing surgery, because of more non–lung cancer deaths after SBRT, indicating patient selection. It is difficult to compare these patient populations (clinical vs pathologic staging, differences in assessment of local control, prospective vs retrospective collection of data, and so forth), but this study suggests that SBRT may be a reasonable alternative for patients who would otherwise undergo a wedge resection for stage I NSCLC.

Two phase II trials have completed accrual formally evaluating the role of SBRT in an operable population. Preliminary outcomes from the Japanese Clinical Oncology Group 0403 study have been presented demonstrating 3-year progression-free and overall survival rates of 55% and 76%, respectively.[43] RTOG 0618 has also completed enrollment and results are pending.

Randomized trials have also been designed to compare surgery with SBRT. Because of various factors, including long established standards of care, lack of equipoise among specialists, and, in particular, patient randomization to a surgical versus nonsurgical treatment, these trials are expected to be difficult to complete. The Randomized Clinical Trial of Either Surgery or Stereotactic Radiotherapy for Early Stage (IA) Lung Cancer trial was initiated in the Netherlands but closed prematurely because of slow accrual. A CyberKnife (Accuray, Sunnyvale, CA) trial sponsored by Accuray is comparing SBRT with lobectomy and is currently enrolling participants. The American College of Surgeons Oncology Group and RTOG have opened a study for high-risk operable patients comparing sublobar resection and SBRT.

Optimal Dose-Fractionation Scheme

A variety of dose-fractionation schemes have been evaluated in prospective trials (see **Table 1**). In clinical practice, the size of the tumor, the location in the chest, and other factors have an influence on the treatment prescription. A randomized phase II study by the RTOG (0915) has completed accrual comparing 34 Gy in one fraction with 48 Gy in 4 fractions. The less toxic regimen will be compared with the 18 Gy × 3 regimen, which was standardized by the prospective studies at Indiana University and RTOG 0236.

Excess toxicity has been encountered when intense treatment regimens (18 Gy × 3) are used for central tumors.[18] RTOG 0813 is a dose-escalation study attempting to define the maximally tolerated dose for tumors that arise within 2 cm of the tracheobronchial tree.

Systemic Therapy

Finally, patterns of failure show that distant metastases are the primary cause of treatment failure after SBRT (see **Fig. 3**). Incorporation of systemic therapies to decrease this risk seems rational but may be difficult in patients who are medically inoperable. Multiple studies have been proposed but none are completed to date.

SBRT: PULMONARY METASTASES
Rationale for Treatment of Limited Metastatic Disease

Because SBRT has been shown to be an effective local therapy for early stage NSCLC, it has also been investigated as a treatment of pulmonary,[44,45] hepatic,[46–48] adrenal,[49,50] retroperitoneal,[51] spinal,[52,53] and multiple organ[26,51,54,55] metastases. Initial studies investigating pulmonary SBRT included patients with both primary tumors and metastases[56–61] because it was assumed that treatment-related toxicity would be similar for both. Since these early retrospective reports, prospective phase I/II studies have shown that SBRT can be used safely and effectively as a noninvasive procedure for many metastatic sites[45,46,48,55,62] with outcomes similar to surgical metastasectomy. Investigations continue to further refine patient selection criteria, optimize radiation-dosing schedules, and understand how to integrate this technology with systemic therapy.

Hellman and Weichselbaum[63,64] proposed a distinct clinical state of oligometastases to provide a framework to guide further research and understanding of potentially curable patients with limited metastatic disease. They postulated that cancer was a spectrum of disease including those that were localized to their original site that would not spread and, on the other extreme, those that had spread with many metastases in many destination organs. Contained within this spectrum was a state with metastatic tumors limited in number and destination organ. For some of these patients, it was proposed that progression may not be widespread in the course of their disease. These patients were designated as having de novo *oligometastases*. Alternatively, a more widely metastatic state could be converted to a limited metastatic burden or *induced oligometastatic state* following the administration of effective systemic therapy. As imaging and systemic therapy improve, the detection of patients with limited metastatic disease (patients with potential de novo oligometastases) as well as the potential for induced oligometastases should be increasing. Promising outcomes of patients following the surgical removal of pulmonary,[65] hepatic,[66] intracranial,[67,68] and multiple organ metastases,[69] with a 5-year survival approaching 25%, supports the prediction from the oligometastatic hypothesis that metastasis-directed therapy can result in long-term disease control.

Radiation therapy can also be used as an effective means to aggressively treat metastatic disease. Although radiation is typically reserved for palliation of hemoptysis, dyspnea, dysphagia, cough, neurologic symptoms, and pain[70] in patients with metastatic cancer, it can also be delivered with the intent of improving overall survival.[71] RTOG 9508 randomized patients with 1 to 3 brain metastases to either whole brain radiotherapy or whole brain radiotherapy and stereotactic radiosurgery. Survival was significantly improved with the addition of SRS in patients with one metastasis, those with squamous or non–small cell histology, and in those in recursive partitioning analysis (RPA) class 1 (good performance status, controlled primary tumors, aged <65 years, and no extracranial disease),[71] similar to results seen following surgical resection of brain metastases.[67,68] These data suggest that for patients who are not technically resectable or medically fit for surgery, aggressive radiation (SBRT) offers a viable alternative for effective metastasis-directed therapy.

For pulmonary metastases, SBRT has been shown to be an effective metastasis-directed therapy for patients with low-volume disease.[44,45,60] The peripheral location and well-circumscribed morphology of many pulmonary metastases allow for delivery of SBRT with a low probability for treatment-related toxicity. Large series reporting on the treatment of pulmonary metastases with SBRT are limited because of the recent development and widespread application of the technique. Selected series are shown in **Tables 2** and **3**. Control of treated pulmonary metastases with SBRT is promising, approaching 70% to 90% at 2 years, comparable with that of pulmonary metastasectomy.[65]

When using SBRT for the treatment of limited metastatic pulmonary disease, patient selection is critical to the success of the procedure. In general, SBRT is best for patients with 1 to 5 sites of low-volume asymptomatic metastatic cancer because these are patients who are most likely to have truly oligometastatic disease and have no or slow disease progression.[72] Recent data have suggested that patients with good performance status, no prior systemic therapy, lack of progression on systemic therapy, and 1 to 3 metastases have better outcomes.[72] An analysis of patients with limited metastatic disease treated with SBRT revealed that those with true oligometastatic disease, defined as either no progression or progression in limited number and destination organs, were more likely to overexpress microRNA 200c.[73] Further study in larger patient numbers is needed to confirm this finding.

As mentioned earlier, SBRT is an exacting, time-intensive technique often necessitated by the close proximity of metastases to critical normal organs. Therefore, patients must be able to lie still for the duration of treatment and should be able to comply with directions for respiratory motion management as well as pretreatment imaging. Ideal candidates are those with small, well-circumscribed lesions surrounded by lung parenchyma. It follows that patients who are symptomatic from pulmonary obstruction, hemoptysis, chest wall invasion, hepatic capsular invasion, osseous destruction, or vascular compression are not good SBRT candidates. Additionally, because radiation planning for the delivery of SBRT for metastases typically takes 1 to 2 weeks from the time of the radiation treatment planning CT scan, patients with spinal cord compression from local tumor extension are also not good candidates for SBRT. Most of the large series reporting on the use of SBRT for metastases across all organs, including pulmonary metastases, typically allowed 1 to 5 metastases to be treated, with the median of 2 treated metastases.[45,48,51,55]

SBRT doses used to treat pulmonary metastases have varied from single large doses (as high as 30 Gy) to 3, 5, 8, 10, and 20 dose regimens.

Smaller metastases that are peripherally located can typically be treated with higher doses because they are usually well separated from the tracheobronchial tree, esophagus, and other normal tissues. Larger tumors, or those in closer proximity to sensitive organs, typically must be treated with smaller doses per treatment. No prospective comparison of dose-fractionation schemes has been performed in patients with pulmonary metastases. Therefore, the selection of radiation dose is reliant on data from phase I and II studies and retrospective series listed in **Tables 2** and **3**.

Studies investigating single fractions have generally included patients with one metastasis.[74,75] From these investigations, single doses greater than 24 Gy are required to achieve treated metastasis control and lesions treated with doses of 26 Gy or more are unlikely to progress. Using a 3-fraction regimen, a phase I/II study determined that 60 Gy in three 20-Gy doses was associated with high rates of pulmonary control and minimal toxicity.[45] However, the most complete study of this regimen treated only 2 metastases per patient, and the treated metastases were generally small. Therefore, it is reasonable to consider this treatment schedule for 1 to 2 peripherally located, small-volume metastases. A pooled analysis of patients treated for primary or metastatic pulmonary and hepatic metastases found that a radiation dose greater than 54 Gy in 3 fractions and smaller tumor volume was associated with improved outcomes,[76] suggesting this as a lower dose limit. However, for larger metastases, or those close to central lung structures, alternative dosing schedules should be considered. Ten dose regimens,[44] typically delivering a total of 50 Gy,

Table 2
Select single-institution series of SBRT for primary pulmonary malignancies and pulmonary metastases

Author, Institution	Year	N	Median f/u (Months)	Primary, Mets, Both	Total Dose (Gy)	Number of Doses	Local Control	OS
Uematsu et al, National Defense Medical College, Japan[91]	1998	45 P: 23 M: 22	11	B	30–75	5–15	B: 97%	—
Nagata et al, Kyoto University, Japan[58]	2002	40 P: 31 M: 9	16	B	40–48	4	T1a: 100% T1b: 93% Mets: 67%	1 y: 87%
Yoon et al, Asan Medical Center, South Korea[92]	2006	91 P: 38 M: 53	14	B	30–48	3–4	2 y: P: 81% M: 80%	2 y: P: 51% M: NS
Blomgren et al, Karolinska Hospital, Sweden[57]	1998	31 M: 5	8.2	B	Mean 40	1–3	92% crude	11 mo (mean)
Wulf et al, University of Wuerzburg, Germany[56]	2005	81 P: 36 M: 45	14	B	30.0–37.5	3	1 y P: 92% M: 72%	1 y P: 52% M: 85%
Le et al, Stanford University, United States[60]	2006	32 P: 20 M: 12	18	B	15–30 Gy	1	1 y P: 78% M: 58%	1 y P: 85% M: 56%
Hamamoto et al, Shikoku Cancer Center, Japan[90]	2010	62 P: 52 M: 10	14	B	48 Gy	4	2 y: P: 88% M: 25%	2 y: P: 96% M: 86%
Takeda et al, Ofuna Chuo Hospital, Japan[87]	2011	217 P: 183 M: 35	15–29	B	50 Gy	5	2 y: P: 93% M: 82%	NS

Abbreviations: B, both; f/u, follow-up; M, metastases; Mets, metastases; NS, not significant; OS, overall survival; P, primary.

Table 3
Select series of SBRT for pulmonary metastases

Author Institution	Year	N	Median f/u (Months)	Total Dose (Gy)	Number of Doses	Local Control	OS
Zhang et al, Chinese Academy of Medical Sciences, China[82]	2011	71	24.7	30–60	2–12	3 y: 75.4%	3 y: 40.8%
Ricardi et al, University Hospital S. Giovanni Battista di Torino, Italy[83]	2012	61	20.4	26–45	1–4	2 y: 89%	2 y: 66.5%
Norihisa et al, Kyoto University Graduate School of Medicine, Japan[93]	2008	34	27.0	48–60	4–5	2 y: 90%	2 y: 84.3%
Rusthoven et al, Multi-institutional, United States[45]	2009	38	15.4	48–60	3	2 y: 96%	2 y: 39%
Okunieff et al, University of Rochester, United States[44]	2006	30	18.7	50–55	10	3 y: 91%	2 y: 38%

Abbreviations: f/u, follow-up; OS, overall survival.

have also achieved high rates of treated metastases control (91%) for both small- and large-volume pulmonary metastases (>50 cm³).[77] Furthermore, because 10 fraction radiation schedules are routinely used for palliation, the tolerance of tumor-free lung and surrounding tissues to these regimens are more easily predicted.

Few prospective studies have included the treatment of pulmonary metastases with SBRT concurrently with SBRT delivered to other metastatic sites. Regimens tested in this setting include 3 fractions and 10 fractions. When a 3-fraction regimen is used, a dose-finding study determined that 48 Gy in 3 fractions could be delivered.[51] Alternatively, a prospective single-institution study in patients with multiple organ (including pulmonary) metastases demonstrated the efficacy of 50 Gy in 10 fractions.[55]

Toxicity following SBRT for pulmonary metastases has been limited; it is typically radiation-induced dyspnea or pneumonitis, pleural effusion, rib fracture, and chest wall/skin desquamation, as mentioned earlier. Vertebral body collapse has been seen following SBRT for pulmonary metastases, indicating a need to restrict the dose to the spine when possible.[78] Different from primary lung tumors, SBRT is often used to treat multiple pulmonary metastases simultaneously. Although the treatment of multiple pulmonary metastases theoretically increases the risk of pulmonary toxicity over primary NSCLC SBRT because it inherently requires greater lung irradiation, this has not been reported in published series, with toxicity comparably low in both cases.[79] Recent analyses of patients treated for multiple pulmonary metastases have elucidated relationships predictive of toxicity that should be considered when selecting radiation doses.[80,81] These factors should be incorporated into the decision to treat patients with pulmonary metastases with SBRT.

Because radiation therapy–induced pulmonary toxicity using conventional fractionation schemes has been associated with the volume of tumor-free lung irradiated, attempts have been made to try to correlate lung exposure in patients treated with

SBRT for pulmonary metastases. Similar to conventionally treated patients, increasing mean radiation doses to tumor-free lung, the mean normalized total dose (NTDmean), was associated with an increasing incidence of radiation-induced pulmonary toxicity.[80] In patients with a grade 2 or higher pulmonary toxicity, the NTDmean was 15.0 Gy compared with 8.5 Gy in those with lower-grade pulmonary toxicity. Additionally, a trend toward higher-grade pulmonary toxicity has been seen with less conformal radiation distribution when targeting multiple metastases. Therefore, careful planning should be performed to ensure tightly wrapped radiation dose distribution and as low a mean lung dose as possible.

Many series have reported prognostic factors for patients with pulmonary metastases treated with SBRT. A disease-free interval of greater than 1 year from the last therapy to SBRT, good performance status and no extrathoracic metastases have been associated with improved outcomes.[82] Additionally, although some studies have shown that smaller tumors are associated with improved survival,[82,83] other studies have also shown excellent control of larger tumors.[77]

Many different histologies have been treated with SBRT; these include lung cancer,[72] sarcoma,[84] renal cell carcinoma,[85] colorectal,[26] and gynecologic[51] malignancies. SBRT has specifically been used to treat pulmonary metastases typically considered radioresistant to conventionally fractionated radiation therapy, such as melanoma[86] and renal cell carcinoma,[85] with high rates of tumor control. Although some series suggest that certain histologies are associated with worse outcomes,[87] others series have not found histology to be an important determinant of treated metastasis control.[56,76]

Following SBRT, the most common pattern of progression is new sites of metastatic disease, which occur in 46% to 77% of patients.[44,45,75] The median time to progression is 4 to 11 months. Overall survival approaches 40% to 66% at 2 years.[45,79,83] It is interesting to note that a significant fraction of patients progress in a limited number and location of metastases so that a repeat course of metastasis-directed therapy can be considered.[51,83] SBRT can be given a second time for new or recurrent metastases,[88,89] but care should be taken when considering re-SBRT with 3 to 5 fractions for central metastases because they are associated with an increased risk of grade 5 toxicity.[88]

Although survival is numerically lower than reported following surgical resection[65] (2-year overall survival of ~75%), patient selection, medical comorbidities, treated histology, and extent of metastatic disease likely contribute. Patients with fewer metastases[74] and initial presentation with a solitary metastasis have better outcomes, similar to patients treated surgically. Further follow-up is necessary to determine if the promising outcomes for these patients will persist because the largest series using SBRT for pulmonary metastasis have relatively short follow-up (14–19 months) compared with the series reporting on surgical resection for metastases. However, for patients who are not medically fit for surgery or technically resectable, SBRT is a valuable tool for metastasis-directed therapy.

Integrating SBRT for Pulmonary Metastases with Systemic Therapy

There is currently no consensus on how to integrate metastasis-directed SBRT and systemic therapy. It is clear that the primary pattern of progression following SBRT is both new intrathoracic and extrathoracic metastases.[51] It is unknown if the addition of systemic therapy immediately before or following SBRT will decrease this risk. To date, only one study has been published specifically looking at the integration of a systemic agent with SBRT. Although not limited to patients with pulmonary malignancies, a phase I study conducted at Mount Sinai Medical Center (New York) determined the maximum tolerated dose of the multi-targeted kinase inhibitor sunitinib to be 37.5 mg by mouth daily in combination with SBRT (50 Gy delivered in 5-Gy fractions).[54] Studies are currently underway in patients with limited NSCLC metastases to determine the role of SBRT in conjunction with standard systemic therapy, and more are planned in patients with oligometastatic breast cancer.

Differences Between SBRT for Primary Pulmonary Malignancies and Pulmonary Metastases

Although there are many similarities between the treatment of primary pulmonary tumors and pulmonary metastases with SBRT, there are some important differences. Although both have high rates of treated tumor control, some,[60,87,90] but not all,[56] series have reported higher control of primary pulmonary tumors (85%–95%) than for pulmonary metastases (70%–90%) (see **Table 2**). If this is a true finding, the reason for the difference in treated tumor control between primary pulmonary tumors and pulmonary metastases following SBRT is not known. Possible explanations could include the differing biology of primary and metastatic tumors as well as possible differences in tumor size, location, and the radiation dosing schedule used.

Pulmonary toxicity following SBRT for pulmonary metastases may vary from those treated for metastatic disease. A large proportion of patients who are treated with SBRT for primary pulmonary tumors receive this treatment because they are medically inoperable because of poor cardiopulmonary reserve. However, the same cannot be said for patients with limited pulmonary metastases, except for those patients with tobacco-related malignancies. Thus, patients with pulmonary metastases may be more likely to have preserved pulmonary function before cancer diagnosis, although this may decline because of the direct effects of systemic therapy and performance status changes.

Although the SBRT methods used to plan and treat patients with metastatic tumors are similar to those with primary tumors, the planning and delivery of SBRT for metastatic patients may require more time and effort depending on the location, size, and number of metastases being treated. Although less of a concern when metastases are widely separated (eg, small right upper lobe and left lower lobe metastases), a much different situation is faced when metastases are in close proximity. In these cases, careful planning needs to be performed to ensure that the exit dose from one metastasis is accounted for in the planning of others (**Fig. 4**). Additionally, limiting the cumulative dose to surrounding normal structures is more challenging as the number of targets increases.

Finally, the selection of patients for SBRT with medically inoperable NSCLC is relatively straightforward. However, selecting patients with limited metastatic disease for SBRT is less so. In patients who are medically fit for resection, and who have limited or no extrathoracic disease, SBRT should be seen as complementary to surgery and used to treat metastases that are not technically resectable or those whereby surgical removal would cripple lung function. For patients who are *not* medically fit for surgery, SBRT is a reasonable alternative. Expectations of survival and control can be based on surgical results indicating most favorable outcomes in those with a long disease-free interval and only one metastasis, with less favorable results in those with a shorter disease-free interval and increasing number of metastases,[65] adjusting for associated comorbidity. In patients with greater than 3 pulmonary metastases, the time required for SBRT planning and patient time on the treatment table becomes prohibitive. Additionally, SBRT is useful for patients with limited metastatic disease in a few organs where metastasis-directed therapy is desired, but surgical recovery would delay the quick initiation of systemic therapy. When delivered, small peripheral tumors

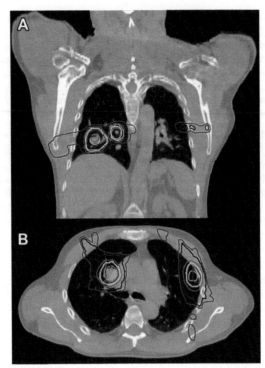

Fig. 4. Radiation dose distribution of a patient with 3 melanoma pulmonary metastases in coronal (A) and axial (B) planes.

should receive at least 24 Gy in a single fraction, 54 Gy in 3 fractions, or 50 Gy in 10 fractions.

SUMMARY

SBRT has become a standard treatment of medically inoperable patients with early stage NSCLC, given the high rates of tumor control and limited reports of toxicity. The application of SBRT to medically operable patients is being actively investigated, with comparisons to both sublobar and lobar resections. For patients with limited pulmonary metastases, SBRT has been shown to result in high rates of treated metastasis control, also with limited toxicity. Studies are ongoing to identify patients who can benefit the most from this treatment as well as to integrate SBRT with standard systemic therapies.

REFERENCES

1. Potters L, Steinberg M, Rose C, et al. American Society for Therapeutic Radiology and Oncology and American College of Radiology practice guideline for the performance of stereotactic body radiation therapy. Int J Radiat Oncol Biol Phys 2004;60:1026–32.
2. Palma D, Visser O, Lagerwaard FJ, et al. Impact of introducing stereotactic lung radiotherapy for elderly patients with stage I non-small-cell lung cancer: a population-based time-trend analysis. J Clin Oncol 2010;28:5153–9.

3. Wisnivesky JP, Halm E, Bonomi M, et al. Effectiveness of radiation therapy for elderly patients with unresected stage I and II non-small cell lung cancer. Am J Respir Crit Care Med 2010;181:264–9.
4. McGarry RC, Song G, des Rosiers P, et al. Observation-only management of early stage, medically inoperable lung cancer: poor outcome. Chest 2002;121:1155–8.
5. Kelsey CR, Marks LB, Hollis D, et al. Local recurrence after surgery for early stage lung cancer: an 11-year experience with 975 patients. Cancer 2009;115:5218–27.
6. Ginsberg RJ, Rubinstein LV. Randomized trial of lobectomy versus limited resection for T1 N0 non-small cell lung cancer. Lung Cancer Study Group. Ann Thorac Surg 1995;60:615–22 [discussion: 622–3].
7. Harpole DH Jr, Herndon JE 2nd, Young WG Jr, et al. Stage I nonsmall cell lung cancer. A multivariate analysis of treatment methods and patterns of recurrence. Cancer 1995;76:787–96.
8. Warren WH, Faber LP. Segmentectomy versus lobectomy in patients with stage I pulmonary carcinoma. Five-year survival and patterns of intrathoracic recurrence. J Thorac Cardiovasc Surg 1994;107:1087–93 [discussion: 1093–4].
9. Lee JH, Machtay M, Kaiser LR, et al. Non-small cell lung cancer: prognostic factors in patients treated with surgery and postoperative radiation therapy. Radiology 1999;213:845–52.
10. Martini N, Bains MS, Burt ME, et al. Incidence of local recurrence and second primary tumors in resected stage I lung cancer. J Thorac Cardiovasc Surg 1995;109:120–9.
11. Dosoretz DE, Galmarini D, Rubenstein JH, et al. Local control in medically inoperable lung cancer: an analysis of its importance in outcome and factors determining the probability of tumor eradication. Int J Radiat Oncol Biol Phys 1993;27:507–16.
12. Graham PH, Gebski VJ, Langlands AO. Radical radiotherapy for early nonsmall cell lung cancer. Int J Radiat Oncol Biol Phys 1995;31:261–6.
13. Krol AD, Aussems P, Noordijk EM, et al. Local irradiation alone for peripheral stage I lung cancer: could we omit the elective regional nodal irradiation? Int J Radiat Oncol Biol Phys 1996;34:297–302.
14. Morita K, Fuwa N, Suzuki Y, et al. Radical radiotherapy for medically inoperable non-small cell lung cancer in clinical stage I: a retrospective analysis of 149 patients. Radiother Oncol 1997;42:31–6.
15. Sibley GS, Jamieson TA, Marks LB, et al. Radiotherapy alone for medically inoperable stage I non-small-cell lung cancer: the Duke experience. Int J Radiat Oncol Biol Phys 1998;40:149–54.
16. Timmerman R, Papiez L, McGarry R, et al. Extracranial stereotactic radioablation: results of a phase I study in medically inoperable stage I non-small cell lung cancer. Chest 2003;124:1946–55.
17. Fakiris AJ, McGarry RC, Yiannoutsos CT, et al. Stereotactic body radiation therapy for early-stage non-small-cell lung carcinoma: four-year results of a prospective phase II study. Int J Radiat Oncol Biol Phys 2009;75:677–82.
18. Timmerman R, McGarry R, Yiannoutsos C, et al. Excessive toxicity when treating central tumors in a phase II study of stereotactic body radiation therapy for medically inoperable early-stage lung cancer. J Clin Oncol 2006;24:4833–9.
19. Timmerman R, Paulus R, Galvin J, et al. Stereotactic body radiation therapy for inoperable early stage lung cancer. JAMA 2010;303:1070–6.
20. Xiao Y, Papiez L, Paulus R, et al. Dosimetric evaluation of heterogeneity corrections for RTOG 0236: stereotactic body radiotherapy of inoperable stage I-II non-small-cell lung cancer. Int J Radiat Oncol Biol Phys 2009;73:1235–42.

21. Olsen JR, Robinson CG, El Naqa I, et al. Dose-response for stereotactic body radiotherapy in early-stage non-small-cell lung cancer. Int J Radiat Oncol Biol Phys 2011;81:e299–303.
22. Onishi H, Shirato H, Nagata Y, et al. Hypofractionated stereotactic radiotherapy (HypoFXSRT) for stage I non-small cell lung cancer: updated results of 257 patients in a Japanese multi-institutional study. J Thorac Oncol 2007;2:S94–100.
23. Grutters JP, Kessels AG, Pijls-Johannesma M, et al. Comparison of the effectiveness of radiotherapy with photons, protons and carbon-ions for non-small cell lung cancer: a meta-analysis. Radiother Oncol 2010;95:32–40.
24. Baumann P, Nyman J, Hoyer M, et al. Outcome in a prospective phase II trial of medically inoperable stage I non-small-cell lung cancer patients treated with stereotactic body radiotherapy. J Clin Oncol 2009;27:3290–6.
25. Bral S, Gevaert T, Linthout N, et al. Prospective, risk-adapted strategy of stereotactic body radiotherapy for early-stage non-small-cell lung cancer: results of a phase II trial. Int J Radiat Oncol Biol Phys 2011;80:1343–9.
26. Hoyer M, Roed H, Hansen AT, et al. Prospective study on stereotactic radiotherapy of limited-stage non-small-cell lung cancer. Int J Radiat Oncol Biol Phys 2006;66:S128–35.
27. Nagata Y, Takayama K, Matsuo Y, et al. Clinical outcomes of a phase I/II study of 48 Gy of stereotactic body radiotherapy in 4 fractions for primary lung cancer using a stereotactic body frame. Int J Radiat Oncol Biol Phys 2005;63:1427–31.
28. Ricardi U, Filippi AR, Guarneri A, et al. Stereotactic body radiation therapy for early stage non-small cell lung cancer: results of a prospective trial. Lung Cancer 2009;68(1):72–7.
29. Kaskowitz L, Graham MV, Emami B, et al. Radiation therapy alone for stage I non-small cell lung cancer. Int J Radiat Oncol Biol Phys 1993;27:517–23.
30. Sandler HM, Curran WJ Jr, Turrisi AT 3rd. The influence of tumor size and pretreatment staging on outcome following radiation therapy alone for stage I non-small cell lung cancer. Int J Radiat Oncol Biol Phys 1990;19:9–13.
31. Fang LC, Komaki R, Allen P, et al. Comparison of outcomes for patients with medically inoperable stage I non-small-cell lung cancer treated with two-dimensional vs. three-dimensional radiotherapy. Int J Radiat Oncol Biol Phys 2006;66:108–16.
32. Hof H, Herfarth KK, Munter M, et al. Stereotactic single-dose radiotherapy of stage I non-small-cell lung cancer (NSCLC). Int J Radiat Oncol Biol Phys 2003;56:335–41.
33. Kyas I, Hof H, Debus J, et al. Prediction of radiation-induced changes in the lung after stereotactic body radiation therapy of non-small-cell lung cancer. Int J Radiat Oncol Biol Phys 2007;67:768–74.
34. Stephans KL, Djemil T, Reddy CA, et al. Comprehensive analysis of pulmonary function test (PFT) changes after stereotactic body radiotherapy (SBRT) for stage I lung cancer in medically inoperable patients. J Thorac Oncol 2009;4:838–44.
35. Overgaard M. Spontaneous radiation-induced rib fractures in breast cancer patients treated with postmastectomy irradiation. A clinical radiobiological analysis of the influence of fraction size and dose-response relationships on late bone damage. Acta Oncol 1988;27:117–22.
36. Dunlap NE, Cai J, Biedermann GB, et al. Chest wall volume receiving >30 Gy predicts risk of severe pain and/or rib fracture after lung stereotactic body radiotherapy. Int J Radiat Oncol Biol Phys 2010;76:796–801.
37. Pettersson N, Nyman J, Johansson KA. Radiation-induced rib fractures after hypofractionated stereotactic body radiation therapy of non-small cell lung cancer: a dose- and volume-response analysis. Radiother Oncol 2009;91:360–8.

38. Voroney JP, Hope A, Dahele MR, et al. Chest wall pain and rib fracture after stereotactic radiotherapy for peripheral non-small cell lung cancer. J Thorac Oncol 2009;4:1035–7.

39. Welsh J, Thomas J, Shah D, et al. Obesity increases the risk of chest wall pain from thoracic stereotactic body radiation therapy. Int J Radiat Oncol Biol Phys 2011;81:91–6.

40. Hoppe BS, Laser B, Kowalski AV, et al. Acute skin toxicity following stereotactic body radiation therapy for stage I non-small-cell lung cancer: who's at risk? Int J Radiat Oncol Biol Phys 2008;72:1283–6.

41. Forquer JA, Fakiris AJ, Timmerman RD, et al. Brachial plexopathy from stereotactic body radiotherapy in early-stage NSCLC: dose-limiting toxicity in apical tumor sites. Radiother Oncol 2009;93:408–13.

42. Grills IS, Mangona VS, Welsh R, et al. Outcomes after stereotactic lung radiotherapy or wedge resection for stage I non-small-cell lung cancer. J Clin Oncol 2010;28:928–35.

43. Nagata Y, Hiraoka M, Shibata T, et al. A phase II trial of stereotactic body radiation therapy for operable T1N0M0 non-small cell lung cancer: Japan Clinical Oncology Group (JCOG0403). Proceedings of ASTRO. Int J Radiat Oncol Biol Phys 2010;78:S27–8.

44. Okunieff P, Petersen AL, Philip A, et al. Stereotactic body radiation therapy (SBRT) for lung metastases. Acta Oncol 2006;45:808–17.

45. Rusthoven KE, Kavanagh BD, Burri SH, et al. Multi-institutional phase I/II trial of stereotactic body radiation therapy for lung metastases. J Clin Oncol 2009;27:1579–84.

46. Katz AW, Carey-Sampson M, Muhs AG, et al. Hypofractionated stereotactic body radiation therapy (SBRT) for limited hepatic metastases. Int J Radiat Oncol Biol Phys 2007;67:793–8.

47. Lee MT, Kim JJ, Dinniwell R, et al. Phase I study of individualized stereotactic body radiotherapy of liver metastases. J Clin Oncol 2009;27:1585–91.

48. Rusthoven KE, Kavanagh BD, Cardenes H, et al. Multi-institutional phase I/II trial of stereotactic body radiation therapy for liver metastases. J Clin Oncol 2009;27:1572–8.

49. Chawla S, Chen Y, Katz AW, et al. Stereotactic body radiotherapy for treatment of adrenal metastases. Int J Radiat Oncol Biol Phys 2009;75(1):71–5.

50. Torok J, Wegner RE, Burton SA, et al. Stereotactic body radiation therapy for adrenal metastases: a retrospective review of a noninvasive therapeutic strategy. Future Oncol 2011;7:145–51.

51. Salama JK, Hasselle MD, Chmura SJ, et al. Stereotactic body radiotherapy for multisite extracranial oligometastases: final report of a dose escalation trial in patients with 1 to 5 sites of metastatic disease. Cancer 2012;118:2962–70.

52. Chang EL, Shiu AS, Mendel E, et al. Phase I/II study of stereotactic body radiotherapy for spinal metastasis and its pattern of failure. J Neurosurg Spine 2007;7:151–60.

53. Chawla S, Schell MC, Milano MT. Stereotactic body radiation for the spine: a review. Am J Clin Oncol 2011. [Epub ahead of print].

54. Kao J, Packer S, Vu HL, et al. Phase 1 study of concurrent sunitinib and image-guided radiotherapy followed by maintenance sunitinib for patients with oligometastases: acute toxicity and preliminary response. Cancer 2009;115:3571–80.

55. Milano MT, Katz AW, Zhang H, et al. Oligometastases treated with stereotactic body radiotherapy: long-term follow-up of prospective study. Int J Radiat Oncol Biol Phys 2012;83:878–86.

56. Wulf J, Baier K, Mueller G, et al. Dose-response in stereotactic irradiation of lung tumors. Radiother Oncol 2005;77:83–7.

57. Blomgren H, Lax I, Naslund I, et al. Stereotactic high dose fraction radiation therapy of extracranial tumors using an accelerator. Clinical experience of the first thirty-one patients. Acta Oncol 1995;34:861–70.

58. Nagata Y, Negoro Y, Aoki T, et al. Clinical outcomes of 3D conformal hypofractionated single high-dose radiotherapy for one or two lung tumors using a stereotactic body frame. Int J Radiat Oncol Biol Phys 2002;52:1041–6.

59. Whyte RI, Crownover R, Murphy MJ, et al. Stereotactic radiosurgery for lung tumors: preliminary report of a phase I trial. Ann Thorac Surg 2003;75:1097–101.

60. Le QT, Loo BW, Ho A, et al. Results of a phase I dose-escalation study using single-fraction stereotactic radiotherapy for lung tumors. J Thorac Oncol 2006;1:802–9.

61. Lee SW, Choi EK, Park HJ, et al. Stereotactic body frame based fractionated radiosurgery on consecutive days for primary or metastatic tumors in the lung. Lung Cancer 2003;40:309–15.

62. Goodman KA, Wiegner EA, Maturen KE, et al. Dose-escalation study of single-fraction stereotactic body radiotherapy for liver malignancies. Int J Radiat Oncol Biol Phys 2010;78:486–93.

63. Hellman S, Weichselbaum RR. Oligometastases. J Clin Oncol 1995;13:8–10.

64. Weichselbaum RR, Hellman S. Oligometastases revisited. Nat Rev Clin Oncol 2011;8(6):378–82.

65. Long-term results of lung metastasectomy: prognostic analyses based on 5206 cases. The International Registry of Lung Metastases. J Thorac Cardiovasc Surg 1997;113:37–49.

66. Fong Y, Cohen AM, Fortner JG, et al. Liver resection for colorectal metastases. J Clin Oncol 1997;15:938–46.

67. Patchell RA, Tibbs PA, Regine WF, et al. Postoperative radiotherapy in the treatment of single metastases to the brain: a randomized trial. JAMA 1998;280:1485–9.

68. Patchell RA, Tibbs PA, Walsh JW, et al. A randomized trial of surgery in the treatment of single metastases to the brain. N Engl J Med 1990;322:494–500.

69. Miller G, Biernacki P, Kemeny NE, et al. Outcomes after resection of synchronous or metachronous hepatic and pulmonary colorectal metastases. J Am Coll Surg 2007;205:231–8.

70. Bezjak A. Palliative therapy for lung cancer. Semin Surg Oncol 2003;21:138–47.

71. Andrews DW, Scott CB, Sperduto PW, et al. Whole brain radiation therapy with or without stereotactic radiosurgery boost for patients with one to three brain metastases: phase III results of the RTOG 9508 randomised trial. Lancet 2004;363:1665–72.

72. Hasselle MD, Haraf DJ, Rusthoven KE, et al. Hypofractionated image-guided radiation therapy for patients with limited volume metastatic non-small cell lung cancer. J Thorac Oncol 2012;7:376–81.

73. Lussier YA, Xing HR, Salama JK, et al. MicroRNA expression characterizes oligometastasis(es). PLoS One 2011;6:e28650.

74. Hof H, Hoess A, Oetzel D, et al. Stereotactic single-dose radiotherapy of lung metastases. Strahlenther Onkol 2007;183:673–8.

75. Wulf J, Haedinger U, Oppitz U, et al. Stereotactic radiotherapy for primary lung cancer and pulmonary metastases: a noninvasive treatment approach in medically inoperable patients. Int J Radiat Oncol Biol Phys 2004;60:186–96.

76. McCammon R, Schefter TE, Gaspar LE, et al. Observation of a dose-control relationship for lung and liver tumors after stereotactic body radiation therapy. Int J Radiat Oncol Biol Phys 2009;73:112–8.

77. Corbin K, Ranck M, Hasselle M, et al. Feasibility and toxicity of hypofractionated image-guided radiotherapy for large volume limited metastatic disease. Pract Radiat Oncol 2012, in press.
78. Rodriguez-Ruiz ME, San Miguel I, Gil-Bazo I, et al. Pathological vertebral fracture after stereotactic body radiation therapy for lung metastases. Case report and literature review. Radiat Oncol 2012;7:50.
79. Siva S, MacManus M, Ball D. Stereotactic radiotherapy for pulmonary oligometastases: a systematic review. J Thorac Oncol 2010;5:1091–9.
80. Yenice KM, Partouche J, Cunliffe A, et al. Analysis of radiation pneumonitis (RP) incidence in a phase I stereotactic body radiotherapy (SBRT) dose escalation study for multiple metastases [abstract 53]. Int J Radiat Oncol Biol Phys 2010;78:S25.
81. Guckenberger M, Baier K, Polat B, et al. Dose-response relationship for radiation-induced pneumonitis after pulmonary stereotactic body radiotherapy. Radiother Oncol 2010;97:65–70.
82. Zhang Y, Xiao JP, Zhang HZ, et al. Stereotactic body radiation therapy favors long-term overall survival in patients with lung metastases: five-year experience of a single-institution. Chin Med J 2011;124:4132–7.
83. Ricardi U, Filippi AR, Guarneri A, et al. Stereotactic body radiation therapy for lung metastases. Lung Cancer 2012;75:77–81.
84. Dhakal S, Corbin KS, Milano MT, et al. Stereotactic body radiotherapy for pulmonary metastases from soft-tissue sarcomas: excellent local lesion control and improved patient survival. Int J Radiat Oncol Biol Phys 2012;82:940–5.
85. Ranck M, Golden D, Corbin K, et al. Stereotactic body radiotherapy for the treatment of oligometastatic renal cell carcinoma. Am J Clin Oncol 2012. [Epub ahead of print].
86. Stinauer MA, Kavanagh BD, Schefter TE, et al. Stereotactic body radiation therapy for melanoma and renal cell carcinoma: impact of single fraction equivalent dose on local control. Radiat Oncol 2011;6:34.
87. Takeda A, Kunieda E, Ohashi T, et al. Stereotactic body radiotherapy (SBRT) for oligometastatic lung tumors from colorectal cancer and other primary cancers in comparison with primary lung cancer. Radiother Oncol 2011;101:255–9.
88. Peulen H, Karlsson K, Lindberg K, et al. Toxicity after reirradiation of pulmonary tumours with stereotactic body radiotherapy. Radiother Oncol 2011;101:260–6.
89. Milano MT, Philip A, Okunieff P. Analysis of patients with oligometastases undergoing two or more curative-intent stereotactic radiotherapy courses. Int J Radiat Oncol Biol Phys 2009;73:832–7.
90. Hamamoto Y, Kataoka M, Yamashita M, et al. Local control of metastatic lung tumors treated with SBRT of 48 Gy in four fractions: in comparison with primary lung cancer. Jpn J Clin Oncol 2010;40:125–9.
91. Uematsu M, Shioda A, Tahara K, et al. Focal, high dose, and fractionated modified stereotactic radiation therapy for lung carcinoma patients: a preliminary experience. Cancer 1998;82:1062–70.
92. Yoon SM, Choi EK, Lee SW, et al. Clinical results of stereotactic body frame based fractionated radiation therapy for primary or metastatic thoracic tumors. Acta Oncol 2006;45:1108–14.
93. Norihisa Y, Nagata Y, Takayama K, et al. Stereotactic body radiotherapy for oligometastatic lung tumors. Int J Radiat Oncol Biol Phys 2008;72:398–403.

Radiation Therapy for Prostate Cancer

Bridget F. Koontz, MD*, W. Robert Lee, MD, MEd, MS

KEYWORDS

- Radiotherapy • Brachytherapy • IMRT • Postoperative • Palliation

KEY POINTS

- Choice of definitive radiation modality (eg, brachytherapy, external beam radiotherapy, use of concurrent androgen suppression) is tailored to the "risk" categorization using clinical characteristics.
- Postoperative prostate bed radiotherapy improves overall survival for patients with adverse pathologic features.
- Radiotherapy, either through x-ray or radiopharmaceutical, is a very effective palliative treatment for bony metastases.

INTRODUCTION

Prostate cancer is the most common cancer diagnosis in men after skin cancer, with more than 240,000 estimated cases in 2012. It is also the second leading cause of cancer death in men (28,000 estimated for 2012).[1] Most prostate cancers are diagnosed at an early stage, allowing for the high rate of success with localized treatment. Between 30% and 45% of men receive radiation as their primary treatment for prostate cancer depending on their age at diagnosis.[2,3]

Both external beam radiotherapy (EBRT) and brachytherapy can be used for the treatment of prostate cancer. The differences and roles of these 2 techniques rely on the physical properties of the radiation and its delivery method. In this article, we review the role of radiation in definitive management, salvage treatment, and palliation for prostate cancer. Although this review is by necessity a brief overview of the extensive literature regarding the use of radiation in prostate cancer management, we rely primarily on "gold standard" clinical trials as well as other reports that offer key findings.

Financial Disclosure: Dr Koontz receives royalties from her role as an author for UpToDate. She has received unrestricted travel grant from Precision X-Ray (North Branford CT). Dr Lee receives a stipend in his role as Editor-in-Chief of Practical Radiation Oncology. Dr Lee receives royalties from his role as Section Editor of Up-to-Date. Dr Lee is a Scientific Advisor to Augmenix.
Department of Radiation Oncology, Duke University Medical Center, DUMC Box 3085, Durham, NC 27710, USA
* Corresponding author.
E-mail address: bridget.koontz@duke.edu

RADIATION AS DEFINITIVE MANAGEMENT
Brachytherapy

"Brachy" is Greek for "short," and brachytherapy is thus a general term for the placement of a radioactive source into or near a tumor. The radioactive sources chosen for brachytherapy typically have a very short effective dose range, allowing for normal tissue sparing. For prostate cancer, either permanent radioactive seeds are placed within the prostate to deliver their dose over weeks to months ("low dose rate" or LDR), or temporary hollow catheters are placed within the prostate allowing for movement of a single source through the catheters delivering the prescribed dose within minutes ("high dose rate" or HDR).

Brachytherapy as monotherapy is most effective in low-risk prostate cancer, commonly defined using National Comprehensive Cancer Network criteria (**Table 1**). Other eligibility criteria include (1) prostate size smaller than 60 mL, (2) none to mild urinary obstructive symptoms (International Prostate Symptom Score of 18 or less),[4] and (3) no history of previous pelvic radiotherapy or transurethral resection of the prostate.[5]

Sources

LDR sources in use include Iodine-125, Palladium-103, and Cesium-131. HDR brachytherapy uses Iridium-192. Half-life, energy characteristics, and prescription doses are described in **Table 2**. The dose varies by source because the biologic response of prostate cancer cells and normal tissues varies based on the dose delivery rate.

Procedure

Brachytherapy planning, whether LDR or HDR, requires 3-dimensional (3-D) understanding of prostate size and shape, typically based on serial axial transrectal ultrasound images. Seed (or iridium source "dwell") locations are designed to provide coverage of the prostate and 2 to 3 mm of extraprostatic tissue while partially sparing the urethra. **Fig. 1** depicts a single axial level of an LDR plan with isodose curves depicting the predicted prostate coverage based on seed placement.

Once a plan has been approved as providing appropriate prostate coverage and minimizing urethral and rectal dose, the seeds (or catheters) are placed into the prostate under imaging guidance. This is performed under anesthesia in the lithotomy position, with placement needles entering through the perineum guided by transrectal ultrasound visualization. For LDR, seed placement can be observed in real time, and if necessary, later seeds adjusted as needed to improve prostate coverage. If HDR is being performed, once all catheters are in place, the plan is confirmed and adjusted based on the actual catheter location in the prostate. Then the Iridium-192 source is robotically advanced sequentially into each catheter, remaining at a given "dwell" position for the amount of time calculated in the plan. HDR treatment can be given as a single fraction or repeated fractions over 24 to 40 hours. Recovery is straightforward, although some men develop prostatic edema requiring Foley catheter

Table 1 National Comprehensive Cancer Network risk criteria		
Low Risk	**Intermediate Risk**	**High Risk**
T1-T2a	T2b-c	T3-4
GS ≤6	GS 7	GS 8–10
PSA <10 ng/mL	PSA 10–20 ng/mL	PSA >20 ng/mL

Abbreviations: GS, gleason score; PSA, prostate-specific antigen.

Table 2
Characteristics of brachytherapy sources

Source	Half-life, d	Energy, kV	Definitive Dose	Dose with 40–50 Gy EBRT
Iodine-125 (LDR)	60	27	145 Gy	110 Gy
Palladium-103 (LDR)	17	23	125 Gy	90–100 Gy
Cesium-131 (LDR)	10	29	1115 Gy (LDR)	85 Gy
Iridium-192 (HDR)	n/a	380	10.5 Gy × 3 9.5 Gy × 4	15 Gy × 1 8.5–10.5 Gy × 2 7.5 Gy × 3 5 Gy × 4

Abbreviations: EBRT, external beam radiotherapy; HDR, high dose rate; LDR, low dose rate.

placement for 24 to 72 hours. Posttreatment imaging is required of LDR treatment to document adequate seed position.

Results

Because implantation of the periprostatic tissue is difficult, brachytherapy is most efficacious in low-risk prostate cancer, although it has been used successfully in cancers more likely to have extraprostatic spread when combined with EBRT.[6,7] The cumulative rates of biochemical recurrence, local failure, distant failure, and overall survival at 8 years were 8%, 6%, 1%, and 88% in a national cooperative group trial of LDR brachytherapy for low-risk prostate cancer.[8] A Radiation Therapy Oncology Group trial of combination brachytherapy and external beam radiation for higher-risk patients has reported 8-year biochemical recurrence rates of 18%.[9]

As stated previously, acute toxicity includes irritative symptoms of the bladder and rectum, which can be managed with alpha blockade, phenazopyridine, and topical hydrocortisone. Rarely, urinary retention can occur, requiring temporary Foley catheter placement. Late toxicity most commonly involves radiation proctitis and/or urethral stricture. Long-term follow-up of LDR brachytherapy studies described

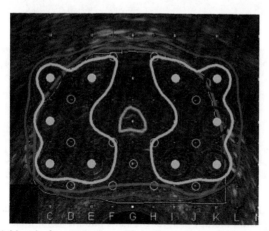

Fig. 1. A single axial level of an LDR plan with isodose curves depicting the predicted prostate coverage based on seed placement. The prostate is contoured in red and the urethra in dark green. Lines demarcating dose show 100% (*pink*), 150% (*green*), and 200% (*blue*). Note coverage of the entire prostate with the 150% isodose line sparing the urethra.

actuarial grade 2+ bladder and rectal late toxicity rates of 25% to 30% and 5% to 7% at 5 years.[8,10,11] Rectal fistula development is a severe but extremely rare side effect of prostate radiotherapy (<1%) that is most likely when brachytherapy and external beam radiation are combined.[12] One potential advantage of brachytherapy is that reported rates of erectile dysfunction (ED) are lower in brachytherapy,[13] although this may be confounded by other inequalities between brachytherapy and external beam radiation.

EBRT

EBRT most commonly uses megavoltage (4–20 MV) photon therapy generated by linear accelerators, although it can also be delivered by protons generated by a particle accelerator (**Fig. 2**). It is used as monotherapy for low-risk prostate cancer, in conjunction with androgen deprivation and/or brachytherapy for intermediate-risk and high-risk cancers, and after prostatectomy for patients with high-risk features or a detectable prostate-specific antigen (PSA).

Dose and schedule

For definitive management of prostate cancer, dose escalation to doses higher than 75 Gy has been found to improve biochemical control for all risk categories in multiple randomized trials and a large meta-analysis.[14] These doses are delivered in 1.8-Gy to 2.0-Gy fractions delivered daily over 8 to 9 weeks.

More recently, hypofractionated regimens have been evaluated, with either moderate hypofractionation (4–5 weeks of daily treatment) or extreme hypofractionation, or

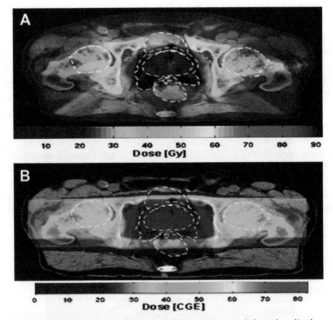

Fig. 2. Example of dose distribution from an (*A*) intensity-modulated radiotherapy plan and (*B*) 3-D conformal proton therapy plan for the same patient. Color indicates dose delivered, whereas the dashed white lines show the contours of the prostate, planning target volume, rectum, bladder, and femoral heads. (*From* Trofimov A, Nguyen PL, Coen JJ, et al. Radiotherapy treatment of early-stage prostate cancer with IMRT and protons: a treatment planning comparison. Int J Radiat Oncol Biol Phys 2007;69(2):444–53; with permission.)

stereotactic body radiotherapy, which consists of 4 to 7 treatments over 1 to 2 weeks. Older studies found mixed results, although they used standard fractionation doses lower than contemporary standards.[15,16] A more recent randomized trial compared 80 Gy in 40 fractions over 8 weeks versus 62 Gy in 20 fractions over 5 weeks. Reported 5-year freedom from biochemical failure was 85% in the hypofractionated arm compared with 79% in the conventional arm ($P = .065$); 3-year genitourinary (GU) and gastrointestinal (GI) toxicity were 16% and 17%, and not statistically different from the conventional fractionation arm.[17] Other moderate hypofractionation trials are pending full results.[18,19] Extreme hypofractionation cohort studies are promising, but the duration of follow-up is short. The reported rates of biochemical progression-free survival are 90% to 95% at 3 to 5 years.[20,21]

Procedure

Intensity modulated radiotherapy (IMRT) is the photon delivery standard of care for definitive radiotherapy of prostate cancer.[22] IMRT treatment plans vary the dose delivered within each treatment field, a characteristic that can be used to create concave treatment plans or escalate dose to certain areas within the target. Therefore IMRT's advantage over 3-D conformal therapy is the ability to lower dose delivered to normal tissues, even while escalating dose to the prostate.[23] IMRT requires high-quality imaging, computerized planning, and quality assurance testing. In addition, a strategy for target localization is necessary to address prostate motion, because IMRT dose drops sharply outside of the planned target area.[24,25]

A planning computed tomography (CT) scan with the patient in the treatment position on a table simulating the treatment couch is required for prostate EBRT planning. Pelvic magnetic resonance (MR) images can be useful to guide prostate delineation. If used, fiducial markers are placed in the prostate by transrectal ultrasound guidance before imaging.[26] These markers can be visualized immediately before each daily treatment. Other methods of prostate localization include transabdominal ultrasound imaging,[27] implanted electromagnetic wireless transponders,[28] and soft tissue on-board localization, which involves CT imaging of the prostate on the treatment equipment.[29,30]

IMRT treatment planning requires delineation of the anatomic regions at risk for disease, an expanded volume that takes into account the potential for set-up and target motion, and avoidance of organs (ie, rectum, bladder, femoral heads, penile bulb, and bowel). Development of the plan involves optimizing 5 to 9 circumferentially placed beams to achieve the minimum and maximum doses prescribed to each structure. Quality assurance is then performed to ensure that the plan can be delivered accurately on the treatment machine.[31–33]

Proton planning is similar to photons, except that most centers use 2 parallel opposed beams entering laterally. Dose coverage of the target and avoidance structures is again optimized through the treatment-planning software.[34]

Monotherapy

EBRT is most commonly used in older men who wish to avoid or have contraindications to an invasive procedure.[2] Dose-escalated EBRT can be quite effective for low-risk cancer with reported 10-year biochemical relapse-free survival of 80% to 90%.[35–37] However, men with intermediate-risk or high-risk cancer experience 10-year biochemical relapse-free survival of approximately 65% and 25% respectively when treated with EBRT alone.[38,39]

EBRT combined with androgen deprivation therapy

Because of the poor results of EBRT monotherapy in higher-risk prostate cancer, concurrent androgen deprivation therapy (ADT) is used to assist in both radiosensitization and treatment of micrometastatic disease. As shown in multiple randomized controlled trials (**Table 3**), the addition of androgen deprivation to radiotherapy improves overall survival for both intermediate-risk and low-risk disease.[38,40] Studies for intermediate disease have evaluated between 3 and 8 months, finding that ADT for at least 6 months provides survival benefit. For high-risk disease, studies have used between 6 months and lifelong ADT; one study comparing 6 months to 3 years found inferior survival with the short ADT arm.[41] Some have reported increased cardiac morbidity with ADT,[42,43] although other large randomized studies of EBRT with ADT have not corroborated this finding.[41,44]

Toxicity

Acute toxicity from IMRT is often quite minimal, with up to 40% having no acute symptoms from prostate irradiation. Many have minor irritative symptoms, but rates of Gr2 GI and GU acute morbidity are very low (2%–10%) with rarely reported more severe toxicity.[45] Late grade 2+ rectal toxicity also remains low with IMRT, 5% to 10% at 10 years,[23] although GU toxicity is more variable depending on the amount of bladder in the treatment volume (2%–20%).[23,46] Finally, ED is actually the most common late effect from prostate radiation.[13] Frequency of ED is variable depending on the patient's age, functional status before treatment, use of ADT, and radiation dose.[47] One prospective study of potent men aged 70+ showed that ED rates increases from 4% immediately after radiotherapy to 47% 5 years after radiation.[48]

SALVAGE THERAPY
Brachytherapy After Definitive Radiation

Although prostate brachytherapy is predominantly used for definitive therapy either alone or as an EBRT boost, brachytherapy can also be used as salvage treatment for local recurrence after primary radiation therapy. Although such a procedure is complex with potential for significant morbidity, several small studies from experienced centers have shown biochemical control between 30% and 65% 5 years after salvage implant.[49,50] Crude rates of grade 3+ were 11% at median 8.6 years of follow-up.[49]

EBRT After Prostatectomy

EBRT can be quite effective at treating patients with local failure or at high risk of local failure after prostatectomy. Certain pathologic features and PSA kinetics are

Table 3
Randomized studies of external beam radiotherapy with or without androgen deprivation

	N	Median FU, y	Length of ADT, mo	Results
Intermediate Risk				
86-10[39]	456	12.5	0 vs 4	36% vs 23% (10-y DSM)
D'Amico[69]	206	7.6	0 vs 6	61% vs 74% (8-y OS)
94-08[40]	1979	9.1	0 vs 4	57% vs 62% (10-y OS)
High Risk				
85-31[70]	977	7.6	0 vs 24	39% vs 49% (10-y OS)
92-02[71]	1554	11.3	4 vs 28	40% vs 45%[a] (10-y OS)
EORTC 22863[38]	415	9.1	0 vs 36	40% vs 58% (10-y OS)
EORTC 22961[41]	970	6.4	6 vs 36	81% vs 85% (5-y OS)

Abbreviations: ADT, androgen deprivation therapy; DSM, disease-specific mortality; EORTC, European Organisation for Research and Treatment of Cancer; FU, follow-up; OS, overall survival.
    [a] For GS8–10 subgroup only.

predictive of durable biochemical control with postoperative radiotherapy, including T3 disease and positive margins.[51-53] Depending on the study, both aggressive and nonaggressive cancers (defined by doubling time and Gleason score) benefit from postoperative therapy.[52,53]

The use of postoperative radiation therapy is supported by 3 randomized control trials (**Table 4**). All 3 required adverse postoperative features, including positive margins or T3 disease. European Organisation for Research and Treatment of Cancer (EORTC) 22911 and Southwest Oncology Group (SWOG) 8794 allowed detectable PSA (present in 30% and 50%, respectively),[54,55] whereas the German ARO (arbeitsgemeinschaft radiologische onkologie) 96-02 excluded those with postoperative detectable PSA.[56] All 3 studies showed improved biochemical relapse-free survival and the SWOG showed an overall survival benefit favoring adjuvant radiotherapy at 10 years (66% vs 74%, $P = .023$). Unplanned subanalysis of the EORTC data found that when pathology was centrally reviewed, extracapsular extension in the setting of negative margins did not have a statistical benefit from adjuvant radiotherapy.[57] Subset analysis of SWOG confirmed that high Gleason grade, extracapsular extension with positive margins, and seminal vesicle invasion did maintain a survival benefit with immediate postoperative radiation.[55]

PALLIATION OF METASTATIC DISEASE
EBRT

EBRT is extremely effective at reducing pain from bone metastases due to prostate cancer, with partial to complete pain relief in 80% of patients.[58] Hypofractionated regimens can be used to reduce the treatment time, with very similar effects. Single-fraction and short-fraction courses carry a 20% risk of requiring retreatment for patients who survive to longer follow-up.[58-60]

EBRT can also be used to palliate local obstructive symptoms or hematuria. Because of the palliative nature of these treatments, they are typically hypofractionated to some degree to a lower dose than is prescribed for curative purposes. Excellent palliation has been reported by series using 2.5-Gy fractions to 50 to 60 Gy.[61,62]

Radiopharmaceuticals

Radioactive compounds trophic to bone have been used to simultaneously treat a large number of blastic bone metastases, which make them well suited to palliative use in prostate cancer. Both Strontium-89[63] and Samarium-153[64] have been in use since the late 1990s. More recently, Radium-223 is under review by the Food and Drug Administration for use in metastatic castrate-resistant prostate cancer based on phase III data showing an improvement in overall survival with Radium-223 compared with placebo (median 14.0 vs 11.2 months, hazard ratio 0.70). Treatment

Table 4				
Randomized studies of immediate postoperative radiotherapy for adverse pathologic features				
		Median FU, y	Radiation Dose, Gy	BRFS, actuarial y, RT vs Observation (FU)
EORTC	1005	10.6	60	61% vs 41% (10)
SWOG	425	12.6	60–64	73% vs 63% (10)
German	385	4.5	60	72% vs 54% (5)

Abbreviations: BRFS, biochemical relapse free survival; EORTC, European Organisation for Research and Treatment of Cancer; FU, follow-up; RT, radiation therapy; SWOG, Southwest Oncology Group.

was well tolerated with mild myelosuppression.[65] These agents are not suitable for patients with bone marrow or renal impairment, pending fracture or cord compression, or men with few, asymptomatic, or predominantly lytic bone metastases.

SUMMARY

Radiation therapy is very well tolerated and can be highly effective in treating prostate cancer, when the appropriate modality is applied based on the stage of disease. Although randomized studies comparing surgical and radiation therapy for localized prostate cancer have failed to accrue,[66] comparison of surgical and nonsurgical trials with similar eligibility show similar results.[67,68] Choice of therapy is ultimately based on stage and toxicity profile of the therapy. Finally, given the overall good outcome for men undergoing surveillance, judicious use of treatment is warranted to minimize any quality-of-life changes based on therapy.

REFERENCES

1. American Cancer Society. Cancer facts and figures 2012. Available at: http://www. cancer.org/acs/groups/content/@epidemiologysurveilance/documents/document/ acspc-031941.pdf. Accessed February 28, 2012.
2. Meltzer D, Egleston B, Abdalla I. Patterns of prostate cancer treatment by clinical stage and age. Am J Public Health 2001;91(1):126–8.
3. Dinan MA, Robinson TJ, Zagar TM, et al. Changes in initial treatment for prostate cancer among Medicare beneficiaries, 1999-2007. Int J Radiat Oncol Biol Phys 2012;82(5):e781–6.
4. Bucci J, Morris WJ, Keyes M, et al. Predictive factors of urinary retention following prostate brachytherapy. Int J Radiat Oncol Biol Phys 2002;53(1):91–8.
5. Nag S, Beyer D, Friedland J, et al. American Brachytherapy Society (ABS) recommendations for transperineal permanent brachytherapy of prostate cancer. Int J Radiat Oncol Biol Phys 1999;44(4):789–99.
6. Potters L, Morgenstern C, Calugaru E, et al. 12-year outcomes following permanent prostate brachytherapy in patients with clinically localized prostate cancer. J Urol 2008;179(Suppl 5):S20–4.
7. Koontz BF, Chino J, Lee WR, et al. Morbidity and prostate-specific antigen control of external beam radiation therapy plus low-dose-rate brachytherapy boost for low, intermediate, and high-risk prostate cancer. Brachytherapy 2009; 8(2):191–6.
8. Lawton CA, Hunt D, Lee WR, et al. Long-term results of a phase II trial of ultrasound-guided radioactive implantation of the prostate for definitive management of localized adenocarcinoma of the prostate (RTOG 98-05). Int J Radiat Oncol Biol Phys 2011;81(1):1–7.
9. Lawton CA, Yan Y, Lee WR, et al. Long-term results of an RTOG Phase II trial (00-19) of external-beam radiation therapy combined with permanent source brachytherapy for intermediate-risk clinically localized adenocarcinoma of the prostate. Int J Radiat Oncol Biol Phys 2012;82(5):e795–801.
10. Keyes M, Miller S, Moravan V, et al. Predictive factors for acute and late urinary toxicity after permanent prostate brachytherapy: long-term outcome in 712 consecutive patients. Int J Radiat Oncol Biol Phys 2009;73(4):1023–32.
11. Keyes M, Spadinger I, Liu M, et al. Rectal toxicity and rectal dosimetry in low-dose-rate (125)I permanent prostate implants: a long-term study in 1006 patients. Brachytherapy 2012;11(3):199–208.

12. Theodorescu D, Gillenwater JY, Koutrouvelis PG. Prostatourethral-rectal fistula after prostate brachytherapy. Cancer 2000;89(10):2085–91.
13. Sanda MG, Dunn RL, Michalski J, et al. Quality of life and satisfaction with outcome among prostate-cancer survivors. N Engl J Med 2008;358(12):1250–61.
14. Viani GA, Stefano EJ, Afonso SL. Higher-than-conventional radiation doses in localized prostate cancer treatment: a meta-analysis of randomized, controlled trials. Int J Radiat Oncol Biol Phys 2009;74(5):1405–18.
15. Lukka H, Hayter C, Julian JA, et al. Randomized trial comparing two fractionation schedules for patients with localized prostate cancer. J Clin Oncol 2005;23(25): 6132–8.
16. Yeoh EE, Fraser RJ, McGowan RE, et al. Evidence for efficacy without increased toxicity of hypofractionated radiotherapy for prostate carcinoma: early results of a Phase III randomized trial. Int J Radiat Oncol Biol Phys 2003;55(4):943–55.
17. Arcangeli G, Fowler J, Gomellini S, et al. Acute and late toxicity in a randomized trial of conventional versus hypofractionated three-dimensional conformal radiotherapy for prostate cancer. Int J Radiat Oncol Biol Phys 2011;79(4):1013–21.
18. Pollack A, Walker G, Buyyounouski MK, et al. Five year results of a randomized external beam radiotherapy hypofractionation trial for prostate cancer. Int J Radiat Oncol Biol Phys 2011;81(2):S1.
19. Kuban DA, Nogueras-Gonzalez GM, Hamblin L, et al. Preliminary report of a randomized dose escalation trial for prostate cancer using hypofraction. Int J Radiat Oncol Biol Phys 2010;78(3):S58–9.
20. Freeman DE, King CR. Stereotactic body radiotherapy for low-risk prostate cancer: five-year outcomes. Radiat Oncol 2011;6:3.
21. Boike TP, Lotan Y, Cho LC, et al. Phase I dose-escalation study of stereotactic body radiation therapy for low- and intermediate-risk prostate cancer. J Clin Oncol 2011;29(15):2020–6.
22. Sheets NC, Goldin GH, Meyer AM, et al. Intensity-modulated radiation therapy, proton therapy, or conformal radiation therapy and morbidity and disease control in localized prostate cancer. JAMA 2012;307(15):1611–20.
23. Zelefsky MJ, Levin EJ, Hunt M, et al. Incidence of late rectal and urinary toxicities after three-dimensional conformal radiotherapy and intensity-modulated radiotherapy for localized prostate cancer. Int J Radiat Oncol Biol Phys 2008;70(4): 1124–9.
24. Bortfeld T. IMRT: a review and preview. Phys Med Biol 2006;51(13):R363–79.
25. Webb S. The physical basis of IMRT and inverse planning. Br J Radiol 2003; 76(910):678–89.
26. Middleton M, Frantzis J, Healy B, et al. Successful implementation of image-guided radiation therapy quality assurance in the Trans Tasman Radiation Oncology Group 08.01 PROFIT Study. Int J Radiat Oncol Biol Phys 2011;81:1576–81.
27. Trichter F, Ennis RD. Prostate localization using transabdominal ultrasound imaging. Int J Radiat Oncol Biol Phys 2003;56(5):1225–33.
28. Quigley MM, Mate TP, Sylvester JE. Prostate tumor alignment and continuous, real-time adaptive radiation therapy using electromagnetic fiducials: clinical and cost-utility analyses. Urol Oncol 2009;27(5):473–82.
29. Barney BM, Lee RJ, Handrahan D, et al. Image-guided radiotherapy (IGRT) for prostate cancer comparing kV imaging of fiducial markers with cone beam computed tomography (CBCT). Int J Radiat Oncol Biol Phys 2011;80:301–5.
30. van Zijtveld M, Dirkx M, Breuers M, et al. Evaluation of the 'dose of the day' for IMRT prostate cancer patients derived from portal dose measurements and cone-beam CT. Radiother Oncol 2010;96(2):172–7.

31. Ezzell GA, Burmeister JW, Dogan N, et al. IMRT commissioning: multiple institution planning and dosimetry comparisons, a report from AAPM Task Group 119. Med Phys 2009;36(11):5359–73.

32. Ezzell GA, Galvin JM, Low D, et al. Guidance document on delivery, treatment planning, and clinical implementation of IMRT: report of the IMRT Subcommittee of the AAPM Radiation Therapy Committee. Med Phys 2003;30(8):2089–115.

33. Klein EE, Hanley J, Bayouth J, et al. Task Group 142 report: quality assurance of medical accelerators. Med Phys 2009;36(9):4197–212.

34. Trofimov A, Nguyen PL, Coen JJ, et al. Radiotherapy treatment of early-stage prostate cancer with IMRT and protons: a treatment planning comparison. Int J Radiat Oncol Biol Phys 2007;69(2):444–53.

35. Alicikus ZA, Yamada Y, Zhang Z, et al. Ten-year outcomes of high-dose, intensity-modulated radiotherapy for localized prostate cancer. Cancer 2011;117: 1429–37.

36. Zelefsky MJ, Yamada Y, Fuks Z, et al. Long-term results of conformal radiotherapy for prostate cancer: impact of dose escalation on biochemical tumor control and distant metastases-free survival outcomes. Int J Radiat Oncol Biol Phys 2008;71(4):1028–33.

37. Zietman AL, Bae K, Slater JD, et al. Randomized trial comparing conventional-dose with high-dose conformal radiation therapy in early-stage adenocarcinoma of the prostate: long-term results from Proton Radiation Oncology Group/American College of Radiology 95-09. J Clin Oncol 2010;28(7):1106–11.

38. Bolla M, Van Tienhoven G, Warde P, et al. External irradiation with or without long-term androgen suppression for prostate cancer with high metastatic risk: 10-year results of an EORTC randomised study. Lancet Oncol 2010;11(11): 1066–73.

39. Roach M 3rd, Bae K, Speight J, et al. Short-term neoadjuvant androgen deprivation therapy and external-beam radiotherapy for locally advanced prostate cancer: long-term results of RTOG 8610. J Clin Oncol 2008;26(4):585–91.

40. Jones CU, Hunt D, McGowan DG, et al. Radiotherapy and short-term androgen deprivation for localized prostate cancer. N Engl J Med 2011;365(2):107–18.

41. Bolla M, de Reijke TM, Van Tienhoven G, et al. Duration of androgen suppression in the treatment of prostate cancer. N Engl J Med 2009;360(24):2516–27.

42. D'Amico AV, Denham JW, Crook J, et al. Influence of androgen suppression therapy for prostate cancer on the frequency and timing of fatal myocardial infarctions. J Clin Oncol 2007;25(17):2420–5.

43. Keating NL, O'Malley AJ, Smith MR. Diabetes and cardiovascular disease during androgen deprivation therapy for prostate cancer. J Clin Oncol 2006;24(27): 4448–56.

44. Efstathiou JA, Bae K, Shipley WU, et al. Cardiovascular mortality after androgen deprivation therapy for locally advanced prostate cancer: RTOG 85-31. J Clin Oncol 2009;27(1):92–9.

45. Takeda K, Takai Y, Narazaki K, et al. Treatment outcome of high-dose image-guided intensity-modulated radiotherapy using intraprostate fiducial markers for localized prostate cancer at a single institute in Japan. Radiat Oncol 2012; 7(1):105.

46. Morgan PB, Ruth K, Horwitz EM, et al. A matched pair comparison of intensity modulated radiotherapy and three-dimensional conformal radiotherapy for prostate cancer: toxicity and outcomes. Int J Radiat Oncol Biol Phys 2007;69(3):S319.

47. Alemozaffar M, Regan MM, Cooperberg MR, et al. Prediction of erectile function following treatment for prostate cancer. JAMA 2011;306(11):1205–14.

48. Mantz CA, Nautiyal J, Awan A, et al. Potency preservation following conformal radiotherapy for localized prostate cancer: impact of neoadjuvant androgen blockade, treatment technique, and patient-related factors. Cancer J Sci Am 1999;5(4):230–6.
49. Burri RJ, Stone NN, Unger P, et al. Long-term outcome and toxicity of salvage brachytherapy for local failure after initial radiotherapy for prostate cancer. Int J Radiat Oncol Biol Phys 2010;77(5):1338–44.
50. Grado GL, Collins JM, Kriegshauser JS, et al. Salvage brachytherapy for localized prostate cancer after radiotherapy failure. Urology 1999;53(1):2–10.
51. Anscher MS, Prosnitz LR. Postoperative radiotherapy for patients with carcinoma of the prostate undergoing radical prostatectomy with positive surgical margins, seminal vesicle involvement and/or penetration through the capsule. J Urol 1987; 138(6):1407–12.
52. Stephenson AJ, Scardino PT, Kattan MW, et al. Predicting the outcome of salvage radiation therapy for recurrent prostate cancer after radical prostatectomy. J Clin Oncol 2007;25(15):2035–41.
53. Trock BJ, Han M, Freedland SJ, et al. Prostate cancer-specific survival following salvage radiotherapy vs observation in men with biochemical recurrence after radical prostatectomy. JAMA 2008;299(23):2760–9.
54. Bolla M, Van Poppel H, Tombal B, et al. 10-year results of adjuvant radiotherapy after radical prostatectomy in pT3N0 prostate cancer (EORTC 22911). Int J Radiat Oncol Biol Phys 2010;78(3):S29.
55. Thompson IM, Tangen CM, Paradelo J, et al. Adjuvant radiotherapy for pathological T3N0M0 prostate cancer significantly reduces risk of metastases and improves survival: long-term followup of a randomized clinical trial. J Urol 2009; 181(3):956–62.
56. Wiegel T, Bottke D, Steiner U, et al. Phase III postoperative adjuvant radiotherapy after radical prostatectomy compared with radical prostatectomy alone in pT3 prostate cancer with postoperative undetectable prostate-specific antigen: ARO 96-02/AUO AP 09/95. J Clin Oncol 2009;27(18):2924–30.
57. Van der Kwast TH, Bolla M, Van Poppel H, et al. Identification of patients with prostate cancer who benefit from immediate postoperative radiotherapy: EORTC 22911. J Clin Oncol 2007;25(27):4178–86.
58. van der Linden YM, Lok JJ, Steenland E, et al. Single fraction radiotherapy is efficacious: a further analysis of the Dutch Bone Metastasis Study controlling for the influence of retreatment. Int J Radiat Oncol Biol Phys 2004;59(2):528–37.
59. Hartsell WF, Scott CB, Bruner DW, et al. Randomized trial of short- versus long-course radiotherapy for palliation of painful bone metastases. J Natl Cancer Inst 2005;97(11):798–804.
60. 8 Gy single fraction radiotherapy for the treatment of metastatic skeletal pain: randomised comparison with a multifraction schedule over 12 months of patient follow-up. Bone Pain Trial Working Party. Radiother Oncol 1999;52(2): 111–21.
61. Gogna NK, Baxi S, Hickey B, et al. Split-course, high-dose palliative pelvic radiotherapy for locally progressive hormone-refractory prostate cancer. Int J Radiat Oncol Biol Phys 2012;83(2):e205–11.
62. Spanos WJ Jr, Clery M, Perez CA, et al. Late effect of multiple daily fraction palliation schedule for advanced pelvic malignancies (RTOG 8502). Int J Radiat Oncol Biol Phys 1994;29(5):961–7.
63. Porter AT, McEwan AJ, Powe JE, et al. Results of a randomized phase-III trial to evaluate the efficacy of strontium-89 adjuvant to local field external beam

irradiation in the management of endocrine resistant metastatic prostate cancer. Int J Radiat Oncol Biol Phys 1993;25(5):805–13.

64. Sartor O, Reid RH, Hoskin PJ, et al. Samarium-153-Lexidronam complex for treatment of painful bone metastases in hormone-refractory prostate cancer. Urology 2004;63(5):940–5.

65. Parker C, Heinrich D, O'Sullivan JM, et al. Overall survival benefit and safety profile of radium-223 chloride, a first-in-class alpha pharmaceutical: results from a phase III randomized trial (ALSYMPCA) in patients with castration-resistant prostate cancer (CRPC) with bone metastases. J Clin Oncol 2012; 30(5S). abstract 8.

66. Wallace K, Fleshner N, Jewett M, et al. Impact of a multi-disciplinary patient education session on accrual to a difficult clinical trial: the Toronto experience with the surgical prostatectomy versus interstitial radiation intervention trial. J Clin Oncol 2006;24(25):4158–62.

67. Vicini FA, Martinez A, Hanks G, et al. An interinstitutional and interspecialty comparison of treatment outcome data for patients with prostate carcinoma based on predefined prognostic categories and minimum follow-up. Cancer 2002;95(10):2126–35.

68. Grimm P, Billiet I, Bostwick D, et al. Comparative analysis of prostate-specific antigen free survival outcomes for patients with low, intermediate and high risk prostate cancer treatment by radical therapy. Results from the Prostate Cancer Results Study Group. BJU Int 2012;109(Suppl 1):22–9.

69. D'Amico AV, Chen MH, Renshaw AA, et al. Androgen suppression and radiation vs radiation alone for prostate cancer: a randomized trial. JAMA 2008;299(3): 289–95.

70. Pilepich MV, Winter K, Lawton CA, et al. Androgen suppression adjuvant to definitive radiotherapy in prostate carcinoma—long-term results of phase III RTOG 85-31. Int J Radiat Oncol Biol Phys 2005;61(5):1285–90.

71. Horwitz EM, Bae K, Hanks GE, et al. Ten-year follow-up of Radiation Therapy Oncology Group protocol 92-02: a phase III trial of the duration of elective androgen deprivation in locally advanced prostate cancer. J Clin Oncol 2008; 26(15):2497–504.

Image-guided Brachytherapy for Gynecologic Surgeons

Junzo Chino, MD[a],*, Angeles Alvarez Secord, MD[b]

KEYWORDS

- Brachytherapy • MRI • Cervical cancer • Gynecologic oncology • HDR

KEY POINTS

- T2-weighted magnetic resonance imaging (MRI) gives the most specific and detailed measure of disease in the pelvis for most gynecologic malignances.
- A high-risk clinical target volume (HRCTV) may be defined as residual disease on T2-weighted MRI; dose to this volume is highly correlated with control in the pelvis.
- High doses to even small volumes of neighboring critical tissues such as the bladder and rectum are correlated with late toxicity to these organs.
- Modern high-dose-rate applicator design allows optimal coverage of the HRCTV while minimizing normal tissue volumes.
- An international trial (the EMBRACE [European Study on MRI-guided Brachytherapy in Locally Advanced Cervical Cancer] study) is ongoing, designed to assess the exportability of these findings in the broader community.

INTRODUCTION TO BRACHYTHERAPY

Brachytherapy has been an integral portion of the curative treatment of several gynecologic malignancies for more than 100 years, beginning with the use of intracavitary radium for inoperable uterine cancer and cervical cancer in the early 1900s.[1] The advantages of this form of radiation delivery compared with external beam treatment derive primarily from the inverse square law: with movement away from an implanted radioactive source, the dose decreases at the inverse square of the distance:

$$D_a = D_b \times (d_b)^2/(d_a)^2$$

with D_a being the dose at a point d_a far from the source and D_b being the dose at point d_b from the source. Thus the dose at 2 cm from the source is one-quarter that of the dose at 1 cm, whereas the dose at 10 cm is one-hundredth of the same dose.

Disclosures: None.
[a] Department of Radiation Oncology, Duke University Medical Center, Box 3085, Durham, NC 27710, USA; [b] Division of Gynecologic Oncology, Department of Obstetrics and Gynecology, Duke Cancer Institute, Duke University Medical Center, Box 3079, Durham, NC 27710, USA
* Corresponding author.
E-mail address: junzo.chino@duke.edu

Surg Oncol Clin N Am 22 (2013) 495–509
http://dx.doi.org/10.1016/j.soc.2013.02.002
1055-3207/13/$ – see front matter © 2013 Elsevier Inc. All rights reserved.

Therefore, when it is possible to place a source within the target, very high doses are achievable centrally, with a sharp decrease of dose at the target boundary. In addition, because the radioactive sources are placed directly within the tumor, the risk of the target migrating out of the field (or conversely, normal tissue migrating into the field) is essentially eliminated.

FILM-BASED TREATMENT PLANNING

The methods of treatment planning for tandem and ovoid-based brachytherapy for cervical cancer remained unchanged throughout the later portion of the twentieth century. The Manchester, Stockholm, and Paris methods of dose specification and loading patterns for low-dose-rate (LDR) implants were developed in 1927 to 1938, later refined and modernized by Fletcher and colleagues[2] at MD Anderson in the late 1940s.[3–5] These systems were based on imaging technology available at the time of their initial conception and development, namely orthogonal plain films of the pelvis with the implant in place. By necessity, surrogates visible on plain radiographs were used for estimating doses to both the target and to the critical normal tissue. Point A, or the paracentral dose, defined at a point 2 cm superior to the top of the ovoids, and 2 cm lateral to the tandem, evolved into a prescription point in these systems (**Fig. 1**).

Despite these limitations, this method defined effective standardized treatment in which doses could be compared across physician practices, and from which a measure of brachytherapy quality could be extracted. Montana and colleagues[6] showed that dose to point A dose was associated with a reduced 4-year recurrence rate; 34% if point A received less than 65 Gy, 14% in those with a dose greater than 75 Gy. Perez and colleagues[7] similarly found that a rectal point dose greater than 75 Gy was associated with a 9% incidence of moderate to severe late toxicity, compared with 4% if the dose was less than 75 Gy; the bladder point was also associated with moderate to severe late toxicity, with a 2% incidence if the dose was less than 70 Gy and 5% if the dose was greater than 75 Gy.

MODERN IMAGING OF CERVICAL CANCER
Computed Tomography

Computed tomography (CT) was the first modality used to perform image-guided brachytherapy; however, images were limited by the artifacts created by the metal applicator and tungsten shields used in the ovoids (**Fig. 2, Table 1**). Weeks and Montana[8] at Duke developed a CT-compatible LDR applicator, which has recently become commercially available.[8,9] An initial analysis of 27 implants showed systematic underestimation of the maximum bladder and rectal dose by the film-based points.[10] Pelloski[11] at MD Anderson found, in 93 implants using a standard applicator, that although the rectal point on orthogonal films correlated with the rectal D2cc (minimum dose to the 2 cm^2 of rectum receiving the highest dose), there was systematic underestimation of the bladder D2cc using the film-based bladder point.

A team from Loyola examined implants in 19 women. The initial planning and treatment was performed with two-dimensional (2D) methods then reevaluated with CT-based three-dimensional (3D) dose calculation.[12] The CT-defined volume of the cervix varied from 12 to 39 cm^2 among women, and, more importantly, the dose covering 90% of the cervix decreased more than 40% when the 2D plan was used for the largest cervical volumes. Schoeppel and colleagues[13] from Michigan similarly showed that the dose to point A consistently underestimated the dose to the CT-visible cervix in all 10 cases of their initial series.

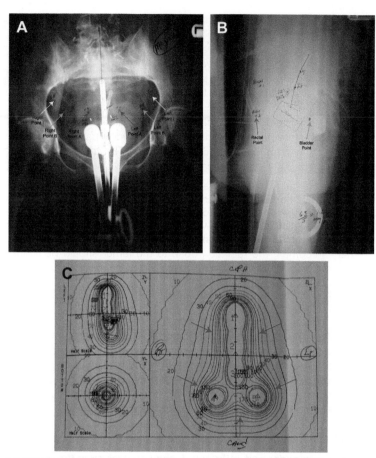

Fig. 1. A treatment plan for IB2 cervical cancer based on orthogonal films. In the anteroposterior radiograph (*A*), right and left points A are seen defined at a point 2 cm superior to the top of the ovoids, and 2 cm lateral to the tandem (*red arrows*). Also note points B defined 5 cm lateral to the tandem (*green arrows*), which were designed as surrogates for the parametrium, and points I (*yellow arrows*) which indicate the pelvic nodes. In the lateral radiograph (*B*), the rectal point is defined 5 mm posterior to the vaginal packing (aided by a rectal tube in this case, *left arrow*), and the bladder point is set at the posterior aspect of the Foley balloon (*right arrow*). Activity of the 5 sources (3 in tandem and 1 in each ovoid) is then varied to arrive at a dose to point A of from 75 to 85 Gy, while limiting the dose to the rectal point to less than 70 to 75 Gy, and to the bladder point to less than 75 to 80 Gy. (*C*) Isodose lines are seen for this case; the prescription was written to the 60 cGy per hour line (the pear-shaped magenta line, *red arrows*).

Thus CT-compatible applicators are better able to define the doses to critical normal tissues and help refine the dose to the cervix. However, CT is not ideal at determining the extent of disease, with only 50% to 65% accuracy at determining size and spread of cancer within the cervix, and 75% to 80% accuracy in evaluation of the parametrium in preoperative studies of early-stage patients.[14,15]

Magnetic Resonance Imaging: T2 Weighted

In these same preoperative studies, magnetic resonance imaging (MRI) was shown to be significantly superior to CT with 75% to 90% accuracy in evaluating the extent of

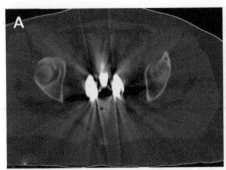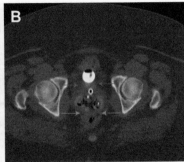

Fig. 2. CT-based image-guided brachytherapy. (*A*) CT images obtained with a conventional Fletcher Suit Delclos LDR applicator, with artifact from the tungsten shielding obscuring the cervix, bladder, and rectum. (*B*) CT images obtained with a CT-compatible Weeks applicator, in which the ovoid shielding is contained within the removable source bucket. The bladder (*upper arrows*) and rectal (*lower arrows*) interfaces are more clearly defined.

disease in the cervix, and 85% to 95% accuracy in evaluation of parametrial spread.[14,15] In a prospective study comparing MRI-based contours with CT in 10 patients, Viswanathan and colleagues[16] found a systematic overestimation of the width of the cervical tumor by CT, by a mean difference of 20%. This significantly affected the potential tumor coverage by brachytherapy planning by up to 35% in this series. This systematic difference in the visualization of the lateral extent of disease between CT and MRI was confirmed by Eskander and colleagues[17] in an additional 11 women, and the MRI volumes also extended further in the superior/ inferior direction compared with CT (**Fig. 3**). Because of these findings, MRI is currently the preferred modality for image-guided brachytherapy.

Emerging Modalities: Metabolic and Functional Imaging

Much work has been performed in the last decade on evaluating the glucose metabolism of cervical cancer. Investigators from Washington University found that a complete metabolic response on fluorodeoxyglucose (FDG) positron emission tomography (PET) obtained 3 months after treatment was highly predictive of progression-free survival (PFS); at 3 years, with complete response, PFS was 78% versus 33% in partial responders, and 0% with PET progression.[18] The same group also investigated the usefulness of FDG-PET obtained during brachytherapy, and found that film-based (2D) plans covered only 70% of the PET-avid regions.[19] However, it remains unexplored how FDG-PET compares with MRI-based plans.

Dynamic contrast-enhanced MRI (DCE-MRI) is a means by which tumor perfusion may be quantified. Because hypoxia and poor perfusion are poor prognostic factors in cervical cancer, decreased and heterogeneous perfusion on DCE-MRI may be associated with poorer outcome.[20] Mayr and colleagues[21] were able to show that the volume of disease with poor perfusion after 2 weeks of therapy was significantly associated with poor local control and disease-specific survival. Although these data have not yet been applied to brachytherapy, DCE-MRI may help define a resistant target volume that may benefit from dose escalation.

Diffusion-weighted MRI (DW-MRI) delineates areas of high cellular density by identifying regions with a low apparent diffusion coefficient (ADC). Danish investigators correlated volumes defined by T2-weighted MRI brachytherapy planning with volumes defined by DW-MRI, finding that, in the high-risk volumes, the ADC was significantly

Table 1
Imaging modalities in cervical cancer and implications for brachytherapy planning

	Standard Modalities			Metabolic and Functional Modalities (Experimental)		
	Plain Films (2D)	CT (3D)	T2 MRI (3D)	FDG-PET	DCE-MRI	DW-MRI
Basis for target delineation	Landmarks based on the applicator	3D x-ray attenuation	3D fluid density	Glucose metabolism	Tumor perfusion (low/heterogeneous = worse outcome)	Cellular density via diffusion restriction
Ability to delineate the primary	Poor	Moderate (overestimates)	Superior	Superior	Uncertain (may identify high-risk volumes)	Uncertain (may identify high-risk volumes)
Ability to delineate normal tissue	Poor	Superior	Superior	Poor	Poor	Poor
Availability	All centers	Most centers	Few centers	Few centers	Few centers	Few centers

Abbreviations: 2D, two-dimensional; 3D, three-dimensional; DCE-MRI, dynamic contrast-enhanced MRI; DW-MRI, diffusion–weighted MRI; FDG-PET, fluorodeoxyglucose positron emission tomography.

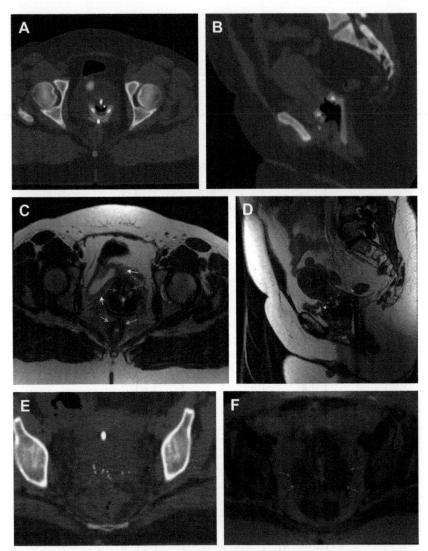

Fig. 3. Two cases studies of CT appearance of disease versus MRI appearance. (*A* and *B*) Axial and sagittal CT reconstructions of a tandem and ring placement for a woman with minimal residual disease at time of brachytherapy. (*C* and *D*) Merged MRI images obtained at the same levels, revealing a small amount of residual hyperintensity in the midcervix (*red arrows*), as well as better delineation of the rectal interface (*green arrows*) and bladder (*yellow arrows*). (*E* and *F*) An axial CT and MRI image obtain at the same level in a patient with residual extensive parametrial involvement at time of brachytherapy apparent on MRI as gray zones (*arrows*). Note the interstitial catheters placed for treatment (bright on CT, dark on MRI) along with the central tandem (more anterior in the fundus).

lower, suggesting that these volumes represent areas at high risk for residual tumor.[22] However, it remains to be seen whether use of DW-MRI in planning can improve outcomes.

One common limitation of these emerging modalities is the lack of normal tissue resolution. Therefore, although these new modalities may aid in the delineation of high-risk areas, either CT or T2-weighted MRI is required for proper avoidance of critical normal tissues.

DEFINING T2-WEIGHTED MRI TARGETS

The Groupe Européen de Curiethérapie and the European Society for Therapeutic Radiology and Oncology (GEC-ESTRO) was charged with determining a consensus method of target delineation on T2-weighted MRI in 2000, and the resulting Gynecologic Working Group published their recommendations in 2005,[23,24] defining the following volumes (**Fig. 4**):

- The gross tumor volume (GTV): this includes all disease visible (high signal intensity on T2 or fast spin echo MRI sequences) at time of brachytherapy.
- The high-risk clinical target volume (HRCTV): this volume includes the GTV, the cervix, and any regions of intermediate signal intensity (so-called gray zones). This volume should receive a dose expected to eliminate macroscopic disease (>75–85 Gy).

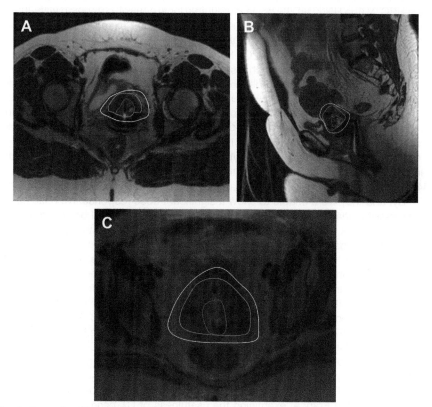

Fig. 4. Example of T2-weighted MRI volume definition using the Groupe Européen de Curiethérapie and the European Society for Therapeutic Radiology and Oncology consensus recommendations in 2 different women (same cases as **Fig. 3**). The gross tumor volume is contoured in red, the high-risk clinical target volume in orange, and the intermediate-risk clinical target volume in yellow. (A and B) Axial and sagittal T2-weighted MR-based contours on a woman with minimal residual disease. (C) Axial T2-weighted MR-based contours in a woman with residual, bilateral parametrial extension.

- The intermediate-risk clinical target volume (IRCTV): this volume includes the HRCTV with a 10-mm margin, restricted in the anterior and posterior direction to 5 mm, along with the original extent of disease before the start of any therapy. This volume should receive a dose expected to eliminate significant microscopic disease (>60–65 Gy).

These volume definitions have since been broadly accepted as the standard in the international community, and serve as a common language moving forward.

CLINICAL RESULTS FOR IMAGE-GUIDED BRACHYTHERAPY

The most mature data for MRI-guided brachytherapy come from investigators in Vienna.[25,26] In their pioneering series, 141 women with International Federation of Gynecology and Obstetrics (FIGO) stage IB to IVA cervical cancer were treated with 45 to 50.4 Gy, and most received concurrent weekly cisplatin (40 mg/m^2). For the first 3 years of the series, although the HRCTV was contoured prospectively, women were treated with point A style 2D plans, whereas, in the last 3 years, plans were optimized to cover the HRCTV. Ninety-six percent of women who received a least 87 Gy to 90% of the HRCTV (the HRCTV D90) achieved durable local control, compared with 80% in those not reaching this dose. There was also a significant association between the minimum dose to 100% of the HRCTV (the HRCTV D100) and local control rates. Those achieving a minimum of 66 Gy had a 93% local control rate compared with 83% local control rate in those with less coverage. The association was maintained even after correcting for larger and more advanced tumors that can lead to compromised dose coverage.

The same group was also able to establish a dose relationship with late toxicity and the dose received from brachytherapy.[27] For the rectum, higher minimum dose to the closest 2 cm^3 (D2cc) was associated with a higher rate of grade 2 to 4 toxicity (5% at 67 Gy, 10% at 78 Gy, and 20% at 90 Gy). There was a similar relationship between the bladder D2cc and late grade 2 to 4 cystitis (5% at 70 Gy, 10% at 101 Gy, and 20% at 134 Gy). In this series, only 3 patients had sigmoid toxicity (with a mean sigmoid D2cc of 77 Gy) and they were unable to show a significant dose response. No relationship was seen with small bowel toxicity. Likely both sigmoid and small bowel are mobile enough that these metrics do not accurately represent the maximum dose to small portions of the organs.

Because of the success of these investigators, a prospective registry trial, the European Study on MRI-guided Brachytherapy in Locally Advanced Cervical Cancer (EMBRACE), was initiated. There are currently 22 institutions participating, including centers in the United States, Asia, and the United Kingdom as well as mainland Europe. This protocol recommends an HRCTV D90 dose of 75 to 96 Gy, and an IRCTV D90 dose of 60 to 75 Gy, as well as limiting the rectal D2cc to less than 70 to 75 Gy, sigmoid D2cc to less than 75 Gy, and bladder D2cc to less than 90 Gy (**Table 2**). The accrual goal is to follow more than 600 patients for 3 years, and they are highly likely to achieve this shortly, perhaps by the time of this publication.

In parallel, the STIC (Soutien aux Techniques Innovantes et Coûteuses) trial was being conducted in France, examining the usefulness of CT-based planning.[28] This prospective but nonrandomized trial accrued 801 women (705 evaluable) treated with either CT-based planning (3D) or film-based plans (2D). The choice depended on the practice of each enrolling center, but the arms were well balanced nonetheless (336 treated 2D, 369 treated 3D). In the group treated with radiation and concurrent chemotherapy, followed by brachytherapy, the local control at 2 years was 73.9% with 2D and 78.5% with 3D (P = .003). In addition, grade 3 to 4 toxicity was

Table 2
Image-guided contours and recommended goals/limits for intracavitary brachytherapy for cervical cancer

Volume	2D Point Analog	3D Dosimetric Measures	Dosimetric Goal/Limit	End Point	Level of Evidence for Goal/Limit
HRCTV (tumor + cervix + parametrial extent at time of implant)	Point A (2 cm superior to ovoids, 2 cm lateral to tandem)	D90 D100	D90>75–85 Gy D100>65 Gy	Pelvic control >90%	Strong
IRCTV (HRCTV + margin + initial extent of disease)	Closest analog is point B (3 cm lateral to point A) for IIB disease	D90	D90>60–75 Gy	Pelvic control (no firm data)	Weak
Bladder	Bladder point (most dependent point of Foley balloon)	D2cc	D2cc<90 Gy	G2–G4 late toxicity <5%–10%	Strong
Rectum	Rectal point (5 mm posterior to vaginal packing)	D2cc	D2cc<75 Gy	G2–G4 late toxicity <5%–10%	Strong
Sigmoid	None	D2cc	D2cc<75 Gy	No firm data	Weak
Small bowel	None	D2cc	D2cc<65 Gy	No firm data	Weak

D## refers to the minimum dose to ##% of the volume (eg, D90 is the minimum dose to 90% of the volume).

D#cc refers to the minimum dose to the #cm² (cc) of volume receiving the highest dose (eg, the D2cc of the bladder refers to the minimum dose to the 2 cm² of bladder receiving the highest dose, or the closest 2 cm² of bladder is receiving at least this dose).

Evidence is strong if it is observed in prospective single-arm studies. Evidence is weak if based on expert opinion.

significantly less in the 3D arm at 2.6% compared with 22.7% in the 2D arm ($P = .002$). Although there are significant caveats with any nonrandomized trial, these are convincing data that CT-based 3D planning can maintain or improve local control while reducing toxicity.

HIGH-DOSE-RATE BRACHYTHERAPY APPLICATIONS

High-dose-rate (HDR) treatment has been available for decades, but it is only recently that applicators compatible with CT and MRI have become commonly available, making possible the previously referenced work. Because of several advantages, HDR has become the most common method of brachytherapy treatment within the United States and internationally (**Table 3**).[29,30] The high specific activity of iridium allows channels of much smaller diameter than was possible with cesium or radium, in turn allowing innovative applicator design. Pulsed dose rate (PDR) is used more frequently in Europe, and is a method of treatment in which HDR applicators are used to deliver hourly pulsed doses to patients admitted to the hospital to mimic the radiobiology of an LDR implant, while retaining some of the advantages of HDR.

The most common variant of these is the tandem and ring applicator, which replaces the lateral ovoids with a single ring channel that, when loaded in its lateral aspects, results in a dose distribution similar to a narrow tandem and ovoid insertion (**Fig. 5**). Perhaps more novel is the introduction of interstitial channels in addition to the ring configuration. This so-called Vienna applicator allows superior coverage of the paracervical and parametrial tissue, of particular importance for those with IIB disease with an incomplete response to initial chemotherapy and radiation.

Table 3
Comparing LDR, HDR, and pulsed-dose-rate (PDR) brachytherapy in cervical cancer

	LDR	HDR	PDR
Sources used	Cesium 137	Iridium 192	Iridium 192
Common treatment schedules	1–2 treatments of 48–72 h (inpatient)	4–6 treatments (may be outpatient)	1–2 treatments of 48–72 h (inpatient, with hourly pulses mimicking LDR schedule)
Imaging compatibility	Film, CT	Film, CT, MRI	Film, CT, MRI
Radiobiology	Preferentially spares normal tissue	No radiobiological advantage	Preferentially spares normal tissue
Planning	Limited by size of source (~1.5 cm) and inventory of treating institution	Single source is stepped through applicator in 5-mm increments. Varying the dwell time allows more flexibility in planning	Single source is stepped through applicator in 5-mm increments. Varying the dwell time allows more flexibility in planning
Radiation safety risk	Exposure to caregivers during inpatient stay. Possible loss of sources	No exposure to caregivers. Source stays in department	No exposure to caregivers (care given between pulses). Source in shielded afterloader near/inside patient room
Availability in the United States	Common	Common	Rare (more common in Europe)

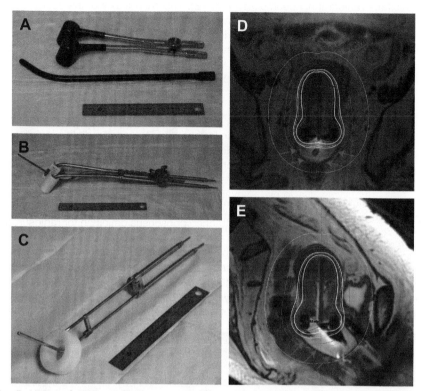

Fig. 5. LDR and HDR applicators compatible with MRI and CT. (*A*) CT-compatible LDR Fletcher Suit Delclos tandem and ovoid set (MRI incompatible). (*B*) HDR tandem and ovoid set compatible with MRI and CT (note the small-diameter tubing). (*C*) HDR tandem and ring set compatible with MRI and CT. (*D* and *E*) A narrow pear-shaped isodose distribution obtained by a tandem and ring in a patient with an excellent response (yellow isodose line is 5.5 Gy). Note the posterior vaginal packing balloon (*red arrows*) moving the rectum out of the high-dose region on the axial view.

Another unique applicator that has recently become available is a multicatheter vaginal balloon (**Fig. 6**). This applicator consists of a vaginal balloon within which 13 catheters are imbedded to allow asymmetric dose distribution within the vagina. Clinical applications include women with thin (<5 mm thick) vaginal lesions, such as recurrent endometrial or primary vaginal cancers.

IMAGE-GUIDED INTERSTITIAL BRACHYTHERAPY

CT and MR guidance have also aided in the planning and delivery of interstitial radiotherapy, either as a primary modality for women with locally advanced cancers with spread beyond what could be covered with an intracavitary implant, or for treatment of recurrent lesions. The use of CT or MRI during planning allows careful contouring of targets and normal tissues, whereas the use of the HDR technique allows a more customized dose distribution given the ability to customize the dwell times every 5 mm in each catheter, rather than being limited to uniform activity in several iridium 192 strands (**Fig. 7**).

Kannan and colleagues[31] from Pittsburgh reported a series of 47 women with cervical cancer treated with CT-based interstitial plans, treating twice a day for

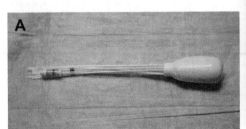

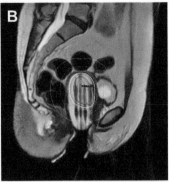

Fig. 6. (*A*) A multicatheter vaginal balloon for HDR treatment of vaginal lesions. (*B*) The applicator in place and an isodose distribution to the anterior vagina in a woman with an isolated local recurrence of endometrial cancer (yellow line = 5 Gy). Note sparing of posterior structures.

5 fractions as inpatients. They were able to achieve reasonable coverage of the HRCTV with a median HRCTV D90 of 76 Gy, while keeping the bladder, rectal, and sigmoid D2cc within tolerance. Their 2-year local control of 61% is reasonable given that these were locally advanced patients, ineligible for standard tandem and ovoid

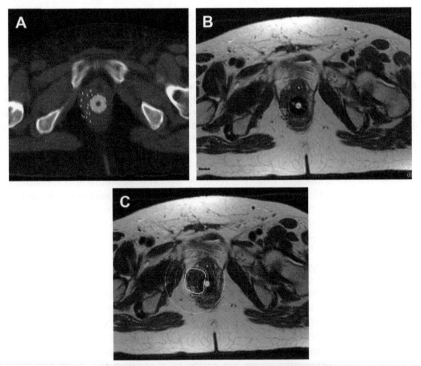

Fig. 7. Image-guided interstitial brachytherapy. (*A*) The CT placement of interstitial catheters for an isolated right vaginal recurrence of endometrial cancer. CT shows poor differentiation between the lesion and normal tissue. (*B*) The same level with a fused MRI obtained during the implantation showing definition of a clear nodule (*arrows*). (*C*) A conformal isodose distribution achievable with HDR (yellow line = 5 Gy).

treatment, and their grade 3 toxicities were 10%. Lee and Viswanathan[32] also explored predictors of toxicity using imaged-guided interstitial treatment (mostly CT-based) in 51 women, finding a slightly lower tolerance to the rectum than is expected from intracavitary treatment, with a 10% risk of grade 2 to 4 toxicity occurring near 62 Gy.

CAUTIONS AND CAVEATS

Although these advances bring significant potential for improving the risk/benefit ratio of brachytherapy, care should be taken in the adoption of these techniques. The increase in complexity and time required cannot be underestimated. A dedicated physics and dosimetry team is required to avoid miscommunication. There is the possibility of new toxicities as treatment plans look less and less like the standard 2D dose clouds. There is also the possibility of worse control in women in whom the dose is significantly lowered because of an excellent MRI response, if microscopic residual disease is not adequately treated.

To help control for these potential issues, it is our practice to start all treatment plans with a dose distribution based on the standard 2D era, and then modify this to match the individual anatomy and disease extent. This treatment is then only be a stepwise variation from previous experience, and is primarily done in response to images in which the normal tissue is clearly moving into the high-dose region, or when obvious disease is not being covered adequately. It is also critical that the treating radiation oncologist thoroughly reviews the applicator reconstruction on the treatment planning system, because a small error in this step of planning can result in large deviations from the intended plan.

In addition, there is an issue of access. Many women diagnosed with this disease have limited access to health care resources. Few radiation oncology departments have dedicated MRI for planning purposes, and transporting a patient to a separate radiology department with an implant in place is a major task. According to a survey from the American Brachytherapy Society in 2007, 55% of respondents were using CT for treatment planning, and only 2% were using MRI in any capacity for planning.[33]

SUMMARY

Despite these caveats, modern imaging and compatible applicators not only allow for the superior visualization of targets but also provide the ability to customize treatment beyond what was possible in the film-based era. This capacity has resulted in unprecedented control of the dose delivered, both in optimizing the coverage of areas of disease and in the avoidance of critical structures. Data are emerging showing significant clinical gain from this dosimetric optimization, and hopes are high that the EMBRACE study will confirm these measures in the wider setting.

REFERENCES

1. Cleaves M. Radium: with a preliminary note on radium rays in the treatment of cancer. Med Rec 1903;601–6.
2. Fletcher GH, Shalek RJ, Wall JA, et al. A physical approach to the design of applicators in radium therapy of cancer of the cervix uteri. Am J Roentgenol Radium Ther Nucl Med 1952;68:935–49.
3. Heyman J. The so-called Stockholm method and results of treatment of uterine cancer at the Radiumhemmet. Acta Radiol 1935;129–47.

4. Lenz M. Radiotherapy of cancer of the cervix at Radium Institute, Paris, France. Am J Roentgenol Radium Ther Nucl Med 1927;335–42.
5. Tod M, Meredith W. A dosage system for use in the treatment of cancer of the uterine cervix. Br J Radiol 1938;809–24.
6. Montana GS, Martz KL, Hanks GE. Patterns and sites of failure in cervix cancer treated in the U.S.A. in 1978. Int J Radiat Oncol Biol Phys 1991;20:87–93.
7. Perez CA, Grigsby PW, Lockett MA, et al. Radiation therapy morbidity in carcinoma of the uterine cervix: dosimetric and clinical correlation. Int J Radiat Oncol Biol Phys 1999;44:855–66.
8. Weeks KJ, Montana GS. Three-dimensional applicator system for carcinoma of the uterine cervix. Int J Radiat Oncol Biol Phys 1997;37:455–63.
9. Adamson J, Newton J, Yang Y, et al. Commissioning a CT-compatible LDR tandem and ovoid applicator using Monte Carlo calculation and 3D dosimetry. Med Phys 2012;39:4515–23.
10. Gebara WJ, Weeks KJ, Hahn CA, et al. Computed axial tomography tandem and ovoids (CATTO) dosimetry: three-dimensional assessment of bladder and rectal doses. Radiat Oncol Investig 1998;6:268–75.
11. Pelloski CE, Palmer M, Chronowski GM, et al. Comparison between CT-based volumetric calculations and ICRU reference-point estimates of radiation doses delivered to bladder and rectum during intracavitary radiotherapy for cervical cancer. In J Radiot Oncol Biol Phys 2005;62:131–7.
12. Gao M, Albuquerque K, Chi A, et al. 3D CT-based volumetric dose assessment of 2D plans using GEC-ESTRO guidelines for cervical cancer brachytherapy. Brachytherapy 2010;9:55–60.
13. Schoeppel SL, LaVigne ML, Martel MK, et al. Three-dimensional treatment planning of intracavitary gynecologic implants: analysis of ten cases and implications for dose specification. Int J Radiat Oncol Biol Phys 1994;28:277–83.
14. Kim SH, Choi BI, Han JK, et al. Preoperative staging of uterine cervical carcinoma: comparison of CT and MRI in 99 patients. J Comput Assist Tomogr 1993;17:633–40.
15. Subak LL, Hricak H, Powell CB, et al. Cervical carcinoma: computed tomography and magnetic resonance imaging for preoperative staging. Obstet Gynecol 1995;86:43–50.
16. Viswanathan AN, Dimopoulos J, Kirisits C, et al. Computed tomography versus magnetic resonance imaging-based contouring in cervical cancer brachytherapy: results of a prospective trial and preliminary guidelines for standardized contours. Int J Radiat Oncol Biol Phys 2007;68:491–8.
17. Eskander RN, Scanderbeg D, Saenz CC, et al. Comparison of computed tomography and magnetic resonance imaging in cervical cancer brachytherapy target and normal tissue contouring. Int J Gynecol Cancer 2010;20:47–53.
18. Schwarz JK, Siegel BA, Dehdashti F, et al. Association of posttherapy positron emission tomography with tumor response and survival in cervical carcinoma. JAMA 2007;298:2289–95.
19. Lin LL, Mutic S, Low DA, et al. Adaptive brachytherapy treatment planning for cervical cancer using FDG-PET. Int J Radiat Oncol Biol Phys 2007;67:91–6.
20. Hockel M, Vorndran B, Schlenger K, et al. Tumor oxygenation: a new predictive parameter in locally advanced cancer of the uterine cervix. Gynecol Oncol 1993;51:141–9.
21. Mayr NA, Huang Z, Wang JZ, et al. Characterizing tumor heterogeneity with functional imaging and quantifying high-risk tumor volume for early prediction of

treatment outcome: cervical cancer as a model. Int J Radiat Oncol Biol Phys 2012;83:972–9.

22. Haack S, Pedersen EM, Jespersen SN, et al. Apparent diffusion coefficients in GEC ESTRO target volumes for image guided adaptive brachytherapy of locally advanced cervical cancer. Acta Oncol 2010;49:978–83.

23. Haie-Meder C, Potter R, Van Limbergen E, et al. Recommendations from Gynaecological (GYN) GEC-ESTRO Working Group (I): concepts and terms in 3D image based 3D treatment planning in cervix cancer brachytherapy with emphasis on MRI assessment of GTV and CTV. Radiother Oncol 2005;74:235–45.

24. Potter R, Haie-Meder C, Van Limbergen E, et al. Recommendations from gynaecological (GYN) GEC ESTRO working group (II): concepts and terms in 3D image-based treatment planning in cervix cancer brachytherapy-3D dose volume parameters and aspects of 3D image-based anatomy, radiation physics, radiobiology. Radiother Oncol 2006;78:67–77.

25. Dimopoulos JC, Potter R, Lang S, et al. Dose-effect relationship for local control of cervical cancer by magnetic resonance image-guided brachytherapy. Radiother Oncol 2009;93:311–5.

26. Dimopoulos JC, Lang S, Kirisits C, et al. Dose-volume histogram parameters and local tumor control in magnetic resonance image-guided cervical cancer brachytherapy. Int J Radiat Oncol Biol Phys 2009;75:56–63.

27. Georg P, Potter R, Georg D, et al. Dose effect relationship for late side effects of the rectum and urinary bladder in magnetic resonance image-guided adaptive cervix cancer brachytherapy. Int J Radiat Oncol Biol Phys 2012;82:653–7.

28. Charra-Brunaud C, Harter V, Delannes M, et al. Impact of 3D image-based PDR brachytherapy on outcome of patients treated for cervix carcinoma in France: results of the French STIC prospective study. Radiother Oncol 2012;103:305–13.

29. Erickson BA, Ho A, Rownd J, et al. Patterns of brachytherapy practice with carcinoma of the cervix (2005–2007): a QRRO study. Int J Radiat Oncol Biol Phys 2011;81:S46–7.

30. Viswanathan AN, Creutzberg CL, Craighead P, et al. International brachytherapy practice patterns: a survey of the Gynecologic Cancer Intergroup (GCIG). Int J Radiat Oncol Biol Phys 2012;82:250–5.

31. Kannan N, Beriwal S, Kim H, et al. High-dose-rate interstitial computed tomography-based brachytherapy for the treatment of cervical cancer: early results. Brachytherapy 2012;11:408–12.

32. Lee LJ, Viswanathan AN. Predictors of toxicity after image-guided high-dose-rate interstitial brachytherapy for gynecologic cancer. Int J Radiat Biol Phys 2012;84:1192–7.

33. Viswanathan AN, Erickson BA. Three-dimensional imaging in gynecologic brachytherapy: a survey of the American Brachytherapy Society. Int J Radiat Oncol Biol Phys 2010;76:104–9.

Chemoradiation Therapy
Localized Esophageal, Gastric, and Pancreatic Cancer

Jennifer L. Pretz, MD[a], Jennifer Y. Wo, MD[b],
Harvey J. Mamon, MD, PhD[c], Lisa A. Kachnic, MD[d],
Theodore S. Hong, MD[b,*]

KEYWORDS

- Gastrointestinal • Cancer • Chemoradiation • Surgery • Targeted therapy

KEY POINTS

- The management of localized gastrointestinal (GI) cancers with definitive intent typically includes multimodality therapy with some combination of surgery, chemotherapy, and radiation.
- In esophageal and gastroesophageal junction (GEJ) cancers, concurrent chemoradiation should be used both in the preoperative setting and the definitive setting.
- Surgery is the mainstay of treatment of gastric cancer, and adjuvant therapy with chemotherapy alone and with chemoradiation are both acceptable standards.
- The role of radiation in pancreatic cancer is controversial, and there are mixed data regarding the role of chemoradiation in both resectable and locally advanced cases.
- Patients with a newly diagnosed GI cancer should be evaluated by a multidisciplinary team to optimize treatment plan and outcomes.

INTRODUCTION

Chemoradiation plays an important role in the management of many localized GI tumors. In most situations, chemoradiation therapy (CRT) is administered adjuvantly to improve local control and, in some situations, to improve overall survival. In anal cancer, CRT alone is often curative. This review presents the current role of CRT in the multidisciplinary management of localized esophageal, gastric, and pancreatic

[a] Harvard Radiation Oncology Program, Harvard Medical School, Boston, MA, USA;
[b] Department of Radiation Oncology, Massachusetts General Hospital, Harvard Medical School, Boston, MA, USA; [c] Department of Radiation Oncology, Brigham and Women's Hospital, Dana Farber Cancer Institute, Harvard Medical School, Boston, MA, USA; [d] Department of Radiation Oncology, Boston Medical Center, Boston University School of Medicine, Boston, MA, USA
* Corresponding author. Massachusetts General Hospital, 100 Blossom Street, Cox 3, Boston, MA 02114.
E-mail address: tshong1@partners.org

Surg Oncol Clin N Am 22 (2013) 511–524
http://dx.doi.org/10.1016/j.soc.2013.02.005
1055-3207/13/$ – see front matter © 2013 Elsevier Inc. All rights reserved.

cancers and discusses future directions for the adjuvant treatment of these selected GI malignancies.

ESOPHAGEAL AND GASTROESOPHAGEAL CANCERS

CRT for esophageal and GEJ cancers is currently used preoperatively for the surgically resectable population as well as definitively in inoperable patients.

Current State: Locally Advanced, Resectable Cancer

The rationale for preoperative therapy in locally advanced, resectable esophageal cancers, American Joint Committee on Cancer 2010 stages IB–III, stems from a high margin positivity rate in the range of 40% to 50%, which subsequently contributes to poor survival.[1] Until recently, however, the data have been mixed regarding the efficacy of this preoperative approach.

Neoadjuvant Chemoradiation

Many studies have evaluated the role of preoperative CRT, referred to as the trimodality approach, versus surgery alone for esophageal and GEJ cancers. Walsh and colleagues[2] originally reported a survival advantage to preoperative CRT compared with surgery alone. The study has been criticized, however, for unexpectedly poor outcomes in the surgery-alone arm (3-year overall survival rate of 6%), possibly due to lack of uniform staging with CT among all patients. Furthermore, subsequent studies failed to consistently confirm a statistically significant benefit to preoperative CRT as opposed to surgery alone (**Table 1**).

The Cancer and Leukemia Group B (CALGB) also attempted to answer the question of whether or not preoperative CRT improved outcomes and reported an improvement in 5-year overall survival rates with the use of CRT from 16% to 39% ($P = .002$).[6] This study was small, however, and closed early due to poor accrual, at only 56 patients. The interpretation of the available data on preoperative therapy in esophageal cancer thus was still considered controversial.

The recently published Chemoradiotherapy for Esophageal Cancer Followed by Surgery Study (CROSS) has provided more convincing data suggesting a benefit to preoperative therapy for locally advanced esophageal and GEJ cancers. This study, the largest randomized controlled trial in esophageal cancer to date, randomized 366 patients to CRT followed by surgery versus surgery alone.[7] This study used weekly carboplatin and paclitaxel as the concurrent preoperative chemotherapy, as opposed

Table 1					
Randomized trials of chemoradiation plus surgery versus surgery alone for esophageal cancer					
Study	N	Randomization	Pathologic CR	3-Y Survival	P Value
Walsh et al,[2] 1996	113	S	25%	6%	$P = .01$
		CRT → S		32%	
Bosset et al,[3] 1997	282	S	26%	37%[a]	$P = .78$
		CRT → S		39%[a]	
Urba et al,[4] 2001	100	S	28%	16%	$P = .15$
		CRT → S		30%	
Burmeister et al,[5] 2005	256	S	16%	36%[a]	$P = .57$
		CRT → S		38%[a]	

Abbreviations: CR, complete response; N, number of patients; S, surgery.
[a] Estimated from survival curve.

to cisplatin-based and 5-fluorouracil (5-FU)–based regimens that were administered in investigations mentioned above. Radiation was prescribed at 41.4 Gy in 23 daily fractions. Of the 366 patients, the majority of patients had adenocarcinoma (266 patients, 75%), with most tumors located in the distal esophagus (58%) or at the GEJ (24%). A pathologic complete response was achieved in 29% of patients who underwent resection after CRT; however, pathologic complete response was more likely to be seen among patients with squamous cell carcinoma than adenocarcinoma (49% vs 23%, P = .008). Treatment with preoperative CRT yielded a significantly higher rate of R0 resection (92% vs 69%, P<.001) and a lower rate of nodal positivity (31% vs 75%, P<.001) compared with the surgery-alone group. With a median follow-up of 45.4 months, preoperative CRT more than doubled the median survival rate compared with surgery alone, at 49 months versus 24 months (P = .003), and the 5-year overall survival rate also significantly improved, at 47% versus 34%. There were no differences in postoperative complications between the 2 arms.

Chemotherapy or Chemoradiation?

Study groups have also looked at the use of preoperative chemotherapy followed by surgery versus surgery alone. In a study by the Radiation Therapy Oncology Group (RTOG) and Intergroup (INT), the RTOG 8911/INT 133 trial, 467 patients with resectable disease were randomized to surgery alone versus preoperative chemotherapy with 3 cycles of cisplatin/5-FU.[1,8] The pathologic complete response rate was disappointing, at 2.5%, and ultimately there was no difference in survival between the 2 groups. The Medical Research Council Esophageal Cancer Working Group also published a study looking at preoperative chemotherapy, randomizing patients to 2 cycles of cisplatin/5-FU before surgery versus surgery alone.[9] Although preoperative chemotherapy in this trial improved the 5-year overall survival rate from 17% to 23%, 9% of patients in both arms also received preoperative radiation, thus making the results difficult to interpret.

Stahl and colleagues[10] looked specifically at the delivery of preoperative chemotherapy versus preoperative CRT in patients with GEJ tumors. In this study, 126 patients were randomized to receive either preoperative chemotherapy with induction cisplatin/5-FU/leucovorin for 3 cycles versus the same induction chemotherapy regimen for 2 cycles followed by preoperative CRT (30 Gy in 15 fractions administered with concurrent cisplatin and etoposide). Treatment with preoperative CRT had a significantly higher probability of pathologic complete response (15.6% vs 2.0%, P = .03) and node negativity (64% vs 38%, P = .01) at the time of resection. The rate of patients without local tumor progression was also better with CRT (76.5% vs 59% at 3 years, P = .06). Although this study closed early due to poor accrual, there was a trend toward a better survival rate with CRT (47% vs 28% at 3 years, P = .07), suggesting the benefit of preoperative CRT.

With the CROSS data now available, the standard of care in patients with locally advanced esophageal or GEJ cancer who are considered surgical candidates has been established as preoperative CRT with carboplatin and paclitaxel followed by surgery. Although the CROSS delivered 41.1 Gy of radiation, in the United States 50.4 Gy has been adopted as standard preoperative dose, per the trial design of CALGB 9781. The most appropriate preoperative radiation dose for resectable disease has yet to be clearly defined.

Current State: Inoperable Cancer

In esophageal or GEJ cancer, patients may be deemed inoperable due to either unfavorable anatomy/local extent of the tumor or medical comorbidities. The RTOG 85-01 study demonstrated that treatment with CRT was superior to radiation alone for this population, with a 5-year overall survival rate of 27% versus 0%.[11–13] Once definitive CRT was established as superior, RTOG 94-05/INT 0123 examined radiation dose escalation in this setting, comparing the conventional 50.4-Gy CRT with CRT at a higher dose of 64.8 Gy.[14] For the 218 eligible patients, there was no significant difference in median survival (13.0 vs 18.1 months), 2-year survival rate (31% vs 40%), or locoregional control (56% vs 52%) between the high-dose and standard-dose arms. This trial was closed early to accrual after interim analysis, due to unexpectedly higher mortality seen in the higher-dose treatment arm (10% in the higher-dose arm vs 2% in the standard arm). The majority of the treatment-related deaths in the higher-dose arm occurred, however, before reaching the standard dose of 50.4 Gy, calling into question whether the treatment-related toxicity was due to the higher treatment dose. Because of these results, 50.4 Gy has been adopted as the standard radiation CRT dose for medically inoperable esophageal or GEJ cancer.

When definitive CRT is delivered in the initially unresectable setting, there may be situations where this treatment converts the disease to resectable status. More recent studies, mostly restricted to squamous cell carcinoma, have shown an equivalence of CRT to CRT followed by surgery in terms of overall survival.[15,16] Surgery seems to offer a local control benefit, however, albeit with a higher treatment-related death rate.

Although it is currently accepted that with inoperable esophageal or GEJ cancer definitive CRT is the treatment of choice, ongoing trials are assessing the optimal chemotherapy regimen for CRT. A recent study of CRT with leucovorin/5-FU/oxaliplatin (FOLFOX) versus CRT with cisplatin/5-FU in the inoperable population showed no difference in survival but had lower treatment-related death rates with FOLFOX.[17] Ultimately, in light of the disappointing outcomes with CRT as definitive therapy, both the optimal chemotherapy type and radiation dose remain unanswered questions.

Future Directions

Although cure rates for esophageal and GEJ cancers have improved over the years, success rates are still modest and further improvements are warranted. As such, the role of targeted agents is under active investigation.

HER2 is a member of the HER receptor family and a transmembrane glycoprotein. It has long been established in breast cancer that, although HER2 overexpression confers a worse prognosis,[18] treatment with trastuzumab (a humanized monoclonal antibody against HER2) yields improved survival.[19–21] It has been recently shown that HER2 is also overexpressed in 20% of GEJ and gastric cancers.[22] Based on encouraging evidence that trastuzumab improves outcomes in GEJ cancers,[23,24] the RTOG has recently initiated a randomized trial, RTOG 10-10, to examine the utility of trastuzumab with CRT in patients with resectable, locally advanced, HER2-positive adenocarcinoma of the esophagus and GEJ.

Epidermal growth factor receptor (EGFR) is, like HER2, a transmembrane protein that when overexpressed portends a poor prognosis. Activation of the EGFR extracellular domain by ligand binding relays growth and division signals to the cell. Cetuximab is a monoclonal antibody directed against EGFR, blocking its signaling. There have been reports of overexpression of EGFR in 30% to 90% of esophageal and gastric cancers[25,26] and several phase II studies have assessed the role of cetuximab with CRT for esophageal cancers.[27–29] Although these trials have shown encouraging pathologic complete response rates of approximately 30%, there have been conflicting data on safety. The Eastern Cooperative Oncology Group (ECOG) 2205 study, which evaluated neoadjuvant CRT with cetuximab and 5-FU/oxaliplatin, closed early after an excessive number of early treatment-related deaths: 4 of 18 patients died postoperatively of acute respiratory distress syndrome.[29] The RTOG also initiated a randomized phase III trial, RTOG 04-36, assessing the potential benefit of adding cetuximab to cisplatin/paclitaxel and 50.4 Gy of radiation in inoperable esophageal cancer. After a planned interim analysis in the spring of 2012, however, the study failed to show superiority in survival with cetuximab and was closed to further enrollment.

The role of targeted therapies with CRT for esophageal cancer continues to evolve. Although HER2 may prove an effective target for esophageal and GEJ cancers, it is overexpressed in only a minority of patients. The disappointing early data with anti-EGFR therapy makes it unlikely that this strategy will be further developed in the setting of esophageal or GEJ cancer. Alternative biologic pathways, such as HGF/MET, Hsp90, and Hedgehog, may represent promising new targets to further explore.

In addition to targeted therapy, the United States is investigating the utility of positron emission tomography scans to assess response and direct adjuvant therapy in patients with esophageal cancer and with GEJ cancer who are receiving CRT. This interest is based on data from Germany that demonstrate the usefulness of early metabolic response evaluation.[30] The CALGB 80803 phase II trial assessing pathologic complete response rate in positron emission tomography scan nonresponders after induction CRT is currently open to accrual.

GASTRIC CANCER

Surgery has been, and continues to be, a critical component in the treatment of locally advanced American Joint Committee on Cancer 2010 stages IB–III gastric cancer. Historically, however, despite aggressive surgery, gastric cancer is associated with high locoregional and distant metastatic failure rates.[31] How and when to use chemotherapy or CRT remain topics of controversy for the adjuvant management of gastric cancer.

Current State

Surgery is the cornerstone of treatment of nonmetastatic gastric cancer. The extent of surgical resection for gastric cancers depends on the location of the primary tumor. In addition to removal of the primary disease, the associated lymph node dissection can range in extensiveness. The D1 dissection involves complete removal of the perigastric lymph nodes, whereas D2 dissection also removes of the nodes around the branches of the celiac trunk. Despite meticulous surgical technique and investigation into the safest and most effective type of lymph node dissection, in Western series, the overall survival rates with surgery alone are still poor, ranging from approximately 20% to 40%.[32–36] These unsatisfactory outcomes have prompted studies evaluating adjuvant therapy in the management of patients with locally advanced gastric cancer.

To date, research groups have examined both adjuvant chemotherapy and adjuvant CRT. In the United States, adjuvant therapy has been informed by the INT-0116 trial.[37] In this study, 556 patients were randomized after surgery to adjuvant chemotherapy and CRT versus observation. The adjuvant arm administered 5-FU for 1 cycle, followed by CRT to 45 Gy with concurrent 5-FU, which was followed by 2 additional cycles of 5-FU. The 3-year overall survival rate was significantly improved with adjuvant CRT, at 50% versus 41% ($P = .005$). This study was criticized, however, because 54% of patients had a D0 lymph node dissection (meaning not all of the perigastric nodes were removed). This raises the question of whether the adjuvant therapy was only compensating for inadequate surgery. Also, the radiation field design was deemed inadequate and necessitated modification in more than half of the patients in the adjuvant arm, highlighting the need for high-quality radiation field design.

During the same period that the INT-0116 trial was accruing patients for adjuvant CRT, the Europeans were investigating the use of perioperative chemotherapy. The results of this were published in the medical research council adjuvant gastric infusional chemotherapy (MAGIC) trial.[38] Patients were treated either with perioperative chemotherapy using a multiagent chemotherapy regimen of epirubicin/cisplatin/5-FU (ECF) or with surgery alone. A 5-year survival benefit was achieved in the perioperative chemotherapy arm of 36% versus 23% ($P = .009$).

Until recently, there were no published randomized comparisons between postoperative CRT and perioperative chemotherapy, and both the INT-0116 and the MAGIC regimens have been considered acceptable standards. More recently, the adjuvant chemoradiation therapy in stomach cancer (ARTIST) trial was published,[39] which randomized D2-resected gastric cancers to adjuvant multiagent chemotherapy versus adjuvant chemotherapy plus CRT. The chemotherapy-alone arm consisted of capecitabine/cisplatin for 6 cycles. The CRT arm administered capecitabine/cisplatin for 2 cycles, followed by CRT with 45 Gy/capecitabine and 2 additional cycles of capecitabine/cisplatin. In this study, there was no significant difference in the disease-free survival rate at 3 years (74% with adjuvant chemotherapy vs 78% with adjuvant chemotherapy plus CRT, $P = .0862$). In a subgroup analysis of patients with positive lymph nodes (which included 85% and 88% of patients in each arm), however, the 3-year disease-free survival rate was improved with the addition of CRT (72% vs 78%, $P = .0365$). Although this result suggests that patients with more extensive locoregional disease at the time of surgery benefit from additional local therapy with radiation, locoregional recurrences were not statistically different between the 2 study arms (8% vs 5%, $P = .3533$). The investigators of this trial indicated they are planning a follow-up study to specifically explore the utility of CRT in node-positive gastric cancer patients.

For the postoperative adjuvant CRT approach, trials continue to examine the optimal chemotherapy regimen. Fuchs and colleagues,[40] in the randomized phase III CALGB 80101 trial, randomized patients with resected gastric or GEJ cancers to adjuvant therapy that either included chemotherapy with 5-FU/leucovorin or ECF, administered before and after CRT with 45 Gy/5-FU. They have, thus far, found no statistically significant differences between the chemotherapy regimens in terms of median or 3-year overall survival.

Ultimately, the optimal strategy for adjuvant therapy in resected locally advanced gastric cancer is under debate. The INT-0116 trial showed that single-agent chemotherapy with radiation was better than observation, and the MAGIC study proved that perioperative multiagent chemotherapy alone was better than observation. The most recent randomized study, the capecitabine and oxaliplatin adjuvant study in stomach Cancer (CLASSIC) trial,[41] evaluated adjuvant-only multiagent chemotherapy (with capecitabine/oxaliplatin) versus observation and also demonstrated a 3-year disease-free survival benefit to chemotherapy. The ARTIST study failed to definitely prove, however, that, in the setting of multiagent chemotherapy, adding radiation further improved outcomes. Given the ARTIST subgroup analysis that indicated radiation was beneficial in node-positive patients, the tendency, at least in the United States, is still to use both chemotherapy and radiation in the adjuvant setting.

Future Directions

Given the recent randomized controlled trials on adjuvant therapy, there remains uncertainty on the optimal adjuvant management for resected gastric cancer. Open questions include the optimal chemotherapy regimen and the role of radiation therapy in the setting of perioperative multiagent chemotherapy. The Dutch chemoradiotherapy after induction chemotherapy in cancer of the stomach (CRITICS) study is a randomized trial that is examining perioperative epirubicin/cisplatin/capecitabine (ECX) chemotherapy versus preoperative ECX and postoperative CRT.[42] Results of this trial may help answer some of these questions. Furthermore, given that large radiation fields are necessary in the postoperative setting, there is increasing interest in using radiation preoperatively.[43–45] Preoperative radiation may reduce the toxicity associated with CRT, be associated with improved compliance to the completion of therapy as prescribed, improve the complete resection rate, and, importantly, also allow for the further development of targeted therapies in gastric cancer.

PANCREATIC CANCER

The role of radiation in pancreatic cancer is highly controversial. Modern randomized controlled trials have suggested a mixed benefit to CRT in both resectable and locally advanced cases.

Current State: Resectable

The rationale for postoperative CRT has been driven by the high risk of locoregional failure, related to the high rates of close or positive margins.[46,47] This is largely due to the tight anatomic proximity of major vessels—the superior mesenteric artery, superior mesenteric vein, and inferior vena cava—which, if involved, lead to positive uncinate and/or retroperitoneal margins.

A seminal trial in the 1980s performed by the Gastrointestinal Tumor Study Group (GITSG) suggested a survival benefit of postoperative CRT compared with observation alone.[48] At 5 years, the overall survival rate was 15% versus 5%. Although this trial was small, at the time it established postoperative CRT as the standard of care. In contrast, a follow-up study performed by the European Organisation for Research and Treatment of Cancer failed to redemonstrate a significant survival benefit of postoperative CRT over observation alone,[49] although there was a trend toward improvement in median survival with CRT (17.1 months vs 12.6 months, $P = .099$). This trial, however, was criticized for including periampullary cancers and being statistically underpowered to address the primary endpoint.

In 2001, the European Study Group for Pancreatic Cancer reported, in a randomized trial, that 5 months of postoperative 5-FU chemotherapy alone improved overall survival, whereas postoperative CRT was associated with a survival detriment.[50] Although this study was criticized due to a lack of radiation and pathologic quality assurance, the postoperative regimen of choice in Europe for resected pancreatic cancer became chemotherapy alone.

More recently, a secondary analysis of RTOG 97-04, which compared adjuvant 5-FU and CRT versus adjuvant gemcitabine and CRT, demonstrated that appropriate radiation field design was associated with improved overall survival, highlighting that accurate radiation planning is critical to demonstrating an impact on outcomes.[51,52] These data are concordant with 2 large single-institution series from Johns Hopkins Hospital and Mayo Clinic, suggesting a survival benefit to high-quality postoperative CRT.[53,54] The role of adjuvant radiation for resected pancreatic adenocarcinoma remains controversial, however, and is currently under evaluation in RTOG 08-48 (discussed later).

Current State: Locally Advanced

As with resectable pancreatic cancer, the role of radiation in the management of locally advanced pancreatic cancer is controversial. Early randomized trials suggested mixed benefits with the use of CRT versus chemotherapy or radiation alone.

The trial that initially established CRT as a superior treatment was conducted by the GITSG.[55] This 3-armed trial randomized patients with locally advanced pancreatic cancer to CRT using 40 Gy and 5-FU, CRT using 60 Gy and 5-FU, or radiation alone to 60 Gy. The 2 CRT arms also received maintenance 5-FU. Both arms that delivered CRT were associated with statistically improved median survivals than when radiation alone was administered (42 and 40 weeks vs 23 weeks, respectively). Among those patients who received CRT, there was no survival difference between the 2 radiation doses.

This study was followed by a trial performed by ECOG, where patients with locally advanced pancreatic cancer were randomized between CRT using 40 Gy and 5-FU followed by maintenance 5-FU versus chemotherapy alone with 5-FU.[56] This study did not show any difference in terms of overall survival but was criticized because of unusually poor survivals in both groups (median survival 5.1 months for CRT vs 6.5 months for chemotherapy). In light of these results, the benefit of using radiation for locally advanced pancreatic cancer was brought into question.

With conflicting results from the original GITSG trial and the ECOG study, the GITSG initiated another investigation, randomizing patients into a multidrug chemotherapy regimen alone versus CRT followed by the same multidrug chemotherapy.[57] The multidrug chemotherapy used was streptozocin, mitomycin C, and 5-FU. The concurrent CRT was 54 Gy with 5-FU. The 1-year overall survival rate was significantly improved with the use of CRT (41% vs 19%, $P<.02$). Although this study was small, with only 43 patients enrolled, it suggested CRT was superior to chemotherapy alone in the treatment of locally advanced pancreatic cancer.

Because of the limitations of the aforementioned historical data, more recently, the Fédération Francophone de Cancérologie Digestive and the Société Française de Radiothérapie Oncologique also evaluated the role of CRT in locally advanced pancreatic cancer.[58] In this trial, patients were randomized to receive CRT with 60 Gy/cisplatin/5-FU followed by maintenance gemcitabine or gemcitabine alone. This study was stopped early when an interim analysis showed that the use of CRT was associated with worse outcomes: median survival was 9 months with CRT versus 13 months with gemcitabine alone ($P = .03$). Although this again brought into question the use of CRT for locally advanced disease, flaws with the design of this study make the results difficult to interpret. Both the radiation dose and the types of chemotherapy used were not standard. The 60 Gy of radiation used was higher than tested in most trials and may have contributed to the increased toxicity observed in the CRT arm.

During the same time that the Fédération Francophone de Cancérologie Digestive trial was taking place in Europe, a similar trial in the United States, ECOG 4201, randomized patients with locally advanced pancreatic cancer into gemcitabine alone versus gemcitabine-based CRT followed by gemcitabine.[59] This study closed early at 74 patients due to poor accrual. Despite greater toxicity in the CRT arm (41% and 9% of patients with grade 4 toxicity in the CRT and chemotherapy-alone arms, respectively), however, median survival was improved with CRT (11.1 months vs 9.2 months, $P = .017$). Although this was the first trial to demonstrate a survival benefit with CRT using concurrent gemcitabine, it had a small number of patients and did not demonstrate any difference between the arms in progression-free survival. In addition, because the radiation was used at the beginning of treatment, it failed to address radiation timing issues.

An accepted standard of care for locally advanced pancreatic cancer was not truly established until the Groupe Coopérateur Multidisciplinaire en Oncologie (GERCOR) published a retrospective review of patients prospectively treated in several phase II and III trials evaluating different chemotherapy regimens.[60] Acknowledging the controversial role of radiation therapy, these trials recommended CRT after 3 months of chemotherapy, only if there was no progression of disease during chemotherapy. This choice was at the discretion of physicians, however, and they could instead choose to continue chemotherapy alone instead. Radiation was delivered to 45 Gy with a boost to a total dose of 55 Gy with continuous infusion 5-FU. In a retrospective analysis of 167 patients in these prospective trials, 71% of locally advanced patients did not have progressive disease after 3 months of chemotherapy and remained eligible for CRT. Of the patients eligible for CRT, 56% received CRT and 44% continued chemotherapy. The median progression-free survivals for the CRT and chemotherapy groups were 10.8 months and 7.4 months, respectively ($P = .005$). The median overall survival was 15 months for the CRT group and 11.7 months for the chemotherapy group ($P = .0009$).

Due to the retrospective nature of this study, it was limited by potential patient selection bias. The 2 treatment groups, however, were well balanced for performance status, age, and chemotherapy response, indicating that there may be patients with locally advanced disease likely to benefit from CRT. These findings suggest that an effective strategy for locally advanced pancreatic cancer is to select those patients with aggressive systemic biology who would not benefit from up-front localized CRT. As such, the current practice in the United States is to start patients with systemic therapy and move to CRT only in those who do not progress after several months of chemotherapy.

Future Directions

For pancreatic cancer, there is ongoing investigation into the optimal systemic regimen and the utility of localized therapy with radiation.

For the past 2 decades, gemcitabine (which was used in the GERCOR study) and 5-FU have been the mainstays of systemic therapy. Recently, a combination chemotherapy regimen of leucovorin, 5-FU, irinotecan, and oxaliplatin (FOLFIRINOX) has shown promising results in the metastatic setting and has been increasingly used in locally advanced disease for patients with excellent performance status.[61] Because pancreatic cancer is a disease marked by early metastasis, more effective systemic therapy is needed.

As discussed previously, the use of radiation for both resected and locally advanced cancers remains controversial. As such, there are ongoing trials that hope to address this question. The RTOG 08-48 is a phase III trial evaluating both erlotinib and CRT as adjuvant treatment of patients with resected head of pancreas adenocarcinoma. In this study, patients who have completed surgical resection are first randomized into receiving chemotherapy with gemcitabine or chemotherapy with gemcitabine and erlotinib, each for a total of 5 cycles. If they remain free from progression, they are further randomized into 1 more cycle of chemotherapy or 1 more cycle of chemotherapy followed by CRT. From a radiation perspective, the primary endpoint is to determine whether the use of concurrent CRT, after gemcitabine-based chemotherapy, enhances survival. The LAP 07 trial, currently under way in Europe, is addressing a similar question in the locally advanced setting, comparing CRT after 4 cycles of chemotherapy (either with gemcitabine or gemcitabine/erlotinib) with 2 more cycles of chemotherapy alone.

Although pancreatic cancer is a disease marked by early metastasis, it may also be a locally invasive process. Understanding an individual's tumor biology at the time of diagnosis may help inform treatment decisions regarding systemic versus localized therapy. The deleted in pancreatic cancer locus 4 (DPC4) gene has been shown to correlate with tumor behavior; tumors with DPC4 loss have more widespread disease, and tumors with intact DPC4 have more locally destructive disease.[62] The use of DPC4 status may provide valuable biologic information at the time of diagnosis, when treatment decisions are made. The RTOG is currently in the process of validating the feasibility of a DPC4 assay on fine-needle aspiration samples.

There has been interest as well in the use of stereotactic body radiation therapy (SBRT), whereby higher radiation doses than can be achieved with standard fractionation can be delivered locally. Investigations to date have varied in SBRT timing and dose. A phase I study demonstrated the feasibility and safety of SBRT for locally advanced pancreatic cancer in patients with poor performance status, treating them with escalating doses of 15 Gy, 20 Gy, and 25 Gy in a single fraction.[63] A follow-up phase II study evaluated the role of SBRT to boost conventionally fractionated CRT.[64] Patients were treated with 45 Gy (in the traditional 25 fractions), followed by a single SBRT boost dose of 25 Gy. Of the 16 patients treated in this manner, 15 were free from local progression until death. In a retrospective review, Mahadevan and colleagues[65] reported on patients with locally advanced disease treated with SBRT to 24 Gy to 36 Gy in 3 fractions, after receiving 3 cycles of chemotherapy. Ultimately, 17% of patients developed metastatic disease during chemotherapy and did not receive SBRT. Of those who did, the local control rate was 85%, and late grade 3 toxicity (duodenal bleeding and obstruction) was observed in 9%. Although local control is believed excellent with SBRT, there is a need for strategies to reduce the potential associated duodenal toxicity.[66]

SUMMARY

The management of localized GI cancers is complex and requires integration of multiple specialties. Patients should be evaluated by a multidisciplinary team before surgery to coordinate care to achieve optimal outcomes. For many GI cancers, such as esophageal and GEJ, preoperative CRT is advocated, whereas for gastric cancer, both perioperative chemotherapy and postoperative CRT strategies are endorsed. The role of CRT for localized pancreatic cancer remains ill defined and hopefully will be answered by the ongoing randomized trials. For all localized GI cancers, future research will include optimizing systemic therapy (with radiation and adjuvantly) as well as integrating novel targeted strategies. The ultimate goal is to understand an individual's tumor biology so that the optimal adjuvant therapy can be tailored.

REFERENCES

1. Kelsen DP, Winter KA, Gunderson LL, et al. Long-term results of RTOG trial 8911 (USA Intergroup 113): a random assignment trial comparison of chemotherapy followed by surgery compared with surgery alone for esophageal cancer. J Clin Oncol 2007;25(24):3719–25.
2. Walsh TN, Noonan N, Hollywood D, et al. A comparison of multimodal therapy and surgery for esophageal adenocarcinoma. N Engl J Med 1996;335(7):462–7.
3. Bosset JF, Gignoux M, Triboulet JP, et al. Chemoradiotherapy followed by surgery compared with surgery alone in squamous cell cancer of the esophagus. N Engl J Med 1997;337(3):161–7.
4. Urba SG, Orringer MB, Turrisi A, et al. Randomized trial of preoperative chemoradiation versus surgery alone in patients with locoregional esophageal carcinoma. J Clin Oncol 2001;19(2):305–13.
5. Burmeister BH, Smithers BM, Gebski V, et al. Surgery alone versus chemoradiotherapy followed by surgery for resectable cancer of the oesophagus: a randomised controlled phase III trial. Lancet Oncol 2005;6(9):659–68.

6. Tepper J, Krasna MJ, Niedzwiecki D, et al. Phase III trial of trimodality therapy with cisplatin, fluorouracil, radiotherapy, and surgery compared with surgery alone for esophageal cancer: CALGB 9781. J Clin Oncol 2008; 26(7):1086–92.

7. Van Hagen P, Hulshof MC, van Lanschot JJ, et al. Preoperative chemoradiotherapy for esophageal or junctional cancer. N Engl J Med 2012;366(22):2074–84.

8. Kelsen DP, Ginsberg R, Pajak TF, et al. Chemotherapy followed by surgery compared with surgery alone for localized esophageal cancer. N Engl J Med 1998;339(27):1979–84.

9. Allum WH, Stenning SP, Bancewicz J, et al. Long-term result of a randomized trial of surgery with or without preoperative chemotherapy in esophageal cancer. J Clin Oncol 2009;27(30):5062–7.

10. Stahl M, Walz MK, Stuschke M, et al. Phase III comparison of preoperative chemotherapy compared with chemoradiothearpy in patients with locally advanced adenocarcinoma of the esophagogastric junction. J Clin Oncol 2009; 27(6):851–6.

11. Herskovic A, Martz K, al-Sarraf M, et al. Combined chemotherapy and radiotherapy compared with radiotherapy alone in patients with cancer of the esophagus. N Engl J Med 1992;326(24):1593–8.

12. al-Sarraf M, Martz K, Herskovic A, et al. Progress report of combined chemoradiotherapy versus radiotherapy alone in patients with esophageal cancer: an intergroup study. J Clin Oncol 1997;15(1):277–84.

13. Cooper JS, Guo MD, Herskovic A, et al. Chemoradiotherapy of locally advanced esophageal cancer: long-term follow-up of a prospective randomized trial (RTOG 85-01). Radiation Therapy Oncology Group. JAMA 1999;281(17):1623–7.

14. Minsky BD, Pajak TF, Ginsberg RJ, et al. INT 0123 (Radiation Therapy Oncology Group 94-05) phase III trial of combined-modality therapy for esophageal cancer: high-dose versus standard-dose radiation therapy. J Clin Oncol 2002;20(5): 1167–74.

15. Stahl M, Stuschke M, Lehmann N, et al. Chemoradiation with and without surgery in patients with locally advanced squamous cell carcinoma of the esophagus. J Clin Oncol 2005;23(10):2310–7.

16. Bedenne L, Michel P, Bouche O, et al. Chemoradiation followed by surgery compared with chemoradiation alone in squamous cancer of the esophagus: FFCD 9102. J Clin Oncol 2007;25(10):1160–8.

17. Conroy T, Galais MP, Raoul JL, et al. Phase III randomized trial of definitive chemoradiotherapy (CRT) with FOLFOX or cisplatin and fluorouracil in esophageal cancer (EC): final results of the PRODIGE 5/ACCORD 17 trial [abstract LBA4003]. J Clin Oncol 2012;30.

18. Slamon DJ, Clark GM, Wong SG, et al. Human breast cancer: correlation of relapse and survival with amplification of the HER-2/neu oncogene. Science 1987;235(4785):177–82.

19. Slamon DJ, Leyland-Jones B, Shak S, et al. Use of chemotherapy plus a monoclonal antibody against HER2 for metastatic breast cancer that overexpresses HER2. N Engl J Med 2001;344(11):783–92.

20. Romond EH, Perez EA, Bryant J, et al. Trastuzumab plus adjuvant chemotherapy for operable HER2-positive breast cancer. N Engl J Med 2005; 353(16):1673–84.

21. Piccart-Gebhart MJ, Procter M, Leyland-Jones B, et al. Trastuzumab after adjuvant chemotherapy in HER2-positive breast cancer. N Engl J Med 2005; 353(16):1659–72.

22. Janjigian YY, Werner D, Pauligk C, et al. Prognosis of metastatic gastric and gastroesophageal junction cancer by HER2 status: a European and USA International collaborative analysis. Ann Oncol 2012;23(10):2656–62.

23. Bang YJ, Van Cutsem E, Feyereislova A, et al. Trastuzumab in combination with chemotherapy versus chemotherapy alone for treatment of HER2-positive advanced gastric or gastro-oesophageal junction cancer (ToGA): a phase 3, open-label, randomised controlled trial. Lancet 2010;376(9742):687–97.

24. Safran H, Dipetrillo T, Akerman P, et al. Phase I/II study of trastuzumab, paclitaxel, cisplatin and radiation for locally advanced, HER2 overexpressing, esophageal adenocarcinoma. Int J Radiat Oncol Biol Phys 2007;67(2):405–9.

25. Yonemura Y, Sugiyama K, Fujumura T, et al. Epidermal growth factor receptor status and S-phase fractions in gastric carcinoma. Oncology 1989;46(3): 158–61.

26. Kim JS, Kim MA, Kim TM, et al. Biomarker analysis in stage III-IV (M0) gastric cancer patients who received curative surgery followed by adjuvant 5-fluorouracil and cisplatin chemotherapy: epidermal growth factor receptor (EGFR) associated with favourable survival. Br J Cancer 2009;100(5):732–8.

27. Safran H, Suntharalingam M, Dipretillo T, et al. Cetuximab with concurrent chemoradiation for esophagogastric cancer: assessment of toxicity. Int J Radiat Oncol Biol Phys 2008;70(2):391–5.

28. Ruhstaller T, Pless M, Dietrich D, et al. Cetuximab in combination with chemoradiotherapy before surgery in patients with resectable, locally advanced esophageal carcinoma: a prospective, multicenter phase IB/II trial (SAKK75/06). J Clin Oncol 2011;29(6):626–31.

29. Kleinberg LR, Catalano PJ, Gibson MK, et al. ECOG 2205: a phase II study to measure response rate and toxicity of neo-adjuvant chemoradiotherapy (CRT) (IMRT permitted) with oxaliplatin and infusional 5-fluorouracil plus cetuximab in patients with operable adenocarcinoma of the esophagus: high risk of post-op adult respiratory distress syndrome. Int J Radiat Oncol Biol Phys 2010;78(3):S72.

30. Lordick F, Ott K, Krause BJ, et al. PET to assess early metabolic response and to guide treatment of adenocarcinoma of the oesophagogastric junction: the MUNICON phase II trial. Lancet Oncol 2007;8(9):797–805.

31. Gunderson LL, Sosin H. Adenocarcinoma of the stomach: areas of failure in a re-operation series (second or symptomatic look) clinicopathologic correlation and implications for adjuvant therapy. Int J Radiat Oncol Biol Phys 1982;8(1):1–11.

32. Meyers WC, Damiano RJ Jr, Rotolo FS, et al. Adenocarcinoma of the stomach: changing patterns over the last 4 decades. Ann Surg 1987;205(1):1–8.

33. Cady B, Rossi RL, Silverman ML, et al. Gastric adenocarcinoma: a disease in transition. Arch Surg 1989;124(3):303–8.

34. Noguchi Y, Imada T, Matsumoto A, et al. Radical surgery for gastric cancer: a review of the Japanese experience. Cancer 1989;64(10):2053–62.

35. Songun I, Putter H, Kranenbarg EM, et al. Surgical treatment of gastric cancer: 15-year follow-up results of the randomised nationwide Dutch D1D2 trial. Lancet Oncol 2010;11(5):439–49.

36. Cuschieri A, Weeden S, Fielding J, et al. Patient survival after D1 and D2 resections for gastric cancer: long-term results of the MRC randomized surgical trial. Surgical Co-operative Group. Br J Cancer 1999;79(9–10):1522–30.

37. Macdonald JS, Smalley SR, Benedetti J, et al. Chemoradiotherapy after surgery compared with surgery alone for adenocarcinoma of the stomach or gastro-esophageal junction. N Engl J Med 2001;345(10):725–30.

38. Cunningham D, Allum WH, Stenning SP, et al. Perioperative chemotherapy versus surgery alone for resectable gastroesophageal cancer. N Engl J Med 2006; 355(1):11–20.
39. Lee J, Lim do H, Kim S, et al. Phase III trial comparing capecitabine plus cisplatin versus capecitabine radiotherapy in completely resected gastric cancer with D2 lymph node dissection: the ARTIST trial. J Clin Oncol 2011;30(3):268–73.
40. Fuchs CS, Tepper JE, Niedzwiecki D, et al. Postoperative adjuvant chemoradiation for gastric or gastroesophageal junction (GEJ) adenocarcinoma using epirubicin, cisplatin, and infusional (CI) 5-FU (ECF) before and after CI 5-FU and radiotherapy (CRT) compared with bolus 5-FU/LV before and after CRT: Intergroup trial CALBG 80101 [abstract 4003]. J Clin Oncol 2011;29(Suppl 15).
41. Bang YJ, Kim YW, Yang HK, et al. Adjuvant capecitabine and oxaliplatin for gastric cancer after D2 gastrectomy (CLASSIC): a phase 3 open-label, randomised controlled trial. Lancet 2012;379(9813):315–21.
42. Dikken JL, van Sandick JW, Maurits Swellengrebel HA, et al. Neo-adjuvant chemotherapy followed by surgery and chemotherapy or by surgery and chemoradiotherapy for patients with resectable gastric cancer (CRITICS) [abstract]. BMC Cancer 2011;11:329.
43. Ajani JA, Mansfield PR, Janjan N, et al. Multi-institutional trial of preoperative chemoradiotherapy in patients with potentially resectable gastric carcinoma. J Clin Oncol 2004;22(14):2274–80.
44. Ajani JA, Winter K, Okawara GS, et al. Phase II trial of preoperative chemoradiation in patients with localized gastric adenocarcinoma (RTOG 9904): quality of combined modality therapy and pathologic response. J Clin Oncol 2006; 24(24):3953–8.
45. Ajani JA, Winter K, Komaki R, et al. Phase II randomized trial of two nonoperative regimens of induction chemotherapy followed by chemoradiation in patients with localized carcinoma of the esophagus: RTOG 0113. J Clin Oncol 2008;26(28): 4551–6.
46. Willett CG, Lewandrowski K, Warshaw AL, et al. Resection margins in carcinoma of the head of the pancreas. Implications for radiation therapy. Ann Surg 1993; 217(2):144–8.
47. Yeo CJ, Cameron JL, Lillemoe KD, et al. Pancreaticoduodenectomy for cancer of the head of the pancreas. 201 patients. Ann Surg 1995;221(6):731–3.
48. Kalser MH, Ellenberg SS. Pancreatic Cancer. Adjuvant combined radiation and chemotherapy following curative resection. Arch Surg 1985;120(8):899–903.
49. Klinkenbijl JH, Jeekel J, Sahmoud T, et al. Ajuvant radiotherapy and 5-flurorouracil after curative resection of cancer of the pancreas and periampullary region: phase III trial of the EORTC gastrointestinal tract cancer cooperative group. Ann Surg 1999;230(6):776–82.
50. Neoptolemos JP, Dunn JA, Stocken DD, et al. Adjuvant chemoradiotherapy and chemotherapy in resectable pancreatic cancer: a randomised controlled trial. Lancet 2001;358(9293):1576–85.
51. Regine WF, Winter KA, Abrams RA. Fluorouracil vs gemcitabine chemotherapy before and after fluorouracil-based chemoradiation following resection of pancreatic adenocarcinoma: a randomized controlled trial. JAMA 2008;299(9):1019–26.
52. Abrams RA, Winter KA, Regine WF, et al. Failure to adhere to protocol specified radiation therapy guidelines was associated with decreased survival in RTOG 9704—a phase III trial of adjuvant chemotherapy and chemoradiotherapy for patients with resected adenocarcinoma of the pancreas. Int J Radiat Oncol Biol Phys 2012;82(2):809–16.

53. Herman JM, Swartz MJ, Hsu CC, et al. Analysis of fluorouracil-based adjuvant chemotherapy and radiation after pancreaticoduodenectomy for ductal adenocarcinoma of the pancreas: results of a large, prospectively collected database at the Johns Hopkins Hospital. J Clin Oncol 2008;26(21):3503–10.

54. Corsini MM, Miller RC, Haddock MG, et al. Adjuvant radiotherapy and chemotherapy for pancreatic carcinoma: the Mayo Clinic experience (1975-2005). J Clin Oncol 2008;26(21):3511–6.

55. Moertel CG, Frytak S, Hahn RG, et al. Therapy of locally unresectable pancreatic carcinoma: a randomized comparison of high dose (6000 rads) radiation alone, moderate dose radiation (4000 rads + 5-fluorouracil), and high dose radiation + 5-fluorouracil: the Gastrointestinal Tumor Study Group. Cancer 1981;48(8): 1705–10.

56. Klaassen DJ, MacIntyre JM, Catton GE, et al. Treatment of locally unresectable cancer of the stomach and pancreas: a randomized comparison of 5-fluorouracil alone with radiation plus concurrent and maintenance 5-fluorouracil—an Eastern Cooperative Oncology Group study. J Clin Oncol 1985;3(3):373–8.

57. [No authors listed] Gastrointestinal Tumor Study Group. Treatment of locally unresectable carcinoma of the pancreas: comparison of combined-modality therapy (chemotherapy plus radiotherapy) to chemotherapy alone. Gastrointestinal Tumor Study Group. J Natl Cancer Inst 1988;80(10):751–5.

58. Chauffert B, Mornex F, Bonnetain F, et al. Phase III trial comparing intensive induction chemoradiotherapy (60 Gy, infusional 5-FU and intermittent cisplatin) followed by maintenance gemcitabine with gemcitabine alone for locally advanced unresectable pancreatic cancer. Definitive results of the 2000-01 FFCD/SFRO study. Ann Oncol 2008;19(9):1592–9.

59. Loehrer PJ, Feng Y, Cardenes H, et al. Gemcitabine alone versus gemcitabine plus radiotherapy in patients with locally advanced pancreatic cancer: an Eastern Cooperative Group Oncology trial. J Clin Oncol 2011;26(31):4105–12.

60. Huguet F, Andre T, Hammel P, et al. Impact of chemoradiotherapy after disease control with chemotherapy in locally advanced pancreatic adenocarcinoma in GERCOR phase II and III studies. J Clin Oncol 2007;25(3):326–31.

61. Conroy T, Desseigne R, Ychou M, et al. FOLFIRINOX versus gemcitabine for metastatic pancreatic cancer. N Engl J Med 2011;364(19):1817–25.

62. Lacobuzio-Donahue CA, Fu B, Yachida S, et al. DPC4 gene status of the primary carcinoma correlates with patterns of failure in patients with pancreatic cancer. J Clin Oncol 2009;27:1806–13.

63. Koong AC, Le QT, Ho A, et al. Phase I study of stereotactic radiosurgery in patients with locally advanced pancreatic cancer. Int J Radiat Oncol Biol Phys 2004;58(4):1017–21.

64. Koong AC, Christorfferson E, Le QT, et al. Phase II study to assess the efficacy of conventionally fractionated radiotherapy followed by a stereotactic radiosurgery boost in patients with locally advanced pancreatic cancer. Int J Radiat Oncol Biol Phys 2005;63(2):320–3.

65. Mahadevan A, Miksad R, Goldstein M, et al. Induction gemcitabine and stereotactic body radiotherapy for locally advanced nonmetastatic pancreas cancer. Int J Radiat Oncol Biol Phys 2011;81(4):e615–22.

66. Schellenberg D, Kim J, Christman-Skieller C, et al. Single-fraction stereotactic body radiation therapy and sequential gemcitabine for the treatment of locally advanced pancreatic cancer. Int J Radiat Oncol Biol Phys 2011;81(1):181–8.

Radiation Therapy in Anal and Rectal Cancer

Brian G. Czito, MD[a],*, Jeffrey Meyer, MD[b]

KEYWORDS

- Rectal cancer • Anal cancer • Radiation • Chemotherapy • Targeted drug
- Rectal cancer surgery

KEY POINTS

- The standard therapy for squamous cell carcinoma of the anal canal consists of chemoradiotherapy using mitomycin and 5-fluorouracil. Recent advances consist of the integration of PET scanning into staging and treatment and the use of intensity-modulated radiation therapy. Study is ongoing on novel systemic agents with radiation therapy.
- Stage II and III rectal cancer is primarily approached using neoadjuvant radiation therapy. Radiation options include long-course chemoradiotherapy and short-course radiation therapy alone.
- The integration of novel systemic agents in conjunction with radiation therapy in the preoperative setting of rectal cancer remains a subject of investigation. To date, no agents beyond fluoropyrimidines have shown a definite advantage when combined with radiation therapy in rectal cancer patients.

HISTORICAL PERSPECTIVE OF ANAL CANAL SQUAMOUS CELL CARCINOMA THERAPY

Historically, the treatment of localized squamous cell carcinoma of the anal canal entailed abdominoperineal resection (APR) with resultant permanent colostomy and high rates of urinary and/or sexual dysfunction, wound morbidity, and perioperative mortality. Surgical studies using this approach have reported 5-year survival rates of 30% to 71% with local regional recurrence rates of 19% to 45%, with one large series from the Mayo Clinic reported local recurrence rates of approximately 30% following APR.[1]

In efforts to improve on these results, Norman Nigro (a surgeon from Wayne State University) and colleagues[2] treated three patients with low-dose preoperative radiation therapy (30 Gy) with concurrent infusional 5-fluorouracil (5-FU) and mitomycin

The authors have nothing to disclose.
[a] Department of Radiation Oncology, Duke University Medical Center, Box 3085, Durham, NC 27710, USA; [b] Department of Radiation Oncology, UT Southwestern Medical Center, 5801 Forest Park Road, Dallas, TX 75235, USA
* Corresponding author.
E-mail address: czito001@mc.duke.edu

followed by APR. The surgical specimens of two patients showed no residual disease, whereas the third patient refused surgery and remained disease-free. Further experience using this approach described similar high rates of clinical and pathologic response using preoperative chemoradiotherapy and surgery[3–7] leading to multiple phase II trials evaluating radiation therapy alone or combined chemoradiotherapy without surgery. These studies demonstrated that most subjects treated by these approaches were long-term disease-free survivors.

THE CONTEMPORARY BASIS OF ANAL CANAL SQUAMOUS CELL CARCINOMA THERAPY

The modern treatment of anal cancer is based on results of four randomized trials. During the initial investigations of radiation therapy alone it was appreciated that high rates of local control and disease-free survival could be achieved and the role of concurrent chemotherapy with radiation therapy uncertain. To clarify this, the United Kingdom Coordinating Committee on Cancer Research (UKCCCR) Anal Canal Trial Working Party performed the ACT I trial, randomizing 585 subjects with anal cancer to receive either 45 Gy of radiation therapy alone versus the same regimen with concurrent chemotherapy (continuous infusion 5-FU weeks 1 and 5, and mitomycin week 1). Subjects achieving a good clinical response received a boost dose of radiation therapy while poor responders underwent salvage surgery.[8] Local control was significantly enhanced in the combined modality therapy group (64% vs 41%, $P<.0001$) with a significant improvement in anal-cancer related mortality (28% vs 39%, $P = .02$), although 3-year overall survival did not differ between the arms (65% vs 58%, $P = .25$). The investigators concluded that patients with squamous cell carcinoma of the anal canal should be treated with radiation therapy, 5-FU, and mitomycin, with surgery reserved for salvage. Recently updated results of this trial, with a median follow-up of 13 years, confirmed a locoregional failure rate of 32% at 5 years with combined modality therapy versus 57% in subjects treated with radiation therapy alone.[9]

Similarly, a study by the European Organization for Research and Treatment of Cancer (EORTC) randomized 110 subjects to radiation therapy alone (45 Gy) followed by a boost radiation dose (dose depending on response) versus the same regimen concurrent with 5-FU weeks 1 and 5, and mitomycin week 1. As in the UKCCCR study, subjects undergoing combined modality therapy had a significant improvement in local control and colostomy-free and progression-free survival rates. No significant survival difference was seen between the groups (3-year survival 72% vs 65%, $P = .17$).[10]

Because mitomycin has significant toxicities, including thrombocytopenia, leucopenia, pulmonary toxicity, nephrotoxicity, and hemolytic-uremic syndrome, a third randomized trial from the United States conducted by the Radiation Therapy Oncology Group (RTOG) and Eastern Cooperative Oncology Group (ECOG) evaluated the role of mitomycin in this treatment regimen. Three hundred ten subjects were randomized to receive radiation therapy (45–54.4 Gy) with infusional 5-FU alone weeks 1 and 5 versus the same regimen with infusion of mitomycin weeks 1 and 5. Subjects with biopsy-proven residual disease were eligible to receive additional (salvage) pelvic radiation therapy (9 Gy) with 5-FU and cisplatin chemotherapy. Four-year colostomy-free and disease-free survival rates were significantly improved in subjects receiving mitomycin versus 5-FU alone, with no difference in overall survival observed. However, grade 4-5 toxicities (primarily related to neutropenia and sepsis) were significantly higher in subjects receiving mitomycin. Of subjects with a positive posttreatment biopsy, half were rendered disease-free by salvage chemoradiotherapy.[11]

However, the efficacy of salvage radiation therapy in this setting is unclear, given there are long tumoral regression periods in some patients following chemoradiotherapy (up to 1 year) as well as reports demonstrating many patients with biopsy-established disease in the months following combined modality therapy will experience long-term disease-free survival with no additional therapy. Therefore, it is the authors' general policy that, in the absence of overt disease progression, patients should not be biopsied for at least 3–6 months following treatment completion and/or there is continued disease regression.

In sum, all three randomized trials demonstrated that combined modality therapy with radiation therapy, 5-FU, and mitomycin results in long-term disease-free survival and sphincter preservation in most patients with anal cancer and superior outcomes relative to radiation therapy alone or radiation therapy combined with 5-FU only, albeit at the expense of higher treatment-related morbidity.

Because of the significant toxicities associated with mitomycin and the efficacy of cisplatin-based chemoradiotherapy in squamous cell carcinoma of other sites (head and neck, esophageal, and cervical cancers), there has been interest in substituting cisplatin for mitomycin in the combined modality treatment of anal cancer. Phase II trials from the United States and Europe using this strategy have demonstrated high rates of local control and disease-free survival, with acceptable toxicity rates, including using an approach of induction chemotherapy alone followed by combined chemoradiotherapy. Based on these data, the RTOG conducted a trial randomizing 682 subjects to receive radiation therapy with continuous infusion 5-FU and bolus mitomycin weeks 1 and 5 versus a regimen of continuous infusion 5-FU and bolus cisplatin alone for two cycles, with radiation (45–59 Gy) starting cycle 3 (ie, a neoadjuvant chemotherapy-alone approach). Not unexpectedly, the rate of significant hematologic toxicity was higher in subjects receiving mitomycin (61% vs 42%, $P<.001$). No significant difference was seen in 5-year disease-free survival rates (60% vs 54%, $P = .17$), overall survival rates (75% vs 70%, $P = .10$), or local-regional relapse rates (25% vs 33%, $P = .07$). However, the 5-year colostomy rate was 10% in subjects receiving mitomycin versus 19% in the cisplatin arm ($P = .02$).[12–14] A recent update of these trial results demonstrated a significant improvement in disease-free survival (67.7% vs 57.6%, $P = .005$), overall survival (78.2% vs 70.5%, $P = .02$), and colostomy-free survival (71.8% vs 64.9%, $P = .05$) in the mitomycin containing arm.[15] This study has been criticized for its design, specifically the use of induction chemotherapy, which prolongs the total treatment course and has the potential to limit the efficacy of subsequent RT as a result of tumor clonogen accelerated repopulation. Nonetheless, the results of these four published randomized trials show that the standard of care for anal cancer remains radiation therapy combined with 5-FU and mitomycin.

In a more direct comparison of the roles of cisplatin to mitomycin with radiation therapy, preliminary results of a phase III trial by the UKCCCR (ACT II) were reported in abstract form.[16] In this largest of anal cancer randomized studies, 950 subjects were randomized to the same radiotherapy regimen (50.4 Gy in 1.8 Gy fractions) with either concurrent 5-FU and cisplatin versus 5-FU and mitomycin, followed by a second randomization to receive two cycles of 5-FU or cisplatin or no further therapy following the completion of chemoradiation. With a median follow-up of 3 years, there were no differences in the rates of complete response, recurrence-free survival, overall survival, or colostomy requirements between any of the groups. Acute grade 3 to 4 hematologic toxicity rates were higher in subjects receiving mitomycin versus cisplatin (25% vs 13%). Although no statistical differences were reported in rates of in high-grade, acute nonhematologic toxicities between treatment arms (61% vs 65%), these figures remained high. A summary of randomized studies is presented in **Table 1**.

Table 1
Summary of conclusions from selected randomized trials in anal cancer

Trial (Reference)	Tested Therapies	Results
UKCCCR[8,9] EORTC[10]	1. RT vs 2. RT + 5-FU + MMC	Addition of chemotherapy to radiation therapy improves local disease control
RTOG-ECOG[11]	1. RT + 5-FU vs 2. RT + 5-FU + MMC	Although associated with more toxicity, addition of MMC improves DFS and CFS rates
RTOG 98-11[12–15]	1. Cisplatin/5-FU followed by RT + 5-FU + cisplatin vs 2. RT + 5-FU + MMC	Induction cisplatin–5-FU associated with lower OS, DFS and CFS rates
ACT II[16]	1. RT + 5-FU + MMC vs 2. RT + 5-FU + cisplatin Additional randomization to no further therapy or maintenance 5-FU and cisplatin	Equivalent regimens with respect to disease control; differing toxicities No benefit to maintenance chemotherapy
ACCORD 03[31]	1. 5-FU + cisplatin followed by RT + 5-FU + cisplatin vs 2. 5-FU + cisplatin followed by high-dose RT + 5-FU + cisplatin vs 3. Same as 1 but without induction therapy vs 4. Same as 2 but without induction therapy	Induction therapy and higher radiation dose do not improve disease-related outcomes
EORTC 22011-40014[29]	1. RT + MMC + 5-FU vs 2. RT + MCC + cisplatin	At early follow-up better response rates in the MMC-cisplatin–treated patients, albeit with lower compliance rates

Abbreviations: CFS, colostomy-free survival; DFS, disease-free survival; MMC, mitomycin-C; OS, overall survival; RT, radiation therapy.

ONGOING AREAS OF INVESTIGATION IN ANAL CANAL SQUAMOUS CELL CARCINOMA
Imaging

The introduction of positron emission tomography (PET) and combined PET-CT have improved the staging and treatment of patients with anal cancer. Recent studies have demonstrated that PET-detected nodal metastases occur in 17% to 24% of patients judged to have clinically uninvolved lymph nodes by CT.[17,18] In the absence of PET, these sites would usually receive subclinical doses of radiation therapy (as compared with higher doses used to treat gross disease), thus leading to underdosing and potentially predisposing patients to pelvic failure. To emphasize this point, in one series of subjects with anorectal cancer receiving chemoradiotherapy with PET-CT–based radiation planning, one fourth of subjects had PET-detected metastases resulting in a subsequent change in overall subject management, as well as altering the radiation oncologist's target volumes and radiation treatment plan in a similar percentage of subjects.[19] Similarly, a recent report from Hamburg evaluating pretherapy PET staging in subjects with anal cancer revealed that radiotherapy fields were changed in 23% of contrasted PET-CT subjects versus CT or PET scanning alone.[20] Another report from the Curie Hospital evaluating the role of PET-CT scan reported 36% of subjects had a change in stage as a result of contrast-enhanced PET-CT use compared with either study alone, suggesting a complimentary role of both imaging modalities.[21] Therefore, it is the authors' general practice to obtain contrast-enhanced PET-CT scans for patients with anal cancer during their initial staging evaluation.

In terms of assessing response to therapy, the same report from Curie Hospital evaluating pretherapy and posttherapy PET scan in subjects anal cancer showed that the sensitivity and specificity of PET in detecting persistent or recurrent disease was 93% and 81%, respectively, affecting the management in 20% of subjects.[21] Additional studies have also suggested that subjects achieving less than a complete metabolic response following combined modality therapy may experience significantly decreased disease-related outcomes.[22] The role of PET in this disease remains an active area of investigation.

Chemotherapy

As described previously, results of the RTOG 98-11 trial have not supported the use of induction chemotherapy in the treatment of this malignancy. In many cancers, the overall treatment course duration (including duration of radiation treatment) influences clinical outcomes. In anal cancer, a phase II dose-escalation trial by the RTOG mandating a 2 week treatment break showed inferior outcomes compared with historical controls. The investigators hypothesized that the mandated treatment break negated any benefits of dose escalation.[23] Similarly, other institutional experiences have reported that patients with prolonged treatment breaks or a protracted duration of therapy were more likely to suffer disease failure.[24] A recent analysis of two randomized RTOG trials showed a significant association between overall treatment duration and colostomy failure, local failure, regional failure, and time-to-failure rates. On multivariate analysis, a significant association with local failure and statistical trend toward an association with colostomy failure and overall treatment duration were seen. The investigators concluded that prolonged total treatment time seemed to have a detrimental effect on local failure and colostomy rate in subjects with anal cancer.[25] In this respect, the role of neoadjuvant chemotherapy preceding (and delaying) definitive radiation therapy remains uncertain at best. These inferior results with induction chemotherapy may be due to the development of tumor clonogen–accelerated repopulation, which occurs as treatments progress, and the role of neoadjuvant chemotherapy in upregulating pathways that confer radioresistance remains unknown.[26–28]

As opposed to the previously discussed RTOG and ACT II trials that evaluated cisplatin as a potential substitute for mitomycin, cisplatin has also been studied as an alternative to 5-FU, maintaining mitomycin in the treatment regimen. The EORTC recently terminated a randomized phase II-III trial (EORTC 22001/400014) comparing mitomycin plus weekly cisplatin given concurrently with radiation therapy versus mitomycin and continuous infusion 5-FU given concurrently with radiation therapy. The initial radiation course consisted of 36 Gy delivered for 4 weeks, followed by a 2 week break, followed by an additional 23.4 Gy given over 2.5 weeks, with concurrent chemotherapy delivered during both radiation sessions.[29] Preliminary phase II trial results reported increased high-grade hematologic toxicity rates in the mitomycin and cisplatin group, with subjects in this group less likely to complete all treatments. However, overall response rates (at 8 weeks following therapy completion) were higher in subjects treated with mitomycin and cisplatin. In an even more intensive chemotherapeutic regimen, a UKCCCR Act II pilot study suggested that the use of triple-drug combination of mitomycin, 5-FU and cisplatin was poorly tolerated and associated with significant morbidity, prohibiting this regimen to be taken into a subsequent randomized III trial.[30]

The French Federation Nationale des Centres de Lutte Contre le Cancer conducted the ACCORD 03 trial.[31] Subjects were randomized to one of four study arms. The first arm consisted of neoadjuvant 5-FU and cisplatin alone followed by combined therapy (radiation dose 45 Gy). Subjects then underwent a scheduled treatment break followed by an additional radiation to a dose of 15 Gy as a boost. The second arm was identical to the first but with a boost dose of 20 to 25 Gy. The third arm was identical the first arm but without a neoadjuvant chemotherapy component, and the fourth was identical to the second but, again, without a neoadjuvant chemotherapy component. This study showed that, at a median follow-up-of 50 months, there was no difference between the four arms in 5-year colostomy-free survival rates (ranging from 70%–82% across the four arms). Cause-specific and overall survival rates were also similar. These results again suggest that induction chemotherapy does not improve patient outcomes and question the role of radiation dose escalation in this disease (see **Table 1**).

Examining the role of agents beyond 5-FU, cisplatin, and mitomycin, a phase II trial from the United Kingdom evaluated the oral 5-FU prodrug capecitabine with mitomycin in 31 subjects with anal cancer. Eighteen subjects completed treatment as planned with low rates of high-grade diarrhea and neutropenia. At 1 month, 24 subjects achieved complete clinical response and, at a median follow up of 14 months, three local regional relapses occurred. The investigators concluded that capecitabine with mitomycin with radiation therapy is well tolerated in anal carcinoma patients and should be studied in future national phase III studies.[32] Investigators from MD Anderson Hospital conducted a phase II study of capecitabine and oxaliplatin combined with radiation therapy in subjects with stage II-III anal cancer. Capecitabine was delivered twice daily on weekdays and oxaliplatin was (initially) given weekly. When 5 out of 11 subjects developed high-grade diarrhea, the protocol was modified to eliminate chemotherapy during weeks 3 and 6. Radiation dose was prescribed based on T-stage of the tumor. For the nine subjects enrolled in the modified protocol, one developed grade 3 diarrhea. In a preliminary report, at a median follow-up of 19 months, there were no local recurrences and one subject experienced distant failure of disease.[33]

In terms of other ongoing studies, the AIDS Associated Malignancies Clinical Trials Consortium is conducting a phase II trial combining cisplatin, 5-FU, and the anti-epidermal growth factor receptor monoclonal antibody cetuximab with radiation therapy in HIV-positive subjects with anal cancer. Similarly, the ECOG is also conducting a phase II trial using a similar regimen in non-HIV subjects, while the Federation Nationale des Centers de Lutte Contre le Cancer in France is conducting a multi-institutional phase II study of radiochemotherapy (65 Gy, plus cisplatin plus 5-FU) combined with cetuximab in subjects with locally advanced anal cancer. Similarly, the Grupo Espanol Multidisciplinario del Cancer Digestivo in Spain is conducting a phase II trial to assess the efficacy and safety of chemoradiation with 5-FU, mitomycin, and the anti-epidermal growth factor receptor monoclonal antibody panitumumab. The results of these studies may help further refine the optimal chemotherapy regimen and sequencing in the treatment of this disease, particularly for more advanced lesions.

Radiation Therapy

Although chemotherapy enhances the acute toxicity of radiation therapy in anal cancer therapy, radiation therapy accounts for most acute and chronic therapy-related toxicities. Acute high-grade dermatologic, hematologic, genitourinary and gastrointestinal toxicity are commonly encountered during a course of chemoradio-therapy due to irradiation of a significant amount of perianal and genital skin, bone, pelvic bone marrow, bladder, and bowel. Severe acute toxicity often mandates treatment breaks, which may lead to a protracted treatment course (namely duration of radiation treatment), potentially compromising chemoradiotherapy antitumor efficacy.[23,24] Along these lines, in the previously discussed analysis of two randomized RTOG trials shorter, more intense radiation courses were associated with reduction in colostomy rates.[25]

The previously described randomized trials have primarily relied on two-dimensional (2D)–based radiation therapy planning in which known anatomic (bony) landmarks are used to guide field design using orthogonal x-ray images. Since the late 1980s, conformal (CT-guided or three-dimensional [3D]) radiotherapy-based treatments have been implemented in the clinic, allowing the radiation oncologist to identify normal, as well as target soft-tissue structures, on axial CT images, facilitating improved treatment accuracy and delivery. Both techniques, however, use uniform fields for radiation therapy delivery, inclusive of a significant amount of perianal and genital skin, pelvic bone or bone marrow, bladder, and bowel. Beginning in the late 1990s, intensity-modulated radiation therapy (IMRT) began to be implemented in the clinic. Similar to 3D conformal radiotherapy, IMRT also involves the 3D identification of normal pelvic organs, as well as target structures, including the primary disease and draining lymph nodes. However, in contrast to 3D based planning, where the physician designs treatment fields based on a beams-eye view of the target volumes and normal structures (ie, fields are designed as if one were inside the machine looking into the patient), IMRT-based planning entails setting strict radiation dose constraints to normal organs, prescription doses to varying target volumes, and the use of computer software inverse planning algorithms to design unconventional treatment fields that would not otherwise be possible with standard planning methods. Importantly, IMRT involves partitioning of a given radiation field into multiple smaller fields, which can occur in the form of dynamic IMRT (ie, collimating leaves or blocks move across an active radiation field using highly specific leaf sequences) or a step-and-shoot IMRT (ie, leaves sculpt the field shape while the beam is off). The result is that the intensity of the radiation beam for any one field varies, sometimes significantly. When these fields are summarized, however, the cumulative effect is a radiation dose distribution that closely conforms the prescription radiation dose around the target volumes while significantly reducing the dose to surrounding normal tissues as compared with conventional planning methods. **Fig. 1** shows an example of IMRT-based treatment in a case of anal cancer. The advantage of IMRT techniques is the potential reduction of acute and chronic radiation-related toxicities, which are often significant when using 2D and 3D approaches. Additionally, IMRT may permit safe radiation dose escalation in this disease given that several series have suggested that increasing radiation dose in the treatment of anal cancer may enhance local control and disease-free survival; however, as described previously, the role of radiation dose escalation remains a topic of study.

Recent clinical series of IMRT-based therapy of anal cancer have reported a significant reduction in acute treatment-related toxicity (primarily related to bowel and skin) and similar disease-related outcomes versus historical controls using 2D and 3D planning.[34,35] The RTOG recently completed a prospective phase II study (RTOG 0529) combining 5-FU, mitomycin, and IMRT-based radiotherapy. The primary goal of this study was determination of the feasibility of this approach in a cooperative group setting, as well as determination of treatment-related toxicity and preliminary disease-related outcomes in these subjects. In a preliminary report, subjects were analyzed,

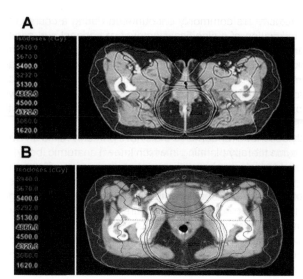

Fig. 1. (*A*) Axial CT view of a 49 year old woman with T2N0 anal canal squamous cell carcinoma treated using IMRT. The colored isodose lines represent varying doses of radiation therapy. Note the conformality of the isodose lines to the anal canal, perianal tissues, and inguinal regions and bending of isodose lines around nearby normal organs, including vulva. (*B*) A more superior axial slice, with sparing of the bladder anteriorly and femoral heads laterally.

comparing toxicity outcomes to subjects treated in RTOG 9811 (described previously) in which conventional radiation planning was used. Rates of greater than or equal to grade 3 dermatologic toxicity were superior in the IMRT study (23% vs 49%, *P*<.0001), as were rates of greater than or equal to grade 3 gastrointestinal toxicity (21% vs 36%, *P* = .0082).[36] This approach also yielded similar 2-year disease-related outcomes compared with RTOG 9811.[37]

One of the most challenging aspects of treating patients with IMRT is the accurate definition of target volumes. With IMRT, there are very precise and conformal high-dose regions enveloping the tumor with a steep dose gradient. If target or desired treatment volumes are not accurately defined, there is the real potential for underdosing of disease and resultant clinical failure.[38] Knowledge of patterns of failure and routes of spread are paramount. Along these lines, real-time quality assurance was performed in RTOG 0529, and a secondary endpoint was whether or not IMRT could be performed in a broader, multi-institutional setting. After the initial quality assurance was performed, contours needed to be modified in 81% of cases, thus illustrating the challenge of implementing this new and complex planning technique in a cooperative group setting and the importance of knowledge of target design using these advanced technologies.[36]

HISTORICAL PERSPECTIVE ON RECTAL ADENOCARCINOMA THERAPY

Surgical intervention remains the foundation of treatment of rectal cancer. Surgery has evolved gradually over the last 100 years, beginning with Miles' introduction of APR in the early twentieth century, followed by subsequent development of anterior resection, with later refinements to include total mesorectal excision (TME).[39,40] Before the era of TME, local-regional tumor failure rates following surgery alone for locally advanced rectal adenocarcinomas were high, occurring in at least 15% to 25% (and often higher) of subjects in many series of resected Dukes B and C (stage II and III) tumors, driving interest in adjuvant pelvic irradiation to reduce these recurrences and their attendant morbidity and mortality.[41,42]

Four randomized American trials conducted between the mid-1970s and the early 1990s evaluated the roles of postoperative chemotherapy and radiotherapy in improving disease outcomes in subjects with operable rectal adenocarcinoma.[42–45] General conclusions from these studies can be summarized as follows: adjuvant pelvic irradiation alone decreases local-regional relapse rates without significant impact on disease-free or overall survival results, whereas adjuvant 5-FU-based chemotherapy improves cause-specific and overall survival outcomes. In a trial conducted by the North Central Cancer Treatment Group (NCCTG), subjects with stage II or III rectal cancer were randomized to receive postoperative radiation alone versus postoperative radiation with concurrent 5-FU plus adjuvant 5-FU and semustine preceding and following chemoradiation.[45] Rates of local recurrence, distant metastasis, and cause-specific and overall survival were significantly improved in the combined-treatment group relative to the adjuvant radiation-alone group.

CONTEMPORARY RECTAL ADENOCARCINOMA RADIATION THERAPY: NEOADJUVANT SHORT-COURSE RADIATION THERAPY AND LONG-COURSE CHEMORADIOTHERAPY

There has been longstanding interest in preoperative, or neoadjuvant, irradiation for rectal tumors in lieu of postoperative irradiation. Several clinical trials conducted over the past 30 years have evaluated a wide variety of neoadjuvant radiation-alone treatment schedules (ie, without concurrent chemotherapy). Swedish investigators conducted a series of studies evaluating the role of short-course (five treatment fractions) radiation therapy, with early indications that this approach improved disease-related outcomes compared with surgery alone in subjects with stage I to III rectal tumors.[46] The Swedish Rectal Cancer Trial randomized over 1000 subjects to short-course neoadjuvant irradiation alone (5 Gy × 5 fractions for a total of 25 Gy) followed by surgery versus surgery alone.[47] Nine hundred eight of the subjects had margin-negative resections and no evidence of distant metastatic disease. Among this group, the 13-year actuarial survival rate was 38% in the radiation-treated subjects versus 30% in the nonirradiated group ($P = .008$). Survival was also improved in the complete cohort of subjects (31% vs 20%, $P = .009$). This improvement in survival seemed to be directly related to the reduction in local recurrence with the use of preoperative irradiation: 9% in the irradiated group versus 26% in surgery-alone subjects ($P<.001$), with no difference between the two groups with respect to rates of distant metastatic disease development.

As surgical techniques advanced, the importance of the circumferential resection margin in local tumor control became apparent through detailed histopathologic analysis of surgical specimens and sharp dissection of the enveloping perirectal fat (ie, mesorectum) emerged as the optimal surgical approach to rectal tumors.[40,48] Surgical series of TME showed significant reductions in local tumor failure relative to older series using conventional blunt dissection of the tissues surrounding the rectum.[41,49] As a result, it was logical to next consider the relevance of irradiation in the context of optimized surgery.

To evaluate this, Dutch investigators conducted a trial of 1861 subjects with stage I-III rectal cancer.[50] Randomization was to preoperative short-course irradiation (5 Gy × 5 fractions) followed by surgery versus surgery alone. TME was mandated for the resections and surgeons were trained in the technique with strict quality assurance monitoring. Results of this study were updated in 2011, demonstrating that subjects receiving preoperative radiation therapy had an improved local control by greater than 50% versus subjects undergoing TME only (10-year local recurrence 5% vs 11%, P<.0001) and a significant improvement in overall tumor recurrence rates (26% vs 32%, P<.05). For subjects with a negative circumferential resection margin, cancer-specific survival was higher in subjects receiving radiation therapy. On subgroup analysis, radiation therapy reduced local recurrence incidence in subjects with negative circumferential resection margins, positive lymph nodes, and in situations in which the tumor was located at greater than 5 cm from the anal verge. In a subgroup analysis of subjects with node-positive disease with uninvolved circumferential resection margins, preoperative radiotherapy improved 10 year survival (41% vs 51%, P = .02). In this trial, however, reduction in local failure did not translate into an overall survival advantage for the entire cohort as it had in the Swedish trial, notably given the low pelvic tumor failure rates following TME in the Dutch study.

In parallel with the use of short-course neoadjuvant radiation-alone regimens, there is also considerable interest in more protracted treatment courses, usually employing doses of 45 to 54 Gy delivered at 1.8 Gy per fraction for 5 to 5.5 weeks in conjunction with concurrently delivered radiosensitizing chemotherapy. 5-FU, the backbone agent of systemic treatment regimens for colon and rectal tumors, has also demonstrated supra-additive interactions when given concurrently with radiation.[51] The Federation Francophone de Cancerologie Digestive (FFCD) group conducted FFCD 9203, which randomized subjects with T3-4 rectal tumors to treatment with radiation alone (45 Gy in 1.8 Gy treatment fractions over 5 weeks) or radiation plus infusional 5-FU and leucovorin (delivered over 5 days during weeks 1 and 5).[52] Seven hundred thirty-three subjects were enrolled with the primary outcome of overall survival. Five-year survival was not significantly different between the two arms, although the rate of complete pathologic response (no residual viable tumor) was higher in the group receiving concurrent chemotherapy (11.4% vs 3.6%, P<.05). Additionally, the 5-year incidence of local tumor failure was lower in the chemoradiotherapy group (8.1% vs 16.5%, (P<.05).

The EORTC also assessed the value of combination chemotherapy and radiation therapy in a four-arm clinical trial (EORTC 22921).[53] TME was documented as the mode of surgery in less than 40% of trial subjects. Subjects with T3 or T4 rectal cancer were randomized to receive (1) radiation (45 Gy) followed by surgery, (2) radiation plus concurrent 5-FU and leucovorin followed by surgery, (3) radiation followed by surgery and postoperative 5-FU and leucovorin, or (4) radiation plus concurrent 5-FU and leucovorin followed by surgery followed by adjuvant 5-FU and leucovorin. One thousand eleven subjects were randomized. However, less than half of the subjects randomized to receive adjuvant chemotherapy received at or near full-intended dose intensity. There was no difference in overall survival between the subjects receiving preoperative radiation alone or chemoradiotherapy (P = .84), and no difference in those randomized to treatment with postoperative chemotherapy or no postoperative chemotherapy (P = .12). However, the 5-year incidence of local failure for the subject group receiving radiation only was 17.1%, whereas it ranged from 7.6% to 9.6% in the three chemotherapy-containing groups.

With both adjuvant and neoadjuvant chemoradiotherapy established as treatment options for patients with rectal adenocarcinoma, randomized clinical trials were conducted to determine the optimal sequencing approach.[54,55] Unlike other studies on this topic, the German CAO/ARO/AIO-94 trial met its accrual goals.[54] Patients were randomized to preoperative radiation (50.4 Gy at 1.8 Gy per fraction over 5.5 weeks) with concurrent 5-FU (delivered as a continuous infusion during weeks 1 and 5), followed by surgery, versus surgery followed by adjuvant radiation (55.8 Gy at 1.8 Gy per fraction) with concurrent infusional 5-FU. The incidence of acute high-grade toxicity was lower in the preoperative group compared with subjects in the postoperative group (27% vs 40%), and more subjects in the postoperative group did not receive the intended course of adjuvant therapy. Five-year overall survival was similar for the two groups (76% preoperative vs 74% postoperative group, $P = .80$) as was disease-free survival (approximately 65% both groups); however, the incidence of 5-year local failure was significantly lower in preoperative subjects at 6% versus 13%. The German trial firmly established neoadjuvant, as opposed to adjuvant, therapy as the standard of care for patients with stage II or III rectal cancer. More recently, another randomized clinical trial further bolstered support for the routine use of neoadjuvant treatment (in the form of short-course irradiation).[56] The MRC CR07/NCIC-CTG C016 trial randomized 1350 subjects with operable rectal adenocarcinoma to preoperative short-course pelvic radiation followed by surgery versus surgery followed by selective postoperative radiation (45 Gy in 25 fractions), concurrent with 5-FU, for subjects with positive radial margins. The actuarial 3-year local failure rates were 4.4% in the preoperative group versus 10.6% in the selective postoperative group. Similarly, a recent report of the American NSABP R-03 study comparing preoperative versus postoperative chemoradiotherapy also demonstrated a significant improvement in disease-free survival (5-year 64.7% vs 53.4%, $P = .011$) and trend toward improved overall survival (5-year overall survival 74.5% vs 65.6%, $P = .065$).[55] These findings have confirmed a new standard of care in the United States and parts of Europe in the treatment of rectal cancer. Results of selected contemporary randomized trials in rectal cancer are shown in **Table 2**.

Table 2
Summary of conclusions from selected randomized neoadjuvant therapy trials in rectal cancer

Trial (Reference)	Tested Therapies	Results
Swedish Trial[47]	1. Short-course RT → surgery vs 2. Surgery	Preoperative radiation improved local control and OS
Dutch Trial[50]	1. Short-course RT → surgery (TME) vs 2. Surgery (TME)	Preoperative radiation improves local control even when optimized surgery is used
MRC Trial[56]	1. Short-course RT → surgery vs 2. Surgery → selective RT + CT	Preoperative radiation improved local control and disease-free survival
German Trial[54]	1. RT + CT → Surgery vs 2. Surgery → RT +CT	Neoadjuvant sequencing better tolerated and yields improved local control
FFCD[52]	1. RT → Surgery vs 2. RT + CT → Surgery	Concurrent chemoradiotherapy improves tumor response and local control relative to radiation alone
EORTC[53]	1. RT → Surgery vs 2. RT + CT → Surgery vs 3. RT → Surgery → CT vs 4. RT + CT → Surgery → CT	Incorporation of chemotherapy with radiation improves tumor response and local control compared with radiation and surgery alone

Abbreviations: CT, chemotherapy; OS, overall survival; RT, radiation therapy.

Although there is a biologic rationale for the possible superiority of preoperative radiation relative to postsurgery treatment, (eg, improved tumor oxygenation or vascular supply in the preoperative setting), it seems that the practical issue of patient tolerability of treatment and thus the ability to receive the full intended course of treatment (superior in the preoperative setting) is an important factor.

One final important area of controversy is the comparison of short-course, neoadjuvant irradiation without chemotherapy (used in many European centers) with long-course, 5-FU–sensitized, neoadjuvant radiation regimens. It is difficult to compare the biologic effectiveness of a short course of 25 Gy in 5 fractions without chemotherapy to 45 to 54 Gy in 25 to 30 fractions with concurrent chemotherapy. There is uncertainty in the fractionation sensitivity of rectal adenocarcinoma as well as the tumor repopulation rate.[57] Bujko and colleagues[58] conducted a randomized trial of 312 subjects with T3 or T4 rectal cancer treated with neoadjuvant radiation alone (25 Gy in 5 fractions) versus chemoradiation (50.4 Gy in 28 fractions with concurrent 5-FU and leucovorin delivered in bolus form). In the short-course arm, surgery (TME) was performed within 1 week of completion of radiation and, in the long-course arm, it was performed 4 to 6 weeks following radiation completion. The primary endpoint of the study was sphincter preservation. Acute toxicity rates were higher in the long-course, chemotherapy-containing group. There was no statistically significant difference in sphincter preservation (61.2% with the short-course treatment vs 58%, $P = .570$), and disease-free and overall survival at 4 years were similar between the two groups. Additionally, there was no difference in sphincter preservation rates in subjects initially deemed to require APR undergoing long-course therapy, despite significant downstaging in subjects receiving combined therapy (which differs from findings in the German rectal cancer study). The incidence of local recurrence was lower in the short-course group, although this did not reach statistical significance (9 vs 14.2%, $P = .17$). Less than 1% of subjects treated with the short-course therapy achieved a pathologic complete response, likely due to the short interval from completion of radiation to the surgery with limited time for tumor regression.

Sphincter preservation in rectal cancer is not only dependent on variables such as tumor location and individual anatomy, but also dependent on both a surgeon's skill and willingness to carry out this operation in light of downstaging or initial surgical impressions. Whether preoperative therapy truly results in improved rates of sphincter preservation is a matter of ongoing debate. Additionally, the impact of a longer break period from completion of short-course therapy to surgery (the standard has been about 1 week) is under investigation in the Stockholm III trial.[59]

As a result of these and other studies, both short-course radiation alone and long-course chemoradiotherapy are established as feasible neoadjuvant regimens. Many oncologists in the United States prefer the latter approach, with investigators further refining chemoradiotherapy regimens (see later discussion).

NEW AND INVESTIGATIONAL CHEMORADIOTHERAPY REGIMENS

Results from the German rectal cancer trial illustrate the critical endpoints (and deficiencies) in the management of operable rectal cancer management, namely disease-free and overall survivals, local control, and tumor response to neoadjuvant therapy. Specifically, pelvic control rates were high (94%), whereas disease-free survival was only 65%, whereas complete tumor sterilization was observed in only 8% of neoadjuvantly treated surgical specimens.

From a local-regional perspective, there is need for further improvement in neoadjuvant approaches for several reasons. First, despite high rates of pelvic tumor control in the setting of neoadjuvant radiation or chemoradiotherapy followed by TME for T3 tumors, local control in patients with T4 and/or low-lying rectal tumors is less optimal.[60] Secondly, there is emerging and provocative data that in well-selected patients with rectal cancer, chemoradiotherapy by itself can serve as radical therapy, obviating surgery.[61] Development of more effective radiation-based treatment regimens may allow for more patients to be treated with this approach. This will likely mandate the introduction of new chemotherapeutic and/or targeted drug agents that have potent radiosensitizing properties. Several agents are under investigation, including capecitabine, oxaliplatin, irinotecan, as well as bevacizumab and cetuximab. The focus of the remainder of this section is on capecitabine, oxaliplatin, and bevacizumab.

Capecitabine is an oral prodrug formulation of 5-FU, which exploits the observation that the enzyme facilitating the last step of its conversion, thymidine phosphorylase, is often upregulated in tumor tissue relative to normal tissue.[62] Phase II studies combining radiation with capecitabine revealed that tumor response rates may be modestly improved relative to those achieved with 5-FU.[63] Recently, results of a phase III German trial comparing capecitabine to 5-FU–based neoadjuvant chemoradiotherapy in subjects with locally advanced rectal cancer suggested capecitabine may serve as a potential replacement for 5-FU in the preoperative treatment of locally advanced rectal cancer, with higher rates of tumor downstaging in subjects receiving capecitabine.[64] The phase III NSABP R-04 and other European randomized trials are, in part, trying to further determine the value of capecitabine relative to more conventional infusional 5-FU.

Oxaliplatin is widely used in the adjuvant treatment of resected advanced-stage colon cancers as well as in the setting of metastatic colon and rectal tumors. Preclinical work also suggested oxaliplatin has radiosensitizing properties.[65] Phase II investigative trials indicated favorable antitumor activity in combination with radiation.[63] Two completed randomized phase III trials (STAR-01 and ACCORD 12/0405 PRODIGE 1), however, did not show major improvements in terms of tumor response over more standard therapy with radiation and 5-FU.[66,67] Toxicity rates, however, did seem to be increased with the addition of oxaliplatin. The NSABP R-04 and several European trials are also investigating the value of oxaliplatin and study results are awaited.

Bevacizumab is an antibody directed against vascular endothelial growth factor (VEGF). Originally designed with the intention of treating systemic disease by inhibiting VEGF-mediated angiogenesis, it also has the potential to sensitize radiation effects. The mechanism of this sensitization is likely multifactorial, including through sensitization of tumor-associated endothelial cells to radiation damage as well as pruning of immature tumor blood vessels with increased oxygen and drug delivery to tumors through the hypothesized process of vascular normalization.[68,69] Two phase II trials have suggested increased tumor response rates and one of these provided direct tissue evidence supporting the concept of vascular normalization.[70,71] Bevacizumab also, however, has the potential to increase treatment-related toxicity, including potentially increasing the risk of postsurgical wound complication rates.[71] ECOG 3204 is a phase II trial investigating the combination of capecitabine, oxaliplatin, and bevacizumab with radiation in the neoadjuvant treatment of rectal cancer. Although analysis revealed good tumor response rates, toxicity rates were also increased.[72]

From the perspective of systemic disease control, there is a clear need for therapeutic improvement because a high proportion of patients will ultimately develop metastatic disease. The value of adjuvant chemotherapy in patients with rectal cancer who have received neoadjuvant chemoradiotherapy remains controversial. The impact of adjuvant chemotherapy may be determined by several factors, including postsurgical treatment delays as well as lack of appropriately intensive or effective treatment regimens. As an alternative to the traditional delivery of chemotherapy in the postoperative setting, Garcia-Aguilar and colleagues[73] are conducted a phase II trial investigating delivery of chemotherapy during the treatment break typical between chemoradiation completion and surgery, with subjects receiving 5-FU, leucovorin, and oxaliplatin (FOLFOX) during the treatment break in an effort to define optimal sequencing of therapy. The value of a more intensive systemic therapy component was attempted to be determined through the ECOG 5204 trial, which randomized subjects who received neoadjuvant chemoradiotherapy and subsequent surgery for rectal cancer to adjuvant therapy with FOLFOX, with or without the addition of bevacizumab. Unfortunately this trial closed prematurely.

IMRT FOR RECTAL CANCER?

As previously discussed, IMRT is an advanced form of radiation treatment planning and delivery that can minimize high-dose irradiation to nontarget critical structures. One of the most important critical structures in rectal cancer treatment is the small intestine. Radiation dose-volume relationships with treatment-induced small intestine toxicity (eg, diarrhea, enteritis, obstruction) have been demonstrated.[74] Although conventional treatment practices (eg, prone patient positioning on a false tabletop, treatment with a full bladder, three-field radiation beam arrangements) can limit small intestine irradiation very effectively, IMRT may yield even further sparing in select circumstances.[75] This is of particular importance because more active, newer-generation chemoradiotherapy regimens have been associated with increased toxicity rates. Other critical structures of interest in pelvic irradiation include the bladder, femurs, and pelvic bone marrow. The potential value of IMRT in rectal cancer treatment is under study in RTOG 0822.

SUMMARY

Although historically managed by surgery, anal cancer is now primarily treated with radiation therapy combined with mitomycin and 5-FU, with surgery reserved for salvage. This regimen results in long-term local control, and colostomy-free and overall survival in most patients. Randomized trials have shown this regimen's superiority to (1) radiation therapy alone, (2) radiation therapy plus 5-FU only, and (3) neoadjuvant cisplatin–5-FU followed by concurrent radiation therapy, cisplatin, and 5-FU. Now, nearly four decades after the pioneering work of Nigro and colleagues,[5] a similar approach continues to be used, albeit with higher radiation doses. Recent advances in anal cancer therapy include the integration of PET into staging, treatment planning, and treatment response evaluation. Acute toxicity in the treatment of anal cancer with chemoradiotherapy undermines the ability to complete therapy in a timely manner and likely compromises disease-related outcomes in some circumstances. Reductions in acute morbidity could potentially result in improved disease-related outcomes by minimizing treatment interruptions. This seems achievable with the use of IMRT, which may also facilitate radiation-dose escalation. Randomized trials have evaluated the role of cisplatin in the neoadjuvant, concurrent, and adjuvant setting as well as the role of radiation dose escalation. Additional phase II trials are evaluating the roles of capecitabine, oxaliplatin, cetuximab, and panitumumab delivered concurrently with radiation therapy. Ultimately, as is increasingly seen in other disease sites in oncology, drug and radiation dosing specific to each individual patient may emerge as the standard treatment approach for this disease.

A similar evolution of therapy has taken place in the management of rectal adenocarcinoma. Clinical studies have demonstrated the ability of both preoperative and postoperative radiation to reduce pelvic tumor failure and that this reduction was still evident even when optimized surgical techniques were used. Broadly speaking, two approaches to neoadjuvant therapy have emerged over time: short-course radiation therapy alone and long-course chemoradiotherapy. A variety of sensitizing chemotherapy agents and targeted drugs have been and continue to be investigated in efforts improve tumor response rates with the goal of continued reductions in local-regional failure, improved sphincter preservation, and potential use of chemoradiotherapy as radical treatment for highly selected rectal adenocarcinoma presentations.

REFERENCES

1. Boman BM, Moertel CG, O'Connell MJ, et al. Carcinoma of the anal canal. A clinical and pathologic study of 188 cases. Cancer 1984;54:114–25.
2. Nigro ND, Vaitkevicius VK, Considine B Jr. Combined therapy for cancer of the anal canal: a preliminary report. Dis Colon Rectum 1974;17:354–6.
3. Buroker TR, Nigro N, Bradley G, et al. Combined therapy for cancer of the anal canal: a follow-up report. Dis Colon Rectum 1977;20:677–8.
4. Michaelson RA, Magill GB, Quan SH, et al. Preoperative chemotherapy and radiation therapy in the management of anal epidermoid carcinoma. Cancer 1983;51: 390–5.
5. Nigro ND, Seydel HG, Considine B, et al. Combined preoperative radiation and chemotherapy for squamous cell carcinoma of the anal canal. Cancer 1983;51: 1826–9.
6. Leichman L, Nigro N, Vaitkevicius VK, et al. Cancer of the anal canal. Model for preoperative adjuvant combined modality therapy. Am J Med 1985;78:211–5.
7. Meeker WR Jr, Sickle-Santanello BJ, Philpott G, et al. Combined chemotherapy, radiation, and surgery for epithelial cancer of the anal canal. Cancer 1986;57: 525–9.
8. Epidermoid anal cancer: results from the UKCCCR randomised trial of radiotherapy alone versus radiotherapy, 5-fluorouracil, and mitomycin. UKCCCR Anal Cancer Trial Working Party. UK Co-ordinating Committee on Cancer Research. Lancet 1996;348:1049–54.
9. Northover J, Glynne-Jones R, Sebag-Montefiore D, et al. Chemoradiation for the treatment of epidermoid anal cancer: 13-year follow-up of the first randomised UKCCCR Anal Cancer Trial (ACT I). Br J Cancer 2010;102:1123–8.
10. Bartelink H, Roelofsen F, Eschwege F, et al. Concomitant radiotherapy and chemotherapy is superior to radiotherapy alone in the treatment of locally advanced anal cancer: results of a phase III randomized trial of the European Organization for Research and Treatment of Cancer Radiotherapy and Gastrointestinal Cooperative Groups. J Clin Oncol 1997;15:2040–9.
11. Flam M, John M, Pajak T, et al. Role of mitomycin in combination with fluorouracil and radiotherapy, and of salvage chemoradiation in the definitive nonsurgical treatment of epidermoid carcinoma of the anal canal: results of a phase III randomized Intergroup study. J Clin Oncol 1996;14:2527–39.
12. Ajani J, Winter K, Gunderson L, et al. Fluorouracil, mitomycin, and radiotherapy vs. fluorouracil, cisplatin, and radiotherapy for carcinoma of the anal canal. a randomized controlled trial. JAMA 2008;299:1914–21.

13. Ajani J, Winter K, Gunderson L, et al. Intergroup RTOG 98-11: a phase III randomized study of 5-fluoruracil (5-FU), mitomycin, and radiotherapy versus 5-fluorouracil, cisplatin and radiotherapy in carcinoma of the anal canal. J Clin Oncol 2006;24:180s.

14. Gunderson LL, Winter K, Ajani J, et al. Intergroup RTOG 9811 phase III comparison of chemoradiation with 5-FU and mitomycin vs. 5-FU and cisplatin for anal canal carcinoma: impact of disease-free, overall and colostomy-free survival [abstract]. Int J Radiat Oncol Biol Phys 2006;66:S24.

15. Gunderson L, Winter K, Ajani JA, et al. Long-term update of U.S. GI Intergroup RTOG-98-11 phase III trial for anal carcinoma: Comparison of concurrent chemoradiation with 5FU mitomycin versus 5FU-cisplatin for disease-free and overall survival. J Clin Oncol 2011;29.

16. James R, Wan S, Glynne-Jones R, et al. A randomized trial of chemoradiation using mitomycin or cisplatin, with or without maintenance cisplatin/5FU in squamous cell carcinoma of the anus (ACT II). J Clin Oncol 2009;27:170s.

17. Trautmann TG, Zuger JH. Positron emission tomography for pretreatment staging and post treatment evaluation in cancer of the anal canal. Mol Imaging Biol 2005; 7:309–13.

18. Cotter SE, Grigsby PW, Siegel BA, et al. FDG-PET/CT in the evaluation of anal carcinoma. Int J Radiat Oncol Biol Phys 2006;65:720–5.

19. Anderson C, Koshy M, Staley C, et al. PET-CT fusion in radiation management of patients with anorectal tumors. Int J Radiat Oncol Biol Phys 2007;69:155–62.

20. Bannas P, Weber C, Adam G, et al. Contrast enhanced fluorodeoxyglucose-positron emission tomography/computed tomography for staging and radiotherapy planning in patients with anal cancer. Int J Radiat Oncol Biol Phys 2011;81(2):445–51.

21. Vercellino L, Montravers F, de Parades V, et al. Impact of FDG PET/CT in the staging and the follow-up of anal carcinoma. Int J Colorectal Dis 2011;26:201–10.

22. Schwarz J, Siegel BA, Dehdashti F, et al. Tumor response and survival predicted by post-therapy FDG-PET/CT in anal cancer. Int J Radiat Oncol Biol Phys 2008; 71(1):180–6.

23. John M, Pajak T, Flam M, et al. Dose escalation in chemoradiation for anal cancer: preliminary results of RTOG 92-08. Cancer J Sci Am 1996;2:194–6.

24. Roohipour R, Patil S, Goodman K, et al. Squamous-cell carcinoma of the anal canal: predictors of treatment outcome. Dis Colon Rectum 2008;51:147–53.

25. Ben-Josef E, Moughan J, Ajani JA, et al. Impact of overall treatment time on survival and local control in patients with anal cancer: a pooled data analysis of Radiation Therapy Oncology Group trials 87-04 and 98-11. J Clin Oncol 2010;28:5061–6.

26. Glynne-Jones R, Hoskin P. Neoadjuvant cisplatin chemotherapy before chemoradiation: a flawed paradigm. J Clin Oncol 2007;25:5281–6.

27. De Ruysscher D, Pijls-Johannesma M, Bentzen SM, et al. Time between the first day of chemotherapy and the last day of chest radiation is the most important predictor of survival in limited-disease small-cell lung cancer. J Clin Oncol 2006;24:1057–63.

28. Brade AM, Tannock IF. Scheduling of radiation and chemotherapy for limited-stage small-cell lung cancer: repopulation as a cause of treatment failure? J Clin Oncol 2006;24:1020–2.

29. Matzinger O, Roelofsen F, Mineur L, et al. Mitomycin C with continuous fluorouracil or with cisplatin in combination with radiotherapy for locally advanced anal cancer (European Organisation for Research and Treatment of Cancer phase II study 22011-40014). Eur J Cancer 2009;45:2782–91.

30. Sebag-Montefiore D, Meadows HM, Cunningham D, et al. Three cytotoxic drugs combined with pelvic radiation and as maintenance chemotherapy for patients with squamous cell carcinoma of the anus (SCCA): long-term follow-up of a phase II pilot study using 5-fluorouracil, mitomycin C and cisplatin. Radiother Oncol 2012;104(2):155–60.
31. Peiffert D, Tournier-Rangeard L, Gerard JP, et al. Induction chemotherapy and dose intensification of the radiation boost in locally advanced anal canal carcinoma: final analysis of the randomized UNICANCER ACCORD 03 trial. J Clin Oncol 2012;30(16):1941–8.
32. Glynne-Jones R, Meadows H, Wan S, et al. EXTRA–a multicenter phase II study of chemoradiation using a 5 day per week oral regimen of capecitabine and intravenous mitomycin C in anal cancer. Int J Radiat Oncol Biol Phys 2008;72: 119–26.
33. Eng C, Chang GJ, Das P, et al. Phase II study of capecitabine and oxaliplatin with concurrent radiation therapy (XELOX-XRT) for squamous cell carcinoma of the anal canal [abstract 4116]. J Clin Oncol 2009;27(Suppl):15s.
34. Salama JK, Mell L, Schomas DA, et al. Concurrent chemotherapy and intensity-modulated radiation therapy for anal canal cancer patients: a multicenter experience. J Clin Oncol 2007;25:4581–6.
35. Pepek JM, Willett CG, Wu QJ, et al. Intensity-modulated radiation therapy for anal malignancies: a preliminary toxicity and disease outcomes analysis. Int J Radiat Oncol Biol Phys 2010;78:1413–9.
36. Kachnic LA, Winter K, Myerson RJ, et al. RTOG 0529: a phase II evaluation of dose-painted intensity modulated radiation therapy in combination with 5-fluorouracil and mitomycin-C for the reduction of acute morbidity in carcinoma of the anal cancer. Int J Radiat Oncol Biol Phys 2012. [Epub ahead of print].
37. Kachnic L, Winter K, Myerson R, et al. Two-year outcomes of RTOG 0529: A phase II evaluation of dose-painted IMRT in combination with 5-fluorouracil and mitomycin-C for the reduction of acute morbidity in carcinoma of the anal canal [abstract 368]. J Clin Oncol 2011;29(Suppl 4).
38. Wright J, Patil S, Temple LK, et al. Squamous cell carcinoma of the anal canal: patterns and predictors of failure and implications for intensity-modulated radiation therapy planning. Int J Radiat Oncol Biol Phys 2010;78(4):1064–72.
39. Miles WE. A method for performing abdomino-perineal excision for carcinoma of the rectum and the terminal portion of the pelvic colon. Lancet 1908;II: 1812–3.
40. Heald RJ, Ryall RD. Recurrence and survival after total mesorectal excision for rectal cancer. Lancet 1986;1(8496):1479–82.
41. McCall JL, Cox MR, Wattchow DA. Analysis of local recurrence rates after surgery alone for rectal cancer. Int J Colorectal Dis 1995;10:126–32.
42. Fisher B, Wolmark N, Rockette H, et al. Postoperative adjuvant chemotherapy or radiation therapy for rectal cancer: Results from NSABP protocol R-01. J Natl Cancer Inst 1988;80:21–9.
43. Wolmark N, Wieand HS, Hyams DM, et al. Randomized trial of postoperative adjuvant chemotherapy with or without radiotherapy for carcinoma of the rectum: National surgical adjuvant breast and bowel project protocol R-02. J Natl Cancer Inst 2000;92:388–96.
44. Gastrointestinal tumor study group. Prolongation of the disease-free interval in surgically treated rectal carcinoma. N Engl J Med 1985;312:1465–72.
45. Krook JE, Moertel CG, Gunderson LL, et al. Effective surgical adjuvant therapy for high-risk rectal carcinoma. N Engl J Med 1991;324:709–15.

46. Stockholm rectal cancer study group. Preoperative short-term radiation therapy in operable rectal carcinoma. A prospective randomized trial. Cancer 1990;66: 49–55.
47. Folkesson J, Birgisson H, Pahlman L, et al. Swedish rectal cancer trial: Long lasting benefits from radiotherapy on survival and local recurrence rate. J Clin Oncol 2005;23:5644–50.
48. Quirke P, Durdey P, Dixon MF, et al. Local recurrence of rectal adenocarcinoma due to inadequate surgical resection. Histopathological study of lateral tumor spread and surgical excision. Lancet 1986;2(8514):996–9.
49. Heald RJ, Moran BJ, Ryall RD, et al. Rectal cancer: the Basingstoke experience of total mesorectal excision, 1978-1997. Arch Surg 1998;133:894–9.
50. van Gijn W, Marijnen CA, Nagtegaal ID, et al. Preoperative radiotherapy combined with total mesorectal excision for resectable rectal cancer: 12-year follow-up of the multicentre, randomised controlled TME trial. Lancet Oncol 2011;12(6):575–82.
51. Shewach DS, Lawrence TS. Antimetabolite radiosensitizers. J Clin Oncol 2007; 25:4043–50.
52. Gerard J-P, Conroy T, Bonnetain F, et al. Preoperative radiotherapy with or without concurrent fluorouracil and leucovorin in T3-4 rectal cancers: Results of FFCD 9203. J Clin Oncol 2006;24:4620–5.
53. Bosset J-F, Collette L, Calais G, et al. Chemotherapy with preoperative radiotherapy in rectal cancer. N Engl J Med 2006;355:1114–23.
54. Sauer R, Becker H, Hohenberger W, et al. Preoperative versus postoperative chemoradiotherapy for rectal cancer. N Engl J Med 2004;351:1731–40.
55. Roh MS, Colangelo LH, O'Connell MJ, et al. Preoperative multimodality therapy improves disease-free survival in patients with carcinoma of the rectum: NSABP R- 03. J Clin Oncol 2009;27:5124–30.
56. Sebag-Montefiore D, Stephens RJ, Steele R, et al. Preoperative radiotherapy versus selective postoperative chemoradiotherapy in patients with rectal cancer (MRC CR07 and NCIC-CTG C-16): a mutlicentre, randomised trial. Lancet 2009; 373:811–20.
57. Suwinski R, Wzietek I, Tarnawski R, et al. Moderately low alpha/beta ratio for rectal cancer may best explain the outcome of three fractionation schedules of preoperative radiotherapy. Int J Radiat Oncol Biol Phys 2007;69:793–9.
58. Bujko K, Nowacki MP, Nasierowska-Guttmejer A, et al. Long-term results of a randomized trial comparing preoperative short-course radiotherapy with preoperative conventionally fractionated chemoradiation for rectal cancer. Br J Surg 2006;93:1215–23.
59. Pettersson D, Cedermark B, Holm T, et al. Interim analysis of the Stockholm III trial of preoperative radiotherapy regimens for rectal cancer. Br J Surg 2010;97:580–7.
60. Sanfilippo NJ, Crane CH, Skibber J, et al. T4 rectal cancer treated with preoperative chemoradiation to the posterior pelvis followed by multivisceral resection: patterns of failure and limitations of treatment. Int J Radiat Oncol Biol Phys 2001;51:176–83.
61. Habr-Gama A, Perez RO, Nadalin W, et al. Operative versus nonoperative treatment for stage 0 distal rectal cancer following chemoradiation therapy: long-term results. Ann Surg 2004;240:711–7.
62. Miwa M, Ura M, Nishida M, et al. Design of a novel fluoropyrimidine carbamate, capecitabine, which generates 5-fluorouracil selectively in tumours by enzymes concentrated in human liver and cancer tissue. Eur J Cancer 1998; 34:1274–81.

63. Patel A, Puthillath A, Yang G, et al. Neoadjuvant chemoradiation for rectal cancer: is more better? Oncology 2008;22:814–26.
64. Hofheinz R, Wenz F, Post S, et al. Chemoradiotherapy with capecitabine versus fluorouracil for locally advanced rectal cancer: a randomised, multi-centre, non-inferiority, phase III trial. Lancet Oncol 2012;13(6):579–88.
65. Hermann RM, Rave-Frank M, Pradier O. Combining radiation with oxaliplatin: a review of experimental results. Cancer Radiother 2008;12:61–7.
66. Gerard JP, Azria D, Gourgou-Bourgade S, et al. Clinical outcome of the ACCORD 12/0405 PRODIGE 2 randomized trial in rectal cancer. J Clin Oncol 2012;30(36): 4558–65.
67. Aschele C, Clonini L, Lonardi S, et al. Primary tumor response to preoperative chemoradiation with or without oxaliplatin in locally advanced rectal cancer: pathologic results of the STAR-01 randomized phase III trial. J Clin Oncol 2011;29(20): 2773–80.
68. Moeller BJ, Cao Y, Li CY, et al. Radiation activates HIF-1 to regulate vascular radiosensitivity in tumors: role of reoxygenation, free radicals, and stress granules. Cancer Cell 2004;5:429–41.
69. Jain RK. Normalization of tumor vasculature: an emerging concept in antiangiogenic therapy. Science 2005;307:58–62.
70. Willett CG, Duda DG, di Tomaso E, et al. Efficacy, safety, and biomarkers of neoadjuvant bevacizumab, radiation therapy, and fluorouracil in rectal cancer: a multidisciplinary phase II study. J Clin Oncol 2009;27:3020–6.
71. Crane CH, Eng C, Feig BW, et al. Phase II trial of neoadjuvant bevacizumab, capecitabine, and radiotherapy for locally advanced rectal cancer. Int J Radiat Oncol Biol Phys 2010;76:824–30.
72. Landry JC, Feng Y, Cohen SJ, et al. Phase II study of preoperative radiation with concurrent capecitabine, oxaliplatin, and bevacizumab followed by surgery and postoperative 5-FU, leucovorin, oxaliplatin (FOLFOX) and bevacizumab in patients with locally advanced rectal cancer: ECOG 3204. Cancer 2013. [Epub ahead of print].
73. Garcia-Aguilar J, Smith DD, Avila K, et al. Optimal timing of surgery after chemoradiation for advanced rectal cancer: preliminary results of a multicenter, non-randomized phase II prospective trial. Ann Surg 2011;254(1):97–102.
74. Baglan KL, Frazier RC, Yan D, et al. The dose-volume relationship of acute small bowel toxicity from concurrent 5-FU-based chemotherapy and radiation therapy for rectal cancer. Int J Radiat Oncol Biol Phys 2002;52:176–83.
75. Kim JY, Kim DY, Kim TH, et al. Intensity-modulated radiotherapy with a belly board for rectal cancer. Int J Colorectal Dis 2007;22:373–9.

Novel Approaches to Treatment of Hepatocellular Carcinoma and Hepatic Metastases Using Thermal Ablation and Thermosensitive Liposomes

Mark W. Dewhirst, DVM, PhD[a,b,c,*], Chelsea D. Landon, MS[b],
Christina L. Hofmann, MS[c], Paul R. Stauffer, MSEE, CCE[a]

KEYWORDS

- Thermal ablation • Thermosensitive liposomes • Hepatocellular carcinoma

KEY POINTS

- Limitations of thermal ablation: this article explains available methods for thermal ablation of hepatocellular carcinomas and emphasizes the limitations, including marginal recurrence of large lesions and tumors near large vessels.
- Combination therapy for thermal ablation and chemotherapeutics: combining thermal ablation with liposomal drugs such as doxorubicin, which behaves synergistically with heat, has shown improvement in coagulation diameter, drug accumulation, and necrosis.
- Thermosensitive liposomes and thermal ablation: development of thermosensitive liposomes has provided a mechanism to combine thermal ablation and drug delivery to maximize drug release at the target site, showing benefits in both preclinical and clinical models.

INTRODUCTION

There is a need for therapies that can effectively treat primary hepatocellular carcinoma (HCC) as well as metastases to the liver. HCC is the fifth most common cancer worldwide and the fourth most common cause for cancer death.[1] Metastasis to the liver occurs commonly from primary cancers of the gastrointestinal track and other solid tumors. Surgical resection is an option for less than 30% of patients presenting

Conflict of Interest Statement: Dr Dewhirst holds stock in the Celsion Corporation.
[a] Radiation Oncology Department, Duke University Medical Center, Durham, NC 27710, USA;
[b] Department of Pathology, Duke University Medical Center, Durham, NC 27710, USA;
[c] Biomedical Engineering Department, Duke University, Durham, NC 27708, USA
* Corresponding author. Radiation Oncology Department, Duke University Medical Center, Box 3455, MSRBI Room 201, Research Drive, Durham, NC 27710.
E-mail address: Mark.dewhirst@duke.edu

with metastases.[1,2] These patients are often not good surgical candidates, because of the location of the tumor or because of intercurrent disease, such as cirrhosis.[2] However, thermal ablation is a cost-effective, nonsurgical option for treatment of patients with HCC and liver metastases[3] and is currently practiced worldwide.

In this review, a new approach is discussed, combining thermal ablation with drug-carrying thermosensitive liposomes. The rationale for this approach is presented and discussed in light of current liposome formulations and methods to achieve thermal ablation. A summary of preclinical and clinical studies that are relevant to treatment of primary and metastatic liver cancer is also presented.

THERMAL ABLATION

There are many technologies capable of thermal ablation treatment of focal liver tumors. Power deposition may be localized in a liver target either with externally applied focused ultrasonography or invasively with 1 of several interstitial heating techniques. The underlying physics for 9 interstitial heating modalities has been reviewed previously.[4] Clinical methodology and results from several of those invasive approaches were highlighted in a special issue on thermal ablation therapy of the *International Journal of Hyperthermia*.[5] For liver tumors, the most common ablative approach involves use of radiofrequency (RF) electrodes inserted percutaneously to the liver target. RF electrodes are available that heat tissue from RF currents between an array of implanted electrodes, along the length of bipolar electrodes, or between implanted electrode(s) and a ground return pad on the skin. Some electrodes include internal cooling to reduce tissue desiccation around the needle, allowing increased power levels and effective treatment volume.[6] To minimize the number of percutaneous insertions and expand the volume of tissue encompassed within an array, RF electrodes are available that deploy multiple tines curving out into surrounding tissue like an umbrella from a central larger electrode.[7]

Although there are fewer clinical systems available, interstitial microwave antennae are increasingly used for thermal ablation of liver tumors,[8,9] to take advantage of increased penetration of power deposition around each implant.[10,11] Laser interstitial thermal therapy is also commonly used for liver ablation,[12] with either ultrasound[13] or magnetic resonance (MR) image guidance.[14] Use of high-intensity focused ultrasonography (HIFU) with MR imaging thermometry has also increased for liver ablation in recent years.[15–17]

Regardless of modality used, power is applied to reach ablative temperatures in the range of 50°C to 100°C. Because of rapid accumulation of lethal thermal dose in this temperature range, ablation generally occurs within minutes. However, this therapy is not without limitations. The risk for marginal recurrence increases when lesions are larger than 3 to 5 cm,[1,18] and when they are located near large, thermally significant vessels, or visceral organs.[18] In addition, long-term patient follow-up has shown high rates of local tumor progression after RF ablation treatment.[3] Thus, there has been interest in combining thermal ablation with treatments that would augment cytotoxicity at the margin of the ablation zone.

THERMAL ABLATION AND CHEMOTHERAPEUTICS

Several techniques have been assessed to overcome these limitations of ablation, including the combination of chemotherapy with RF ablation. Many chemotherapeutic agents, including doxorubicin, are known to interact synergistically with hyperthermia,[19–23] so combining these agents with RF ablation would potentially be effective. For example, Mostafa and colleagues[24] assessed the combination of RF ablation and a chemoembolic mixture, consisting of doxorubicin in iodized oil, in rabbits with hepatic tumors and showed that the combination of local drug delivery and hyperthermia resulted in larger coagulation areas relative to controls.

However, the main dose-limiting factor with chemotherapeutic agents, such as doxorubicin, is normal tissue toxicity, supporting the use of a less toxic liposomal formulation. The first doxorubicin HCl liposome formulation (Doxil, Janssen Products, LP, Horsham, PA, USA), was approved for several clinical indications by equal anti-tumor activity to free drug combined with reduced cardiotoxicity, which is a dose-limiting organ for free doxorubicin.[25,26]

DOXORUBICIN LIPOSOME FORMULATION

Liposomes are spontaneously forming lipid bilayer vesicles containing an aqueous medium.[27] They are nanoscale in size, in the range of 1 to a few hundred nanometers in diameter. They can be unilamellar or multilamellar. The most common types are uni-lamellar formulations, which are formed by passing larger liposomes at high pressure through filters of defined pore diameter or by ultrasonication. Several drugs have been encapsulated into liposomes.[28] For oncologic applications, doxorubicin has been the most widely used drug, because it can be loaded at high concentration. By preloading the liposomes with acid, doxorubicin, which is a weak base, diffuses across the lipid bilayer and reaches such high concentrations inside the liposome that it crystallizes.[29] This review focuses on doxorubicin-containing liposomes, because these are the best-developed formulations and they have been used in clinical trials.

THERMAL ABLATION AND LIPOSOMAL DOXORUBICIN

Several studies have assessed the combination of RF ablation and the nonthermally sensitive liposomal doxorubicin, showing larger ablation zones compared with RF abla-tion alone, both at the preclinical and clinical levels.[30–36] Goldberg and colleagues[34] assessed the combination of RF ablation and Doxil in a rat mammary adenocarcinoma model and observed increased coagulation diameter in the solid tumors compared with RF ablation alone, and in a follow-up study, D'Ippolito and colleagues[33] observed a decrease in tumor growth and potential increase in rat survival. In the same tumor model, Ahmed and colleagues[32] reported that the combination of RF ablation and lipo-somal doxorubicin increased tumor uptake and accumulation of doxorubicin compared with liposomal doxorubicin alone, as well as increased tumor necrosis compared with ablation alone.[31,32] Ahmed and colleagues[30] also studied the combina-tion of RF ablation followed by liposomal doxorubicin treatment in canine sarcomas, rabbit liver and kidneys, and in the thigh muscle of rats. These investigators observed increased coagulation and doxorubicin accumulation after the combined treatment, showing the effectiveness of this treatment in multiple tissue and tumor types. A clinical study conducted by Goldberg and colleagues[35] treated 10 patients presenting with focal hepatic tumors and showed 25% to 30% greater tumor destruction when lipo-somal doxorubicin was combined with RF ablation compared with RF ablation alone.[37]

Several mechanisms have been suggested for the synergistic effect of liposomal doxorubicin and RF ablation.[38] Solazzo and colleagues[39] observed increased markers of DNA breakage, oxidative stress, and apoptosis, as well as increased heat-shock protein 70 in the areas surrounding the ablation zone after combination treatment. In addition, the changes in vasculature caused by ablation may affect liposome accu-mulation within the tumor.[38] Ahmed and colleagues[32] observed increased intratumoral drug uptake and found that less doxorubicin was necessary for tumor destruction after combined RF ablation and Doxil.

Although these studies on the combination of RF ablation and liposomal doxorubicin have shown improvement (ie, increased coagulation and antitumor effect), it has been suggested that optimization is still necessary to improve clinical outcome,[35] particularly if advantage could be taken of the heat produced by ablation. One possible approach is through the use of thermosensitive liposomes, which would take advantage of the more moderate hyperthermic temperatures at the tumor margin, allowing for triggered release of drug at the edge of the heated zone. Gasselhuber and colleagues[40] performed mathematical modeling of drug delivery from low-temperature-sensitive liposomes (LTSL) during RF ablation, which predicted higher drug accumulation with liposomal doxorubicin compared with free drug, as well as lower peak plasma concentration, supporting the use of temperature-sensitive liposomes in combination with RF ablation.

HISTORY OF THERMOSENSITIVE LIPOSOMES LEADING TO DEVELOPMENT OF SECOND-GENERATION FORMULATIONS

Dozens of studies have been published combining nonthermally sensitive liposomes with hyperthermia.[41] The rationale for such combinations emanates from the observation that hyperthermia increases vascular pore sizes in tumor microvessels, leading to enhanced extravasation.[42] Although tumor vasculature is typically more permeable to nanoparticles, this enhanced permeability and retention (EPR) effect is substantially increased with hyperthermia treatment. In this review, these studies are not discussed, because when compared head to head, thermally sensitive liposomes achieve higher drug delivery and better antitumor effect.[42,43] Reviews of previous work with nonthermally sensitive liposomes have been published.[41] Similarly, details of the chemical compositions and physical characterizations of thermosensitive liposomes have been reviewed elsewhere and are not discussed here.[27,44]

In a frozen state, the liposome membrane contains plates of frozen lipid that interface in a pattern that resembles a soccer ball.[27] When the temperature is increased, the junctions between the frozen plates melt first, leading to enhanced permeability.[27] The liposomes are not destroyed during the melting process; they merely go from a frozen to a melted state. Milton Yatvin was the first to recognize that the enhanced permeability of liposomes to aqueous media near their solid-liquid transition could be harnessed as a drug delivery method if it was combined with local application of heat.[45,46] The original formulation contained a mixture of 2 lipids of different melting temperatures; it showed a peak in permeability at 45°C. Yatvin and colleagues published several articles[45,47,48] with this formulation, showing that it could improve antitumor effect of several drugs, when combined with hyperthermia. Yatvin and colleagues[46] surmised that the increased antitumor effect seen with this formulation was the result of several mechanisms: (1) thermally increased perfusion and EPR, (2) enhanced release of bioavailable drug and (3) enhanced transendothelial drug transport.

Although the principle of thermally mediated drug delivery pioneered by Yatvin was brilliant, the earlier formulations[46,49] had 3 important limitations:

1. The liposome was readily taken up by the reticuloendothelial system, as opposed to circulating long enough to be efficiently delivered to the heated tumor. The discovery that the circulation time of liposomes could be prolonged considerably by adding polyethylene glycol (PEG) to the surface was a major achievement; these liposomes could circulate for days, thereby maximizing the EPR effect.[50] Gaber and colleagues[49] PEGylated the Yatvin formulation to yield a long circulating thermosensitive liposome. Hyperthermia treatment induced enhanced liposome accumulation in tumors and increased drug release. The combination of these 2 effects

enhanced delivery of drug to the tumor by nearly 50-fold, compared with administering the liposomes without heating.[51]

2. The temperature for drug release was too high (43°C–45°C). Typical temperatures that can be achieved in patients without pain or risk of thermal injury are in the range of 40°C to 43°C.[52] Thus, there was a mismatch between what temperatures were achievable clinically and what was needed for maximum drug delivery.

3. The time to reach maximal drug release was too slow (>30 minutes) for routine clinical use.[43] If a liposome entered the heated region and did not extravasate into the tumor, then it would not completely release its contents before the blood containing the liposome exited the tumor. As is shown later, the second-generation thermosensitive liposomes were designed to correct these deficiencies.

SECOND-GENERATION THERMOSENSITIVE LIPOSOME FORMULATIONS

David Needham and Mark Dewhirst and colleagues collaborated to develop the first doxorubicin-containing thermosensitive liposome that showed release in the clinically acceptable hyperthermia range.[42,43] In addition to a mixture of 2 double-chain fatty acids, the formulation contained a small percentage of a single chain fatty acid, known as a lysolipid. It also contained PEG to extend the circulation time. The lysolipid provided for a very rapid drug release (<20 seconds).[43] The maximum release rate temperature was 41.3°C (**Fig. 1**), but enhanced release occurred over a range from 39.5°C to 42°C. The circulation time was on the order of 2 hours in humans, which is considerably shorter than Doxil, but of sufficient length to work with a typical hyperthermia treatment, which lasts 30 to 60 minutes.[1] The formulation was given the generic term LTSL. In this review, LTSL-Dox is used to represent the doxorubicin-containing formulation, which is the only drug formulation that has been studied extensively with this type of liposome. The generic term for the commercial doxorubicin-containing LTSL is lysothermosensitive liposomal doxorubicin (LTLD).

Other groups have also developed LTSL formulations. Lindner and colleagues[53] described a long circulating formulation that contains a mixture of natural and synthetic lipids. This liposome achieves maximal release at 42°C. This group has

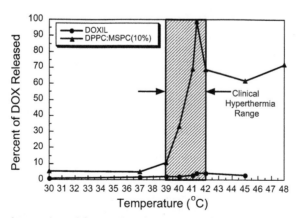

Fig. 1. Percent of Dox released for Doxil and DPPC/MSPC (10%) at t = 4 minutes. Comparison of doxorubicin release after 4 minutes of heating across a range of temperatures for LTSL-Dox (DPPC/MSPC (10%)) versus Doxil. LTSL-Dox releases drug in the temperature range between 39.5°C and 42°C, which is in the range that can be achieved for routine application of hyperthermia. Maximal release occurs at the phase transition temperature of 41.3°C. DPPC - Dipalmitoylphosphatidylcholine; MSPC - Monostearoylphosphatidylcholine.

extensively studied how plasma proteins affect the stability of LTSLs[54] and has recently reported that the stability is affected by both albumin and IgG, the 2 most common proteins found in plasma.[55] Both proteins tend to lower the temperature dependence of drug release from thermosensitive liposomes. The presence of PEG does not seem to protect the liposomes from these effects. It is important to keep such effects in mind in the engineering of LTSLs so that they still perform to expectation when used clinically. In this case, the goal is to have them maintain drug until heated so that release of drug is maximized in the area receiving hyperthermia.

Dicheva and colleagues[56] have recently reported on a new cationic LTSL formulation. The rationale for this design is based on a different principle than LTSL-Dox. In this case, the goal is to permit intracellular uptake of the cationic liposomes by vascular endothelium and tumor cells, before administration of heat. This concept comes from previous observations that cationic liposomes have a greater affinity for endothelial cells and tumor cells than other types of liposomes. There has been some speculation that damage to vascular endothelium by drug-containing cationic liposomes may lead to ischemia and tumor cell death, independent of any direct tumor cell killing caused by drug delivered by the liposomes. Thus, once accumulated, rapid drug release by intracellular cationic liposomes may achieve high intracellular concentrations of drug, thereby maximizing damage to both the endothelial cell and tumor cell compartments (**Fig. 2**). This factor is especially important for this approach, because reliance on the EPR effect alone does not yield uniform drug delivery throughout the tumor (also see **Fig. 3**).[57]

Several other investigators have described liposomes containing polymers that show similar drug release characteristics.[58–62] Thus, there is increasing interest in exploiting this type of drug delivery system.

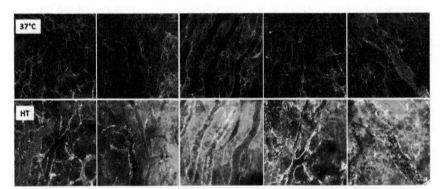

Fig. 2. Performance of cationic thermosensitive liposome. Using the dorsal skin-fold window chamber, the localization and extravasation of the liposomes can be monitored over time. (*Upper panel*) Selected images of cationic thermosensitive liposome accumulation in endothelial cells lining vessel walls of B16 melanoma tumors, 2 hours after administration. Some evidence for extravasation is also observed. (*Bottom panel*) Appearance of window chamber after 1 hour of heating at 43°C. Green represents the presence of carboxyfluorescein, which was previously loaded into the liposomes. The appearance of green signal shows that the contents have been released. Note the lack of green signal in the images taken before heating, which reflects quenching of the fluorescence when calcein is encapsulated inside the liposome (*upper panel*). (*Reprinted from* Dicheva BM, Hagen TL, Li L, et al. Cationic thermosensitive liposomes: a novel dual targeted heat-triggered drug delivery approach for endothelial and tumor cells. Nano Lett 2012; [Epub ahead of print]. Copyright (2012) American Chemical Society; with permission.)

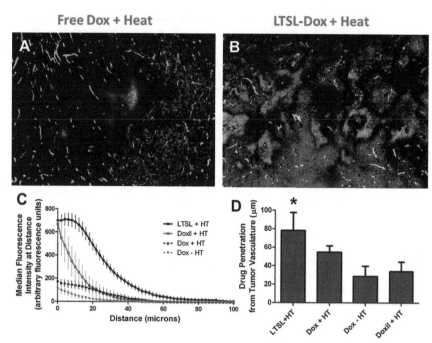

Fig. 3. Comparison of drug penetration distances from nearest blood vessel for free drug ± 42°C heating for 1 hour, LTSL-Dox + heat and Doxil + heat (*A, B*). Green = CD31 for endothelial cells, red = doxorubicin, and yellow = EF5 hypoxia marker. The difference in total amount of drug delivered for free drug versus LTSL drug is obvious, but more importantly is the drug coverage around tumor blood vessels and the encroachment into hypoxic areas. The drug penetration distance was doubled for *P* = .0106, between LTSL + HT and Doxil + HT compared with the other treatment groups (*C, D*). The differences were highly significant. (*From* Manzoor AA, Lindner LH, Landon CD, et al. Overcoming limitations in nanoparticle drug delivery: triggered, intravascular release to improve drug penetration into tumors. Cancer Res 2012;72(21):5573; with permission.)

PRECLINICAL STUDIES WITH LTSL-DOX

The LTSL-Dox formulation developed by Needham and Dewhirst has been tested extensively at the preclinical level. When FaDu head and neck cancer xenografts were heated to 42°C, LTSL-Dox showed 25-fold greater doxorubicin accumulation in the tumor tissue than free drug-treated tumors.[42] It delivered 5-fold more drug than a Doxil formulation and the PEGylated thermosensitive liposome described by Gaber and colleagues[49] (**Fig. 4**). Furthermore, the percentage of drug bound to DNA was substantially greater for LTSL-Dox, compared with the other treatment groups. DNA-bound drug is an important end point for this drug, because DNA damage is a primary mechanism for cell death with doxorubicin.

In 2 separate tumor growth delay studies using the maximum tolerated dose (MTD) of doxorubicin in combination with local hyperthermia to the tumor-bearing limb, the LTSL-Dox formulation yielded a substantial proportion of long-term tumor control up to 60 days after treatment.[42,43] Free drug showed little to no activity, whereas the other liposome formulations yielded some growth delay, but virtually no cures. LTSL-Dox showed superior antitumor activity in several xenograft and allograft tumor models.[63]

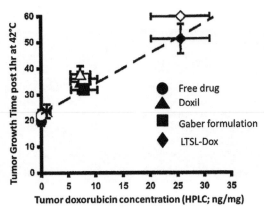

Fig. 4. Relationship between the concentration of doxorubicin achieved in tumor tissue and the tumor growth time for free drug and 3 liposomal formulations. The Gaber formulation[49] is a PEGylated version of the original Yatvin formulation.[46] The open and closed symbols represent replicate experiments. Data were obtained by removing a cohort of animals at the end of treatment from each group and having the tumor analyzed for total doxorubicin concentration, using high-performance liquid chromatography. The remaining animals in each group were followed for tumor regrowth. (*Adapted from* Kong G, Anyarambhatla G, Petros WP, et al. Efficacy of liposomes and hyperthermia in a human tumor xenograft model: importance of triggered drug release. Cancer Res 2000;60:6954; with permission.)

The extent of antitumor effect seen after LTSL-Dox treatment has been proportional to the concentration of drug delivered.[42,63,64] Using noninvasive optical methods to measure doxorubicin concentrations and properties of hemoglobin in the SKOV3 ovarian cancer xenograft, Palmer and colleagues[64] showed that the efficacy of LTSL-Dox with hyperthermia was also influenced by perfusion and hypoxia in addition to drug concentration achieved in each tumor (**Fig. 5**). It is not surprising to see the influence of hypoxia, because the efficacy of this drug has previously been reported to be reduced under hypoxic conditions in some tumor cell lines.[65] The concentration dependence of the observed antitumor effect may reflect variations in the total amount of drug delivered, which is related to efficiency of perfusion. LTSL-Dox cannot show its antitumor activity if the drug is not delivered to all portions of the tumor. These results strongly suggest that measurements of perfusion and hypoxia before treatment with LTSL-Dox might yield important prognostic information about the usefulness of this formulation in individual patients. Alternatively, doxorubicin accumulation could be measured directly by using liposomes that are coloaded with MR contrast agents.[66,67] The ability to measure drug accumulation in tumor tissue in real time while adjusting the heating pattern has been coined drug dose painting. This approach is being pursued by several groups that are involved in the development of HIFU as an alternative method to deliver drugs with thermally ablative temperatures in a variety of tumor sites.[16,68–71]

The combination of hyperthermia with LTSL-Dox yielded higher drug concentrations than the Doxil and Gaber formulations, even although these were of equivalent size to LTSL-Dox. This finding led to the hypothesis that the difference in the achieved drug concentration was caused by intravascular drug release.[42] If such a mechanism were operational, it would drive the drug out of the vasculature down its concentration gradient and into the interstitial space of the tumor. Recently, this theory has been proved.[57] Using a combination of fluorescently labeled liposomes and taking advantage of the natural fluorescence of doxorubicin, Manzoor and colleagues[57] used the

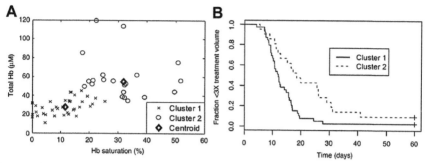

Fig. 5. Relationship between perfusion and extent of tumor hypoxia and duration of local tumor control after treatment with LTSL-Dox and hyperthermia. (*A*) Total hemoglobin (Hb) and Hb saturation (Hbsat) reflect perfusion and extent of hypoxia in individual tumors as measured using a noninvasive optical spectroscopy method. These same tumors were followed for growth time. Cluster analysis revealed 2 separate populations of tumors, which were characterized by relatively low Hb and Hbsat versus the second group, which had higher values of these 2 parameters. (*B*) The time to reach 3 times treatment volume was linked to these values, indicating that the more poorly perfused and hypoxic tumors responded less favorably to the treatment. (*Reproduced from* Palmer GM, Boruta RJ, Viglianti BL, et al. Non-invasive monitoring of intra-tumor drug concentration and therapeutic response using optical spectroscopy. J Control Release 2010;142(3):463; with permission.)

dorsal skin-fold window chamber model to show that liposomal extravasation does not contribute to the enhanced drug delivery with LTSL-Dox when combined with 42°C heating. Instead, nearly 100% of the drug is released intravascularly. This situation creates a local continuous infusion of drug, exclusively in the heated tumor site. The properties of the original LTSL-Dox formulation of Needham and that of Lindner were similar in this respect. The presence of high intravascular drug concentration during heating yields greater perivascular penetration than can be achieved with either free drug or Doxil when they are combined with hyperthermia (see **Fig. 3**).

LTSL-Dox and the cationic thermosensitive formulations show maximal uptake in endothelial cell and pericyte nuclei.[56,57] This uptake was not observed with free doxorubicin. It has previously been shown that LTSL-Dox treatment with 42°C heating can lead to vascular shutdown, whereas neither heat nor LTSL-Dox alone can achieve this type of effect.[72] The antivascular effect may have been the result of endothelial cell damage and death after treatment, driven by the high concentrations of drug found in these cells. It would be interesting to compare the performance of the cationic liposomes, described earlier, with LTSL-Dox, to determine whether they show similar antivascular effects.

CANINE CLINICAL STUDIES WITH LTSL

Before being used in human clinical trials, the LTSL-Dox formulation was tested in a phase I trial of companion dogs with spontaneous tumors.[73] A total of 21 dogs were entered into this study at doses of 0.7, 0.93, and 1.0 mg/kg, with a planned course of 3 cycles every 3 weeks. Histologies included sarcomas and carcinomas. The median tumor volume was 90.6 cm³ (range, 3.1–1747.0 cm³).

The first 4 animals enrolled showed an anaphylactoid reaction during drug infusion. This reaction was typified by hypotension and an increase in end-respiratory pressure. Subsequent studies in normal dogs revealed this reaction to be a result of marked histaminemia. The remaining animals enrolled on the study were premedicated with steroids and antihistamines. No further reactions of this type were encountered. Similar premedication regimens are also being used in subsequent human trials. Dose-limiting toxicities (DLTs) included neutropenia (2 DLTs each at 0.93 and 1.0 mg/kg) and hepatic necrosis in 1 patient at 1.0 mg/kg after the second course. It is not clear whether the necrosis was caused by drug, as there were no increases in liver enzymes in this patient after the first treatment. The median temperature achieved for all cycles was 41.2°C, and the median 10th percentile of the temperature distribution was 39.5°C. Temperatures achieved in the tumors were adequate to initiate drug release from LTSL-Dox. A total of 20 of the dogs had at least 2 cycles of treatment. Of these dogs, 12 achieved stable disease, and 6 had a partial response to treatment.

HUMAN CLINICAL STUDIES WITH LTSL-DOX

The first clinical trials conducted with LTSL-Dox were in patients with liver metastases or HCC.[1,74] Until now, we have focused on developing a drug formulation that performs well for an hour of heating in the temperature range from 39.5°C to 42°C, whereas thermal ablation temperatures are typically more than 50°C for a few minutes. After the publication of the antitumor effects of the LTSL-Dox,[42] Dr Dewhirst was contacted by Bradford Wood, an interventional radiologist at the National Institutes of Health (NIH). Wood suggested that this formulation might have usefulness in the treatment of liver metastases and in primary liver cancer, if it were combined with RF-mediated thermal ablation. The rationale for the combination of thermal ablation with LTSL-Dox comes from the risk of marginal recurrence, as discussed earlier.[1] Temperatures at the margins of lesions greater than 3 cm are not high enough to cause thermal coagulation, but they are in the range for drug release by LTSL-Dox. The concept is that any residual cells not killed directly by ablation would be killed by massive amounts of doxorubicin deposited there.

Subsequently, the first studies on humans were conducted at the NIH, in collaboration with the commercial developer. Later, the phase 1 study was expanded to include a site in Hong Kong, and additional Asian sites were added.[74,75]

Pharmacokinetics properties and MTD were determined in a phase 1 dose escalation study.[75] Based on the plasma concentration–time curve, Poon and colleagues[74] optimized the dose levels and treatment timing so that tumor ablation occurred during the peak plasma concentration. The phase 1 trials clearly showed that residual cancer cells remaining after ablation were killed with LTSL-Dox treatment. First, the imageable lesions tended to become larger after combined treatment (**Fig. 6**), whereas with RF ablation alone, they tended to shrink. In addition, the median time to progression for patients receiving the MTD (50 mg/m^2) was 374 days, versus 80 days for patients receiving less than the MTD ($P = .03$). Lesions smaller than 3 cm are effectively treated with RF ablation alone, and tumors with metastases beyond the liver would not be suitable for a local treatment but are candidates for systemic chemotherapy.

Based on positive phase 1 results, the US Food and Drug Administration permitted the company to move directly to a randomized, double-blind phase 3 trial, which compared RF ablation alone with RF ablation with LTSL-Dox.[76] This trial was completed recently, with 700 patients accrued (NCT00617981).

FUTURE DIRECTIONS

In addition to treating liver cancers, LTSL-Dox has been used in combination with local hyperthermia in 2 phase 1 trials of chest wall recurrences of breast cancer.[77] One trial

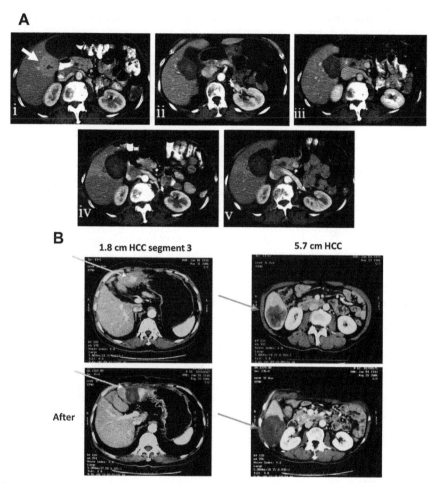

Fig. 6. Contrast-enhanced computed tomography scans of hepatic lesions, before and after RF ablation, combined with LTLD. (*A*) Appearance of metastatic adrenal cell carcinoma, before and several months after thermal ablation. Note that the ablation zone enlarges and stabilizes after treatment. (*i*) Before treatment (*arrow*), (*ii*) 3 days after treatment, (*iii*) 4 weeks after treatment, (*iv*) 11 weeks after treatment, (*v*) 20 weeks after treatment. (*B*) Appearance of 2 primary HCCs, before and after thermal ablation. (*Courtesy of* Brad Wood and Celsion Corporation, Lawrenceville, NJ; Images (*i*), (*ii*), and (*v*) in (*A*) Reprinted from Wood BJ, Poon RT, Locklin JK, et al. Phase I study of heat-deployed liposomal doxorubicin during radiofrequency ablation for hepatic malignancies. J Vasc Interv Radiol 2012;23(2):248–55.e7, with permission from author and publisher; and Images (*iii*) and (*iv*) in (*A*) were kindly provided by the Celsion Corporation.)

was conducted at Duke University, and the second was sponsored by the company that licensed the drug (NCT00826085). Results of those 2 trials are being combined, and a report will be submitted for publication soon. A phase 2 trial is being developed as a follow-on study. Other indications for this drug formulation are being considered. The company recently announced a collaborative agreement with Philips Corporation to test the drug in combination with HIFU for the treatment of bone metastases.

If the LTSL could be used to deliver other common anticancer agents or the newer targeted agents, the applicability of this technology could be expanded. Formulations are typically restricted to drugs that are relatively water-soluble so that the drug can remain encapsulated inside the liposome. We are currently developing LTSL-cisplatin, which could have broader applications in gastrointestinal cancer if it performs as well as LTSL-Dox.

Technologies are available that are capable of heating deep-seated tumors, such as pancreatic and colorectal cancer. The RF phased array systems of the BSD Corporation can heat these deep-seated tumors to the temperature ranges needed for local-regional drug delivery with LTSLs.[78–80] Trials could be envisioned that would combine LTSL-cisplatin with other chemotherapy and radiation for locally advanced rectal cancer and pancreatic cancer, for example. To take full advantage of such promising approaches requires substantial commercial support. This support has been sorely lacking for thermotherapy trials, aside from the phase 3 trial with LTSL-Dox referred to earlier. Lack of strong commercial support has made it challenging to conduct these types of clinical trials in the United States. On the other hand, insurance coverage for this modality is strong in Europe, and several well-organized trials have been completed there.[81–83]

ACKNOWLEDGMENTS

Work supported by a grant from the NIH-NCI CA42745. The author thanks Celsion Corporation for the computed tomography images provided for **Fig. 6**.

REFERENCES

1. Poon R, Borys N. Lyso-thermosensitive liposomal doxorubicin: a novel approach to enhance efficacy of thermal ablation of liver cancer. Expert Opin Pharmacother 2009;10(2):333–43.
2. Lencioni R, Crocetti L, Cioni D, et al. Percutaneous radiofrequency ablation of hepatic colorectal metastases–technique, indications, results, and new promises. Invest Radiol 2004;39(11):689–97.
3. Solbiati L, Livraghi T, Goldberg SN, et al. Percutaneous radio-frequency ablation of hepatic metastases from colorectal cancer: long-term results in 117 patients. Radiology 2001;221(1):159–66.
4. Stauffer PR, Diederich CJ, Seegenschmiedt MH. Interstitial heating technologies. In: Seegenschmiedt MH, Fessenden P, Vernon CC, editors. Thermoradiotherapy and thermochemotherapy: volume 1, biology, physiology and physics. Berlin, New York: Springer-Verlag; 1995. p. 279–320.
5. Stauffer PR, Goldberg SN. Introduction: thermal ablation therapy. Int J Hyperthermia 2004;20(7):671–7.
6. Schirmang TC, Dupuy DE. Image-guided thermal ablation of nonresectable hepatic tumors using the Cool-Tip radiofrequency ablation system. Expert Rev Med Devices 2007;4(6):803–14.
7. Koda M, Tokunaga S, Matono T, et al. Comparison between different thickness umbrella-shaped expandable radiofrequency electrodes (SuperSlim and CoAccess): experimental and clinical study. Exp Ther Med 2011;2(6):1215–20.
8. Lencioni R, Crocetti L. Image-guided ablation for hepatocellular carcinoma. Recent Results Cancer Res 2013;190:181–94.
9. Liu Y, Zheng Y, Li S, et al. Percutaneous microwave ablation of larger hepatocellular carcinoma. Clin Radiol 2013;68(1):21–6.
10. Andreano A, Huang Y, Meloni MF, et al. Microwaves create larger ablations than radiofrequency when controlled for power in ex vivo tissue. Med Phys 2010;37(6): 2967–73.

11. Brace CL. Radiofrequency and microwave ablation of the liver, lung, kidney, and bone: what are the differences? Curr Probl Diagn Radiol 2009;38(3):135–43.
12. Pacella CM, Francica G, Di Costanzo GG. Laser ablation for small hepatocellular carcinoma. Radiol Res Pract 2011;2011:595627.
13. Francica G, Petrolati A, Di Stasio E, et al. Influence of ablative margin on local tumor progression and survival in patients with HCC </=4 cm after laser ablation. Acta Radiol 2012;53(4):394–400.
14. Vogl TJ, Jost A, Nour-Eldin NA, et al. Repeated transarterial chemoembolisation using different chemotherapeutic drug combinations followed by MR-guided laser-induced thermotherapy in patients with liver metastases of colorectal carcinoma. Br J Cancer 2012;106(7):1274–9.
15. Cheung TT, Chu FS, Jenkins CR, et al. Tolerance of high-intensity focused ultrasound ablation in patients with hepatocellular carcinoma. World J Surg 2012; 36(10):2420–7.
16. Staruch R, Chopra R, Hynynen K. Localised drug release using MRI-controlled focused ultrasound hyperthermia. Int J Hyperthermia 2011;27(2):156–71.
17. Wijlemans JW, Bartels LW, Deckers R, et al. Magnetic resonance-guided high-intensity focused ultrasound (MR-HIFU) ablation of liver tumours. Cancer Imaging 2012;12(2):387–94.
18. Widmann G, Schullian P, Haidu M, et al. Stereotactic radiofrequency ablation (SRFA) of liver lesions: technique effectiveness, safety, and interoperator performance. Cardiovasc Intervent Radiol 2012;35(3):570–80.
19. Hahn GM, Strande DP. Cytotoxic effects of hyperthermia and adriamycin on Chinese hamster cells. J Natl Cancer Inst 1976;57(5):1063–7.
20. Overgaard J. Combined adriamycin and hyperthermia treatment of a murine mammary carcinoma in vivo. Cancer Res 1976;36(9 Pt 1):3077–81.
21. Rotstein LE, Daly J, Rozsa P. Systemic thermochemotherapy in a rat model. Can J Surg 1983;26(2):113–6.
22. Haas GP, Klugo RC, Hetzel FW, et al. The synergistic effect of hyperthermia and chemotherapy on murine transitional cell-carcinoma. J Urol 1984;132(4):828–33.
23. Dahl O. Hyperthermic potentiation of doxorubicin and 4'-epi-doxorubicin in a transplantable neurogenic rat tumor (BT4A) in BD IX rats. Int J Radiat Oncol Biol Phys 1983;9(2):203–7.
24. Mostafa EM, Ganguli S, Faintuch S, et al. Optimal strategies for combining transcatheter arterial chemoembolization and radiofrequency ablation in rabbit VX2 hepatic tumors. J Vasc Interv Radiol 2008;19(12):1740–8.
25. Gabizon A, Peretz T, Sulkes A, et al. Systemic administration of doxorubicin-containing liposomes in cancer patients: a phase I study. Eur J Cancer Clin Oncol 1989;25(12):1795–803.
26. Safra T, Muggia F, Jeffers S, et al. Pegylated liposomal doxorubicin (Doxil): reduced clinical cardiotoxicity in patients reaching or exceeding cumulative doses of 500 mg/m(2). Ann Oncol 2000;11(8):1029–33.
27. Landon CD, Park JY, Needham D, et al. Nanoscale drug delivery and dyperthermia: the materials design and preclinical and clinical testing of low temperature-sensitive liposomes used in combination with mild hyperthermia in the treatment of local cancer. Open Nanomed J 2011;3:38–64.
28. Gregoriadis G. Engineering liposomes for drug delivery: progress and problems. Trends Biotechnol 1995;13(12):527–37.
29. Li X, Hirsh DJ, Cabral-Lilly D, et al. Doxorubicin physical state in solution and inside liposomes loaded via a pH gradient. Biochim Biophys Acta 1998; 1415(1):23–40.

30. Ahmed M, Liu Z, Lukyanov AN, et al. Combination radiofrequency ablation with intratumoral liposomal doxorubicin: effect on drug accumulation and coagulation in multiple tissues and tumor types in animals. Radiology 2005;235(2):469–77.

31. Ahmed M, Lukyanov AN, Torchilin V, et al. Combined radiofrequency ablation and adjuvant liposomal chemotherapy: effect of chemotherapeutic agent, nanoparticle size, and circulation time. J Vasc Interv Radiol 2005;16(10):1365–71.

32. Ahmed M, Monsky WE, Girnun G, et al. Radiofrequency thermal ablation sharply increases intratumoral liposomal doxorubicin accumulation and tumor coagulation. Cancer Res 2003;63(19):6327–33.

33. D'Ippolito G, Ahmed M, Girnun GD, et al. Percutaneous tumor ablation: reduced tumor growth with combined radio-frequency ablation and liposomal doxorubicin in a rat breast tumor model. Radiology 2003;228(1):112–8.

34. Goldberg SN, Girnan GD, Lukyanov AN, et al. Percutaneous tumor ablation: increased necrosis with combined radio-frequency ablation and intravenous liposomal doxorubicin in a rat breast tumor model. Radiology 2002;222(3): 797–804.

35. Goldberg SN, Kamel IR, Kruskal JB, et al. Radiofrequency ablation of hepatic tumors: increased tumor destruction with adjuvant liposomal doxorubicin therapy. Am J Roentgenol 2002;179(1):93–101.

36. Solazzo S, Mertyna P, Peddi H, et al. RF ablation with adjuvant therapy: comparison of external beam radiation and liposomal doxorubicin on ablation efficacy in an animal tumor model. Int J Hyperthermia 2008;24(7):560–7.

37. Ahmed M, Goldberg SN. Combination radiofrequency thermal ablation and adjuvant IV liposomal doxorubicin increases tissue coagulation and intratumoural drug accumulation. Int J Hyperthermia 2004;20(7):781–802.

38. Ahmed M, Moussa M, Goldberg SN. Synergy in cancer treatment between liposomal chemotherapeutics and thermal ablation. Chem Phys Lipids 2012;165(4): 424–37.

39. Solazzo SA, Ahmed M, Schor-Bardach R, et al. Liposomal doxorubicin increases radiofrequency ablation-induced tumor destruction by increasing cellular oxidative and nitrative stress and accelerating apoptotic pathways. Radiology 2010; 255(1):62–74.

40. Gasselhuber A, Dreher MR, Negussie A, et al. Mathematical spatio-temporal model of drug delivery from low temperature sensitive liposomes during radiofrequency tumour ablation. Int J Hyperthermia 2010;26(5):499–513.

41. Kong G, Dewhirst MW. Hyperthermia and liposomes. Int J Hyperthermia 1999; 15(5):345–70.

42. Kong G, Anyarambhatla G, Petros WP, et al. Efficacy of liposomes and hyperthermia in a human tumor xenograft model: importance of triggered drug release. Cancer Res 2000;60(24):6950–7.

43. Needham D, Anyarambhatla G, Kong G, et al. A new temperature-sensitive liposome for use with mild hyperthermia: characterization and testing in a human tumor xenograft model. Cancer Res 2000;60(5):1197–201.

44. Koning GA, Eggermont AM, Lindner LH, et al. Hyperthermia and thermosensitive liposomes for improved delivery of chemotherapeutic drugs to solid tumors. Pharm Res 2010;27(8):1750–4.

45. Weinstein JN, Magin RL, Yatvin MB, et al. Liposomes and local hyperthermia: selective delivery of methotrexate to heated tumors. Science 1979;204(4389): 188–91.

46. Yatvin MB, Weinstein JN, Dennis WH, et al. Design of liposomes for enhanced local release of drugs by hyperthermia. Science 1978;202(4374):1290–3.

47. Yatvin MB, Muhlensiepen H, Porschen W, et al. Selective delivery of liposome-associated cis-dichlorodiammineplatinum(II) by heat and its influence on tumor drug uptake and growth. Cancer Res 1981;41(5):1602–7.
48. Yatvin MB, Cree TC, Tegmo-Larsson IM, et al. Liposomes as drug carriers in cancer therapy: hyperthermia and pH sensitivity as modalities for targeting. Strahlentherapie 1984;160(12):732–40.
49. Gaber MH, Hong K, Huang SK, et al. Thermosensitive sterically stabilized liposomes: formulation and in vitro studies on mechanism of doxorubicin release by bovine serum and human plasma. Pharm Res 1995;12(10):1407–16.
50. Papahadjopoulos D, Allen TM, Gabizon A, et al. Sterically stabilized liposomes–improvements in pharmacokinetics and antitumor therapeutic efficacy. Proc Natl Acad Sci U S A 1991;88(24):11460–4.
51. Gaber MH, Wu NZ, Hong K, et al. Thermosensitive liposomes: extravasation and release of contents in tumor microvascular networks. Int J Radiat Oncol Biol Phys 1996;36(5):1177–87.
52. Dewhirst MW, Vujaskovic Z, Jones E, et al. Re-setting the biologic rationale for thermal therapy. Int J Hyperthermia 2005;21(8):779–90.
53. Lindner LH, Eichhorn ME, Eibl H, et al. Novel temperature-sensitive liposomes with prolonged circulation time. Clin Cancer Res 2004;10(6):2168–78.
54. Hossann M, Wiggenhorn M, Schwerdt A, et al. In vitro stability and content release properties of phosphatidylglyceroglycerol containing thermosensitive liposomes. Biochim Biophys Acta 2007;1768(10):2491–9.
55. Hossann M, Syunyaeva Z, Schmidt R, et al. Proteins and cholesterol lipid vesicles are mediators of drug release from thermosensitive liposomes. J Control Release 2012;162(2):400–6.
56. Dicheva BM, Hagen TL, Li L, et al. Cationic thermosensitive liposomes: a novel dual targeted heat-triggered drug delivery approach for endothelial and tumor cells. Nano Lett 2012. [Epub ahead of print].
57. Manzoor AA, Lindner LH, Landon CD, et al. Overcoming limitations in nanoparticle drug delivery: triggered, intravascular release to improve drug penetration into tumors. Cancer Res 2012;72(21):5566–75.
58. Kono K. Thermosensitive polymer-modified liposomes. Adv Drug Deliv Rev 2001; 53(3):307–19.
59. Ruel-Gariepy E, Leclair G, Hildgen P, et al. Thermosensitive chitosan-based hydrogel containing liposomes for the delivery of hydrophilic molecules. J Control Release 2002;82(2–3):373–83.
60. Kono K, Nakai R, Morimoto K, et al. Thermosensitive polymer-modified liposomes that release contents around physiological temperature. Biochim Biophys Acta 1999;1416(1–2):239–50.
61. Pradhan P, Giri J, Rieken F, et al. Targeted temperature sensitive magnetic liposomes for thermo-chemotherapy. J Control Release 2010;142(1):108–21.
62. Unezaki S, Maruyama K, Takahashi N, et al. Enhanced delivery and antitumor-activity of doxorubicin using long-circulating thermosensitive liposomes containing amphipathic polyethylene-glycol in combination with local hyperthermia. Pharm Res 1994;11(8):1180–5.
63. Yarmolenko PS, Zhao Y, Landon C, et al. Comparative effects of thermosensitive doxorubicin-containing liposomes and hyperthermia in human and murine tumours. Int J Hyperthermia 2010;26(5):485–98.
64. Palmer GM, Boruta RJ, Viglianti BL, et al. Non-invasive monitoring of intra-tumor drug concentration and therapeutic response using optical spectroscopy. J Control Release 2010;142(3):457–64.

65. Jung EU, Yoon JH, Lee YJ, et al. Hypoxia and retinoic acid-inducible NDRG1 expression is responsible for doxorubicin and retinoic acid resistance in hepatocellular carcinoma cells. Cancer Lett 2010;298(1):9–15.

66. Ponce AM, Viglianti BL, Yu D, et al. Magnetic resonance imaging of temperature-sensitive liposome release: drug dose painting and antitumor effects. J Natl Cancer Inst 2007;99(1):53–63.

67. Viglianti BL, Ponce AM, Michelich CR, et al. Chemodosimetry of in vivo tumor liposomal drug concentration using MRI. Magn Reson Med 2006;56(5):1011–8.

68. Negussie AH, Yarmolenko PS, Partanen A, et al. Formulation and characterisation of magnetic resonance imageable thermally sensitive liposomes for use with magnetic resonance-guided high intensity focused ultrasound. Int J Hyperthermia 2011;27(2):140–55.

69. de Smet M, Heijman E, Langereis S, et al. Magnetic resonance imaging of high intensity focused ultrasound mediated drug delivery from temperature-sensitive liposomes: an in vivo proof-of-concept study. J Control Release 2011;150(1): 102–10.

70. Peller M, Schwerdt A, Hossann M, et al. MR characterization of mild hyperthermia-induced gadodiamide release from thermosensitive liposomes in solid tumors. Invest Radiol 2008;43(12):877–92.

71. Ranjan A, Jacobs GC, Woods DL, et al. Image-guided drug delivery with magnetic resonance guided high intensity focused ultrasound and temperature sensitive liposomes in a rabbit Vx2 tumor model. J Control Release 2012; 158(3):487–94.

72. Chen Q, Tong S, Dewhirst MW, et al. Targeting tumor microvessels using doxorubicin encapsulated in a novel thermosensitive liposome. Mol Cancer Ther 2004; 3(10):1311–7.

73. Hauck ML, LaRue SM, Petros WP, et al. Phase I trial of doxorubicin-containing low temperature sensitive liposomes in spontaneous canine tumors. Clin Cancer Res 2006;12(13):4004–10.

74. Poon RT, Borys N. Lyso-thermosensitive liposomal doxorubicin: an adjuvant to increase the cure rate of radiofrequency ablation in liver cancer. Future Oncol 2011;7(8):937–45.

75. Wood BJ, Poon RT, Locklin JK, et al. Phase I study of heat-deployed liposomal doxorubicin during radiofrequency ablation for hepatic malignancies. J Vasc Interv Radiol 2012;23(2):248–255.e7.

76. Celsion. Phase 3 study of ThermoDox with radiofrequency ablation (RFA) in treatment of hepatocellular carcinoma (HCC). Bethesda (MD): National Library of Medicine (US); 2011. Available at: ClinicalTrials.gov [Internet] [Accessed June 15, 2012].

77. Celsion. Phase 1/2 study of ThermoDox with approved hyperthermia in treatment of breast cancer recurrence at the chest wall (DIGNITY). Bethesda (MD): National Library of Medicine (US); 2012. Available at: ClinicalTrials.gov [Internet] [Accessed June 15, 2012].

78. Jones EL, Samulski TV, Dewhirst MW, et al. A pilot Phase II trial of concurrent radiotherapy, chemotherapy, and hyperthermia for locally advanced cervical carcinoma. Cancer 2003;98(2):277–82.

79. Rau B, Wust P, Hohenberger P, et al. Preoperative hyperthermia combined with radiochemotherapy in locally advanced rectal cancer: a phase II clinical trial. Ann Surg 1998;227(3):380–9.

80. de Wit R, van der Zee J, van der Burg ME, et al. A phase I/II study of combined weekly systemic cisplatin and locoregional hyperthermia in patients with

previously irradiated recurrent carcinoma of the uterine cervix. Br J Cancer 1999; 80(9):1387–91.

81. van der Zee J, Gonzalez Gonzalez D, van Rhoon GC, et al. Comparison of radiotherapy alone with radiotherapy plus hyperthermia in locally advanced pelvic tumours: a prospective, randomised, multicentre trial. Dutch Deep Hyperthermia Group. Lancet 2000;355(9210):1119–25.

82. Issels RD, Lindner LH, Verweij J, et al. Neo-adjuvant chemotherapy alone or with regional hyperthermia for localised high-risk soft-tissue sarcoma: a randomised phase 3 multicentre study. Lancet Oncol 2010;11(6):561–70.

83. Overgaard J, Gonzalez Gonzalez D, Hulshof MC, et al. Randomised trial of hyperthermia as adjuvant to radiotherapy for recurrent or metastatic malignant melanoma. European Society for Hyperthermic Oncology. Lancet 1995;345(8949): 540–3.

Radiotherapy After Mastectomy

Rachel C. Blitzblau, MD, PhD*, Janet K. Horton, MD

KEYWORDS

- Breast cancer • Mastectomy • Radiotherapy • Biologic subtype

KEY POINTS

- Breast cancer biologic subtype is an important predictor of locoregional recurrence (LRR) and should be considered, along with tumor–node–metastasis (TNM) parameters, in the determination of benefit from postmastectomy radiotherapy (PMRT).
- The biology of node-negative tumors greater than or equal to 5 cm is heterogeneous. Tumor size alone is likely insufficient to estimate degree of benefit from PMRT.
- LRR risk in early-stage patients after mastectomy is generally low. Patients with multiple risk factors, however, in particular those with triple-negative tumors, may derive benefit from PMRT. Clinical trials are needed to establish this benefit.
- Early data link gene expression to risk of LRR and demonstrate promise as a future predictive tool.
- The role of chemotherapy response biomarkers in predicting LRR is incompletely understood. Until additional data are available, a combination of clinical and pathologic staging parameters should be considered.

INTRODUCTION

PMRT has long been a component of comprehensive breast cancer management, particularly in the setting of locally advanced disease. Historic trials from Denmark and British Columbia enrolled a large number of primarily node-positive patients to evaluate the use of PMRT in a randomized fashion. Both local control and overall survival (OS) rates were significantly improved with the use of radiotherapy (RT).[1,2] As described extensively in the past, however, these trials had significant problems that limit their applicability to present-day practice. In particular, modern nodal staging and imaging techniques have resulted in significant stage migration. In combination with advances in cytotoxic chemotherapy and endocrine therapy as well as the advent of targeted therapy, extrapolating the extent of recurrence risk from these landmark trials is difficult.

Department of Radiation Oncology, Duke University Medical Center, Box 3085, Durham, NC 27710, USA
* Corresponding author.
E-mail address: rachel.blitzblau@duke.edu

Surg Oncol Clin N Am 22 (2013) 563–577
http://dx.doi.org/10.1016/j.soc.2013.02.012
1055-3207/13/$ – see front matter © 2013 Elsevier Inc. All rights reserved.

Many subsequent series have suggested that the modern risk of LRR is substantially lower than previously reported in both breast-conserving and postmastectomy settings.[3–6] This is particularly relevant in the ongoing effort to maintain a desirable benefit/risk ratio such that patients obtain maximum tumor control at a minimum cost. RT, however, is also radically different from that used in the classic trials and evidence suggests that morbidity is decreasing.[7,8] The 2005 update of the Early Breast Cancer Trialists' Collaborative Group[8] meta-analysis revealed that the benefit in breast cancer survival attributable to the use of RT has translated into OS, in contrast to prior reports in which the breast cancer–specific survival benefit from RT was offset by a near-equal increase in treatment-related mortality. These data suggest that for every 4 local recurrences that are prevented, 1 life is saved. This supports a more generous use of RT when the locoregional risk is intermediate or high. Even within the context of this positive RT impact, however, the data also suggest that there is a point of diminishing returns (ie, when the local recurrence risk becomes sufficiently low, the benefit of therapy does not outweigh the risks) (**Fig. 1**).

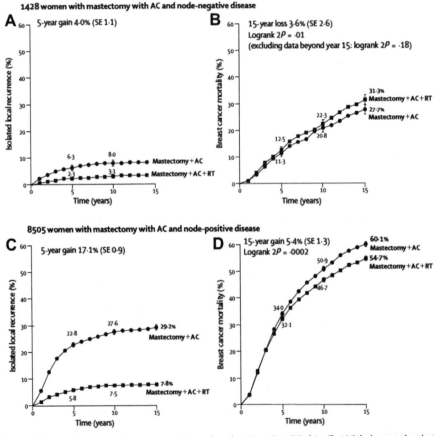

Fig. 1. RT produces consistent proportional reductions in LRR (*A, C*). With large absolute benefits, breast cancer mortality decreases (*D*). Treatment toxicity may outweigh gains, however, in patients with small absolute locoregional benefits (*B*). AC, axillary clearance. (*From* Clarke M, Collins R, Darby S, et al. Effects of radiotherapy and of differences in the extent of surgery for early breast cancer on local recurrence and 15-year survival: an overview of the randomized trials. Lancet 2005;366(9503):2087–106; with permission.)

Therefore, radiation oncologists must carefully estimate a patient's starting risk of LRR in order to ascertain the benefit of therapy. Classically, this risk has been defined largely by TNM parameters. In the past decade, however, understanding of breast cancer biology has radically changed. Tumor size and nodal involvement are now joined by biologic subtypes that drive prognosis and therapy. This section explores the impact of these changes on the prescription of locoregional RT.

CHANGING PARADIGM

In addition to advances in therapeutics, understanding of breast cancer as a disease has been transformed by work published in 2000 by Perou and colleagues.[9] Several distinct subtypes of breast cancer were identified with unique patterns of gene expression. These have subsequently proved both prognostic and predictive.[9] These subtypes have so significantly changed the approach that clinical trials evaluating systemic therapy are often now typically developed for a specific subtype. This has allowed further development of biomarkers, such as chemotherapy response, to be incorporated into routine practice. Although TMN staging remains a critical part of determining outcomes and need for therapy, tumor biology plays an equally important role.

Data have only recently started to emerge, however, on the impact of tumor biology on LRR risk. In 2008, Nguyen and colleagues[10] published one of the first articles addressing the impact of the 4 main breast cancer subtypes on local recurrence after breast-conserving therapy (BCT). Both human epidermal growth factor receptor 2 (HER2)-positive and basal subtypes demonstrated a higher risk of recurrence than the more favorable luminal subtypes. Subsequently, multiple additional series have verified this finding in both postmastectomy and breast conservation scenarios.[10–12] These series seem to suggest that the subtypes may be both prognostic in regards to risk of local recurrence and predictive in evaluating the benefit of RT. Kyndi and coworkers[12] demonstrated that the subgroup of patients with steroid receptor negativity with or without HER2 positivity experienced smaller improvements in local control with the addition of radiation. As a result, the survival benefit attributable to radiation was only seen in the more favorable subgroups. These data predate, however, modern systemic and targeted therapy such that competing systemic risks likely mask any radiation benefit.

A similar effect can be seen in a more modern series evaluating approximately 3000 patients who underwent mastectomy (only 25% received RT) or BCT (all received RT).[11] In patients treated with mastectomy, molecular subtype clearly predicted risk of local recurrence. These differences should largely have disappeared in the breast-conserving group, where all patients received RT, if all of the breast cancer subtypes were equally responsive to RT. Instead, a pattern of subtype-specific locoregional risk persists, suggesting that there are inherent differences in a priori risk as well as variability in radiation response among the breast cancer subtypes (**Fig. 2**).

These data, in conjunction with what has been learned about the impact of biologic subtype on chemotherapy response, suggest that revisiting the approach to PMRT may be in order. The classic distinctions of nodal involvement and tumor size may no longer be sufficient, in isolation, to guide therapeutic decision making. Although it is unlikely that the classic trials will be repeated by specific biologic subtypes, at the least this biologic information needs to be incorporated into future radiation clinical trials. Patients with early-stage disease, previously considered ineligible for PMRT, may benefit at much earlier stages, and some patients with more advanced disease but favorable biology may not require adjuvant RT. In addition, high-risk patients with aggressive biology may require some form of radiosensitization in order to gain

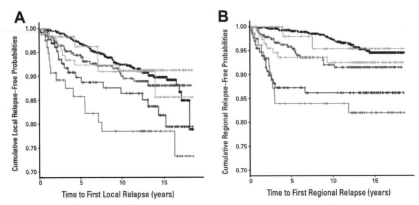

Fig. 2. Risk of local recurrence according to biologic subtype in patients treated with mastectomy (*A*) and BCT (*B*). A clear impact of biologic subtype on recurrence risk is seen, with or without postsurgical radiotherapy. Violet line, luminal A; light blue line, luminal HER2; dark blue line, luminal B; gold line, five-marker–negative phenotype; red line, basal; and beige line, HER2 enriched. (*From* Voduc KD, Cheang MC, Tyldesley S, et al. Breast cancer subtypes and the risk of local and regional relapse. J Clin Oncol 2010;28(10):1684–91; with permission.)

the full benefit of therapy whereas those with favorable biology may benefit from strategies designed to limit radiation toxicity.

RISK STRATIFICATION IN NODE-NEGATIVE CANCER

PMRT has not traditionally been offered for patients with node-negative disease, except in the case of T3/4 tumors or positive margins. A 2005 survey conducted in North America and Europe showed that 88.8% of American Radiation Oncologists and 84.8% of European Radiation Oncologists would offer PMRT to patients with T3N0 breast cancer.[13] Data are available, however, that question both the automatic use of RT in the setting of T3 disease and the automatic exclusion of RT in the setting of T1/2N0 disease with certain biologic risk factors.

T3N0

The T3N0 subgroup of breast cancer patients is small, comprising approximately 1% of new breast cancer diagnoses,[14] so there are few data sets to guide clinical practice. In support of adjuvant therapy, in node-negative patients enrolled in the Danish 82b and 82c postmastectomy radiation trials, PMRT resulted in a substantial reduction in risk of LRR—5% versus 22% in 82b, and 6% versus 23% in 82c.[15,16] One caveat frequently noted regarding these trials, however, is that their overall LRR rates in all subsets are higher than in many modern series. Additionally, the median number of nodes in the axillary dissection was lower than is now considered standard, the systemic therapy was older, and T4 tumors were included. Nonetheless, there was a benefit to RT in this subgroup. Another small study evaluated 38 patients with T3N0 disease and found an overall LRR of 16% at 5 years—9% with RT and 60% without RT.[14] Again this is a small study, as expected with such a limited patient group, so generalizations are difficult.

In contrast, a retrospective analysis of 313 patients with node-negative tumors greater than or equal to 5 cm enrolled in 5 National Surgical Adjuvant Breast and Bowel Project (NSABP) clinical trials, treated from 1981 to 1998 with mastectomy but without RT, noted a low incidence of locoregional failure of 7.1% at

10 years[4]; 74.5% of patients had some form of systemic therapy, and this seemed to decrease LRR risk, because the rate was 12.6% in patients who received no systemic therapy versus 4.6% to 5.6% in patients who received chemotherapy and/or tamoxifen; 24 of 28 recurrences were on the chest wall. Similarly, a multi-institutional retrospective series of patients with node-negative tumors greater than or equal to 5 cm treated from 1981 to 2002 identified 70 patients treated with mastectomy and adjuvant systemic therapy but no RT[17]; 57% of patients had some form of systemic therapy. The investigators noted a 5-year LRR rate of 7.6%, with 4 of 5 failures on the chest wall. Lymphovascular invasion (LVI) was significantly associated with LRR risk as well as with disease-free survival and OS in univariate and multivariate analysis.

Goulart and colleauges[18] reported outcomes for 100 patients with node-negative tumors greater than or equal to 5 cm treated from 1989 to 2000 with mastectomy, with or without PMRT. The cumulative 10-year LRR was 2.3% with PMRT and 8.9% without PMRT. For the subset of patients with grade 3 histology and no PMRT, however, the LRR rate at 10 years was 17%; 4 of 6 recurrences were on the chest wall. Approximately 50% of patients had chemotherapy, and 50% had hormonal therapy. One factor that may limit applicability of these data is that all 3 of these studies were significantly weighted toward the lower end of the size spectrum, with 46%, 34%, and 28% of patients having 5.0 cm tumors, respectively. They highlight, however, a population of large tumors with low LRR rates after PMRT, particularly if systemic therapy is used.

Overall, the conflicting data suggest that the biology of tumors greater than 5 cm varies and that this is a heterogeneous population for which size alone is insufficient to determine LRR risk and benefit of PMRT. Biologically, tumors that grow to a large size without spreading to lymph nodes may in general be less aggressive. Features, such as high grade and LVI, however, may point to a subset with more aggressive biology likely to derive a greater benefit from PMRT. Additionally, PMRT should likely still be strongly considered for patients with tumors significantly larger than 5 cm, because this subset of patients is poorly represented in any data set. Finally, whether or not a patient is eligible for systemic therapy in the form of chemotherapy and/or hormonal therapy should be weighed, because this can mitigate LRR risk as well. In all the data sets, the majority of locoregional failures were confined to the chest wall, suggesting that this is the highest-risk target volume.

T1/2N0

T1/2N0 cancers treated with mastectomy have traditionally been thought of as low risk and, therefore, not warranting consideration of PMRT. A growing set of data question this, however, as an across-the-board approach for all patients. An analysis of women treated from 1981 to 1985, in a randomized trial with mastectomy without PMRT, identified factors associated with LRR in 1275 node-negative patients.[19] Two-thirds of the women received 1 cycle of chemotherapy. In premenopausal women, tumor size greater than 2 cm and vascular invasion (VI) were associated with increased risk for LRR. The LRR rate with no risk factor was 6%, 13% with either factor alone, and 15% with both. In postmenopausal women, VI alone was associated with LRR, with an observed recurrence rate of 6% without VI versus 14% with VI.

Jagsi and colleagues[20] identified 877 patients with T1–T3N0 tumors treated from 1980 to 2000 with mastectomy and axillary node dissection. No patients received PMRT, and T4 tumors were excluded. The cumulative incidence of LRR was 6%. Factors associated with increased LRR risk were tumor size greater than 2 cm, margin less than 2 mm, premenopausal status, and LVI. LRR was 1.2% with no risk factors,

10% with 1 risk factor, 17.9% with 2 risk factors, and 40.6% with 3 risk factors; 80% of failures were on the chest wall. An updated series from the same institution, with 1136 patients treated from 1980 to 2004, showed the association of tumor size greater than 2 cm, LVI, close or positive margin, age less than or equal to 50, and no systemic therapy with increased risk for LRR.[21] LRR was 2.0% with no risk factors versus 19.7% with 3 or more factors. Again, close to 80% of failures were on the chest wall alone.

A series from British Columbia of 1505 women with T1/2N0 cancers treated from 1989 to 1999 with mastectomy and no adjuvant RT reported an overall LRR rate of 7.8%.[22] Approximately half the women had systemic chemotherapy. Histologic grade, LVI, T stage, and systemic therapy use were identified as independent predictors of LRR. High-grade histology as a sole risk factor was associated with an LRR rate of 12.1% versus 5.5% for low grade or intermediate grade. Concomitant LVI increased LRR risk to 21.2%. High tumor grade plus size greater than 2 cm had an LRR of 13.4% with systemic therapy and 23.2% without systemic therapy. To evaluate this further, a subset of 763 women who all received adjuvant systemic therapy after mastectomy was selected from the cohort to evaluate relapse based on the presence or absence of LVI.[23] They found that LVI was associated with significantly higher risk of LRR. If LVI was present in conjunction with age less than 50 years, premenopausal status, grade III histology, or estrogen receptor (ER)-negative disease, the LRR risk increased to 15% to 20%.

Building on these findings, a recent prospective randomized multicenter trial evaluating PMRT restricted eligibility to women with early-stage cancer but triple-negative biology—681 Chinese women were treated with mastectomy plus adjuvant chemotherapy versus chemotherapy plus radiation[24] and 82% of patients had node-negative disease. At a median follow-up of 86.5 months, the recurrence rate with chemotherapy alone was 25.4% versus 11.7% with chemotherapy plus RT. Five-year OS was also significantly improved with the addition of RT, to 90.4% versus 78.7% with chemotherapy alone. Although the degree of radiation benefit likely reflects, in part, a higher-risk patient population (62% of patients were less than or equal to 50 years old, and 18% were node positive) and suboptimal chemotherapy (cyclophosphamide, methotrexate, and 5-fluorouracil), it provides compelling preliminary data for confirmatory clinical trials.

Taken as a whole, the data for T1/2N0 tumors show a low LRR rate when all patients are considered as a group. There are, however, biologic subgroups with significantly higher risk for LRR. A review of the literature and meta-analysis of randomized trials for node-negative tumors treated with mastectomy and no radiation found that LRR risk is increased with grade 3 histology, LVI, tumor size greater than 2 cm, close margins, and premenopausal status or age less than 50,[25] all seen in greater proportions in biologically aggressive tumors. The baseline LRR risk with no risk features is uniformly close to 5% but ranges from 15% to 40% with 2 or more risk factors.

The meta-analysis (discussed previously) showed a large LRR and OS benefit for PMRT. The randomized trials included in the meta-analysis used older or no chemotherapy, lacked data regarding axillary node dissection, or had low median numbers of dissected nodes, and the N0 tumors were often T3. This result is in agreement, however, with the improvement in LRR (and OS) seen in the randomized Chinese trial of adjuvant RT for T1/2N0 triple-negative breast cancer (discussed previously), suggesting that there is a subgroup of node-negative patients who derive significant benefit from PMRT. A majority of LRR seen in all the node-negative data sets are confined to the chest wall, suggesting that treatment of the chest wall alone may be sufficient to mitigate the majority of the LRR risk in these patients.

The biologic factors associated with LRR in node-negative cancers may also be useful for risk stratification in patients with 1 to 3 involved nodes. Several retrospective series have identified features that predict increased LRR risk in patients with 1 to 3 nodes similar to those that predict LRR in node-negative patients,[19,26–31] again supporting the idea that tumor size or nodal status alone is not sufficient to fully define risk. The ongoing Selective Use of Postoperative Radiotherapy after Mastectomy trial randomizes T1/2N0/1 and T3N0 patients with grade 3 histology or LVI to PMRT to the chest wall versus observation. The results of this trial will hopefully yield important information regarding the benefit of PMRT for patients with low-risk T/N stage but high-risk biology as well as the appropriateness of chest wall RT alone.[32]

THE ROLE OF GENOMIC PREDICTION TOOLS

Another developing area of research into prediction of both local and distant recurrence is the use of molecular markers and genomic assays. The data in this area for LRR are still sparse; however, the data for distant recurrence are more mature. The well-known 21-gene assay, Oncotype Dx, has been validated as a prognostic and predictive marker of distant recurrence risk and benefit from chemotherapy.[33,34] This assay is routinely used for decision making regarding use of chemotherapy in node-negative, ER-positive breast cancers. More recent data suggest that this may also be useful in making chemotherapy decisions for node-positive patients.[35] Additionally, a 70-gene assay, called MammaPrint, has been shown predictive of distant recurrence and OS.[36,37] A large randomized multicenter clinical trial is ongoing to validate the use of this assay in predicting benefit of adjuvant chemotherapy.[38]

As the use of such assays has become more prominently used in making systemic therapy decisions, similar markers for LRR are being sought. Chang and colleagues[39] identified 94 patients who were treated with mastectomy without adjuvant RT. They used a subset of the patients as a training cohort and identified a 258-gene profile and a 34-gene profile, which were then validated in a separate cohort. With the 258-gene model, patients with a predictive index of more than 0.8 had a local control probability of 95% versus 46% for those with 0.8 or lower. Using the 34-gene model, the local control probability in patients with a predictive index of more than 0.8 was 91% versus 40% in those with an index of 0.8 or lower. These were both significant, regardless of whether patients were node negative or node positive. The 34-gene model was an independent prognostic factor for LRR in a Cox proportional hazards model, with a hazard ratio of 22 (95% CI, 6–81) in patients with a predictive index of 0.8 or lower.

Nuyten and coworkers[40] also used gene expression profiling to identify genomic signatures that would help predict local recurrence. They used a 70-gene prognosis profile, a wound response signature, and a hypoxia-induced profile. They reported an association of the wound response signature with local recurrence, with a subset of patients with low risk (5%) or high risk (29%) of local recurrence at 10 years. This was an independent predictor of local recurrence on multivariate analysis. A follow-up study that again examined these gene expression profiles, in patients with or without local recurrence after BCT, failed to confirm an association between the wound response signature or any other gene signature tested.[41] The impact of RT on reduction of locoregional risk, however, may have masked the effect of the predictor in this study.

Mamounas and colleauges[42] evaluated the 21-gene recurrence score assay in node-negative, ER-positive breast cancer patients who were enrolled in the NSABP B-14 and B-20 trials. There were 895 tamoxifen-treated patients from the 2 trials,

355 placebo-treated patients from B-14, and 424 chemotherapy plus tamoxifen–treated patients from B-20. They found that in the tamoxifen-treated patients, LRR was significantly associated with recurrence score. Low-risk patients had a recurrence rate of 4.3% versus 7.2% for intermediate-risk scores and 15.8% for those with high-risk scores. The association was also significant in placebo-treated patients and in chemotherapy plus tamoxifen–treated patients, although in the latter group the absolute differences between the groups were smaller due to the impact of systemic therapy on LRR. On multivariate analysis, the recurrence score was an independent predictor of LRR, along with age and type of initial treatment. Correlation with risk score was also noted in the subgroup receiving mastectomy without radiation (**Fig. 3**). Specifically, in mastectomy patients, the 10-year estimates of local recurrence by recurrence score were 2.3% for low-risk patients, 4.7% for intermediate-risk patients, and 16.8% in high-risk patients, with no difference by age.

In patients treated with lumpectomy plus RT, the recurrence score did not correlate well for women older than age 50 (see **Fig. 3**). In these patients with low overall risk, the impact of RT likely obscured any small differences seen among patients with low-risk and high-risk scores. In the younger and, therefore, higher-risk population, however, the recurrence score was successful in predicting locoregional risk. A more recent study of use of biologic subtype and 21-gene recurrence score to predict local recurrence was performed using patients who were enrolled in the randomized Eastern Cooperative Oncology Group E2197 trial comparing 2 adjuvant systemic chemotherapy regimens for patients with BCT.[43] In this study, neither biologic subtype nor 21-gene recurrence score was associated with local recurrence or local regional recurrence on univariate or multivariate analysis in patients receiving modern systemic therapy and BCT.

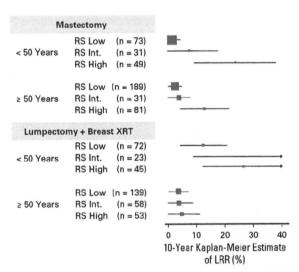

Fig. 3. Kaplan-Meier estimates of 10-year LRR risk by recurrence score (RS), initial local treatment modality, and age in tamoxifen-treated patients enrolled in NASBP B-14 and B-20 trials. After mastectomy, RS correlates with LRR risk at any age. XRT, radiotherapy. (*From* Mamounas EP, Tang G, Fisher B, et al. Association between the 21-gene recurrence score assay and risk of locoregional recurrence in node-negative, estrogen receptor-positive breast cancer: results from NSABP B-14 and NSABP B-20. J Clin Oncol 2010;28(10):1677–83; with permission.)

These studies support the idea that use of a profiling score may be more complicated in the setting of breast conservation with RT and may be further complicated by the impact of modern cytotoxic and targeted therapy. It is unclear how, if at all, this can be extrapolated to the postmastectomy setting. Therefore, additional data exploring this relationship are needed prior to widespread application of these tools. The use of genomic assays shows promise, however, as a future tool for estimating LRR risk and, therefore, RT benefit.

IMPACT OF NEOADJUVANT CHEMOTHERAPY

For many years, patients with breast cancer were treated with surgery first, followed by adjuvant therapy as directed by tumor pathology. This approach has been challenged, however, in recent years. Preoperative, or neoadjuvant, therapy has evolved in an effort to allow a larger percentage of patients to undergo breast-conserving surgery. Although the initial hope for neoadjuvant treatment was to target subclinical micrometastatic disease at an earlier time point and thus improve OS, this concept was not borne out in the earliest randomized trials.[44–46] As a result, in patients who initially desire mastectomy or are deemed ineligible for BCT regardless of treatment response, the role of neoadjuvant chemotherapy is diminished. Nonetheless, some patients undergo neoadjuvant chemotherapy in an unsuccessful attempt at BCT and, in some clinical scenarios, an assessment of response to systemic therapy may be worthwhile.

In these situations, tumor response to neoadjuvant therapy may play a role in determining residual risk of local failure. It has been well documented that pathologic response to chemotherapy identifies a subgroup of patients within the aggressive tumor phenotypes that have more favorable outcomes.[44] As knowledge has evolved about tumor subtypes and their intrinsic response to chemotherapy, some studies have identified a survival benefit for those with greater pathologic complete response rates.[47] In the future, treatment response will likely be used to tailor subsequent therapy. As such, it is likely that neoadjuvant chemotherapy will continue to play a significant role in breast cancer therapy, even for those patients who will not be eligible to keep their breasts.

Therefore, the historic approach to determining the locoregional risk of recurrence must evolve. Classic data reporting the utility of PMRT based on pathologic disease stage are less relevant because patients with HER2-positive and triple-negative breast cancer subtypes can have dramatic responses to chemotherapy, rendering them disease-free and obscuring the initial pathologic stage. The optimal way to interpret clinical and pathologic staging in the determination of LRR remains an area of significant interest and growing data.

Preoperative Nodal Evaluation

Concurrent with the development of neoadjuvant chemotherapy, the approach of preoperative sentinel lymph node evaluation was suggested as a partial solution to obtaining necessary pathologic information for both chemotherapy and RT decision making, while still supporting the major rationale of neoadjuvant chemotherapy (BCT). Those in opposition to this approach, however, argued that the 20% to 40% of women with clearing of axillary disease as a result of neoadjuvant therapy[44] would be committed to an axillary dissection that may not be necessary. Nonetheless, preoperative nodal evaluation was initially highly desirable due to the lack of data on locoregional control after chemotherapy and a greater dependence, at that time, on degree of nodal involvement to determine chemotherapy regimens. As neoadjuvant therapy has matured and significant additional data compiled, the advantages of a preoperative nodal assessment seem less significant. Medical oncologists rely heavily on features of the primary, in particularly biologic subtype and gene expression, to determine their use of cytotoxic treatment. Furthermore, the use of sentinel lymph node evaluation after chemotherapy is becoming more widely accepted.[48] Finally, additional data aiding radiation oncologists in determining risk after chemotherapy response have become available from both institutional reviews and from maturation of randomized trials.[44,49–52] Therefore, in recent years, use of postoperative nodal staging has become more common with incorporation of nodal chemotherapy response into adjuvant RT decision-making.

One critical scenario where this approach can be problematic, however, is when a patient may not otherwise be a candidate for PMRT. For example, consider a patient presenting with a large T2, node-negative, strongly estrogen-driven lobular cancer on preoperative imaging. If the patient were to have either an unsuspected large T3 lesion, as is common in lobular cancers, or nodal involvement not initially detectable on clinical imaging, the patient may require PMRT. In contrast, a patient with a true T2N0 lesion with low-risk biologic features would likely not require treatment. Further complicating this scenario is that the response of lobular carcinomas to neoadjuvant chemotherapy is incompletely understood[53] and, therefore, a large residual cancer burden of unclear significance may be noted at the time of surgical resection. In a strongly ER/PR (progesterone receptor)–positive tumor, this residual cancer burden may or may not be an appropriate biomarker for residual LRR risk but, regardless, leaves radiation oncologists in a difficult situation regarding recommendations for further therapy. As a result, in scenarios where the clinical picture is ambiguous, the benefit from neoadjuvant chemotherapy is less definitive, and the radiation decision is all or nothing, an upfront surgical approach may be desirable. At the least, an initial multidisciplinary evaluation is critical.

Postmastectomy Radiotherapy in the Setting of Neoadjuvant Chemotherapy

The most robust data defining the relationship between chemotherapy response and local control come from the randomized NSABP B-18 and B-27 trials.[54] Briefly, these trials included patients with clinical T1–T3, N0 1 breast tumors. Treatment included neoadjuvant chemotherapy followed by BCT or mastectomy and axillary lymph node dissection. RT was delivered to the breast only after a lumpectomy and was prohibited after mastectomy. Local control, as well as disease-free survival and OS, were comparable in patients treated preoperatively and postoperatively. As with survival outcomes, however, response to chemotherapy was predictive of LRR. Patients with residual nodal disease after chemotherapy had a 14.6% rate of LRR at 8 years, whereas those with no residual nodal disease but residual disease in the breast had an LRR rate of 8.4%, and those with a pathologic complete response had only a 6.6% risk of recurrence. This pattern was true in patients treated with breast-conserving surgery as well as those undergoing mastectomy.

Several other groups have also reported outcomes for their patients undergoing neoadjuvant therapy. In 2006, investigators at MD Anderson Cancer Center formulated a prognostic index that helped identify those at significant residual risk of LRR: clinical N2-3 disease, LVI, residual primary tumor greater than 2 cm, and multifocal residual disease. This mix of clinical and pathologic factors was meaningful in the setting of breast conservation as well as mastectomy.[55]

A separate MD Anderson series looked at those with advanced disease (stage III) who had a complete response to chemotherapy. Although only a few patients fell into this subgroup, the risk of recurrence after mastectomy remained high despite a robust chemotherapy response.[50] Nagar and colleaugues[49] restricted their series to a somewhat lower-risk subgroup, including patients with clinical T3N0 tumors, and evaluated the impact of treatment response in this subgroup. In general, there was a benefit to PMRT in this cohort (24% risk of recurrence in those not receiving treatment vs 4% in those treated), but residual pathologic nodal involvement again predicted for residual risk because those with negative nodes after chemotherapy had only a 14% risk of recurrence. This was reduced to 2% with the use of PMRT, but the improvement was not significant. Similarly, 134 patients at the Institut Curie with clinical stage II/III disease and no residual nodal involvement after neoadjuvant therapy had no significant increase in locoregional control after PMRT.[52]

The validity of chemotherapy response as a biomarker for response in all biologic subtypes must also be considered. Excellent response to chemotherapy may identify a more favorable subset of patients who may not need locoregional treatment but additional data are needed. In contrast, patients with biologically more indolent tumors may not have a robust response to chemotherapy but, nevertheless, their residual risk may not be significant enough to justify the use of PMRT.

In 2008, a National Cancer Institute Statement of the Science Conference was convened to address the controversies surrounding preoperative therapy. Recommendations regarding the use of PMRT after neoadjuvant chemotherapy were formulated at that time and are still relevant. It seems that patients with clinical stage III disease benefit from PMRT regardless of response to chemotherapy. Similarly, the benefits of PMRT seem to outweigh the risks in those with residual nodal involvement after chemotherapy. The benefit of treatment in those with clinical stage II disease and no nodal involvement at the time of surgery, however, is less clear. At present, both clinical and pathologic parameters remain important determinants of treatment benefit. For those with uncertain benefit, treatment in a clinical trial is ideal and, otherwise, must be individually tailored.

SUMMARY

Appropriate selection of patients who derive a significant benefit from PMRT continues to be a challenging and debated topic. The primary driving force for selection of patients is the estimated risk of LRR. Although historical series show a benefit for adjuvant RT in any node-positive patients, more extensive surgical exploration of the axilla and modern systemic therapies seems to have a positive impact on both distant and LRR risk.

There is increasing recognition that the underlying biology of the tumor is one of the strongest predictors of both local and distant recurrence. Therefore, significant retrospective and prospective research is ongoing to determine the optimal use of these subtypes in predicting LRR. Sorting of patients into risk groups and therapy regimens by biologic subtype is a departure from the traditional TNM staging and is likely to result in more appropriate and effective treatments for individual patients.

Finally, there are emerging data regarding the utility of genomic profiling to predict locoregional risk as well. These data are not yet mature enough for daily use in the clinical setting. It is likely, however, to become another tool for prediction of LRR in the near future, as more data to support the utility of genomic assays are reported.

Overall, the use of all these factors in combination can help practicing radiation oncologists to appropriately select patients for therapy by identifying both patients who may not have traditionally been offered postmastectomy therapy but may benefit from it and patients who would have traditionally been offered PMRT but may derive such little benefit that the toxicities of treatment outweigh the reduction in risk.

REFERENCES

1. Ragaz J, Olivotto IA, Spinelli JJ, et al. Locoregional radiation therapy in patients with high-risk breast cancer receiving adjuvant chemotherapy: 20-year results of the British Columbia randomized trial. J Natl Cancer Inst 2005;97(2):116–26.
2. Nielsen HM, Overgaard M, Grau C, et al. Study of failure pattern among high-risk breast cancer patients with or without postmastectomy radiotherapy in addition to adjuvant systemic therapy: long-term results from the Danish Breast Cancer Cooperative Group DBCG 82 b and c randomized studies. J Clin Oncol 2006; 24(15):2268–75.
3. Katz A, Strom EA, Buchholz TA, et al. Locoregional recurrence patterns after mastectomy and doxorubicin-based chemotherapy: implications for postoperative irradiation. J Clin Oncol 2000;18(15):2817–27.
4. Taghian AG, Jeong JH, Mamounas EP, et al. Low locoregional recurrence rate among node-negative breast cancer patients with tumors 5 cm or larger treated by mastectomy, with or without adjuvant systemic therapy and without radiotherapy: results from five national surgical adjuvant breast and bowel project randomized clinical trials. J Clin Oncol 2006;24(24):3927–32.
5. Taghian A, Jeong JH, Mamounas E, et al. Patterns of locoregional failure in patients with operable breast cancer treated by mastectomy and adjuvant chemotherapy with or without tamoxifen and without radiotherapy: results from five National Surgical Adjuvant Breast and Bowel Project randomized clinical trials. J Clin Oncol 2004;22(21):4247–54.
6. Recht A, Gray R, Davidson NE, et al. Locoregional failure 10 years after mastectomy and adjuvant chemotherapy with or without tamoxifen without irradiation: experience of the Eastern Cooperative Oncology Group. J Clin Oncol 1999; 17(6):1689–700.
7. Favourable and unfavourable effects on long-term survival of radiotherapy for early breast cancer: an overview of the randomised trials. Early Breast Cancer Trialists' Collaborative Group. Lancet 2000;355(9217):1757–70.
8. Clarke M, Collins R, Darby S, et al. Effects of radiotherapy and of differences in the extent of surgery for early breast cancer on local recurrence and 15-year survival: an overview of the randomised trials. Lancet 2005;366(9503): 2087–106.
9. Perou CM, Sorlie T, Eisen MB, et al. Molecular portraits of human breast tumours. Nature 2000;406(6797):747–52.
10. Nguyen PL, Taghian AG, Katz MS, et al. Breast cancer subtype approximated by estrogen receptor, progesterone receptor, and HER-2 is associated with local and distant recurrence after breast-conserving therapy. J Clin Oncol 2008; 26(14):2373–8.
11. Voduc KD, Cheang MC, Tyldesley S, et al. Breast cancer subtypes and the risk of local and regional relapse. J Clin Oncol 2010;28(10):1684–91.
12. Kyndi M, Sorensen FB, Knudsen H, et al. Estrogen receptor, progesterone receptor, HER-2, and response to postmastectomy radiotherapy in high-risk breast cancer: the Danish Breast Cancer Cooperative Group. J Clin Oncol 2008;26(9):1419–26.
13. Ceilley E, Jagsi R, Goldberg S, et al. Radiotherapy for invasive breast cancer in North America and Europe: results of a survey. Int J Radiat Oncol Biol Phys 2005; 61(2):365–73.
14. Helinto M, Blomqvist C, Heikkila P, et al. Post-mastectomy radiotherapy in pT3N0M0 breast cancer: is it needed? Radiother Oncol 1999;52(3):213–7.

15. Overgaard M, Hansen PS, Overgaard J, et al. Postoperative radiotherapy in high-risk premenopausal women with breast cancer who receive adjuvant chemotherapy. Danish Breast Cancer Cooperative Group 82b Trial. N Engl J Med 1997;337(14):949–55.

16. Overgaard M, Jensen MB, Overgaard J, et al. Postoperative radiotherapy in high-risk postmenopausal breast-cancer patients given adjuvant tamoxifen: Danish Breast Cancer Cooperative Group DBCG 82c randomised trial. Lancet 1999; 353(9165):1641–8.

17. Floyd SR, Buchholz TA, Haffty BG, et al. Low local recurrence rate without post-mastectomy radiation in node-negative breast cancer patients with tumors 5 cm and larger. Int J Radiat Oncol Biol Phys 2006;66(2):358–64.

18. Goulart J, Truong P, Woods R, et al. Outcomes of node-negative breast cancer 5 centimeters and larger treated with and without postmastectomy radiotherapy. Int J Radiat Oncol Biol Phys 2011;80(3):758–64.

19. Wallgren A, Bonetti M, Gelber RD, et al. Risk factors for locoregional recurrence among breast cancer patients: results from International Breast Cancer Study Group Trials I through VII. J Clin Oncol 2003;21(7):1205–13.

20. Jagsi R, Raad RA, Goldberg S, et al. Locoregional recurrence rates and prognostic factors for failure in node-negative patients treated with mastectomy: implications for postmastectomy radiation. Int J Radiat Oncol Biol Phys 2005;62(4): 1035–9.

21. Abi-Raad R, Boutrus R, Wang R, et al. Patterns and risk factors of locoregional recurrence in T1-T2 node negative breast cancer patients treated with mastectomy: implications for postmastectomy radiotherapy. Int J Radiat Oncol Biol Phys 2011;81(3):e151–7.

22. Truong PT, Lesperance M, Culhaci A, et al. Patient subsets with T1-T2, node-negative breast cancer at high locoregional recurrence risk after mastectomy. Int J Radiat Oncol Biol Phys 2005;62(1):175–82.

23. Truong PT, Yong CM, Abnousi F, et al. Lymphovascular invasion is associated with reduced locoregional control and survival in women with node-negative breast cancer treated with mastectomy and systemic therapy. J Am Coll Surg 2005; 200(6):912–21.

24. Wang J, Shi M, Ling R, et al. Adjuvant chemotherapy and radiotherapy in triple-negative breast carcinoma: a prospective randomized controlled multi-center trial. Radiother Oncol 2011;100(2):200–4.

25. Rowell NP. Radiotherapy to the chest wall following mastectomy for node-negative breast cancer: a systematic review. Radiother Oncol 2009;91(1):23–32.

26. Galper S, Recht A, Silver B, et al. Factors associated with regional nodal failure in patients with early stage breast cancer with 0–3 positive axillary nodes following tangential irradiation alone. Int J Radiat Oncol Biol Phys 1999; 45(5):1157–66.

27. Cheng JC, Chen CM, Liu MC, et al. Locoregional failure of postmastectomy patients with 1–3 positive axillary lymph nodes without adjuvant radiotherapy. Int J Radiat Oncol Biol Phys 2002;52(4):980–8.

28. Woodward WA, Strom EA, Tucker SL, et al. Locoregional recurrence after doxorubicin-based chemotherapy and postmastectomy: implications for breast cancer patients with early-stage disease and predictors for recurrence after postmastectomy radiation. Int J Radiat Oncol Biol Phys 2003;57(2):336–44.

29. Fodor J, Polgar C, Major T, et al. Locoregional failure 15 years after mastectomy in women with one to three positive axillary nodes with or without irradiation the significance of tumor size. Strahlenther Onkol 2003;179(3):197–202.

30. Truong PT, Olivotto IA, Kader HA, et al. Selecting breast cancer patients with T1-T2 tumors and one to three positive axillary nodes at high postmastectomy locoregional recurrence risk for adjuvant radiotherapy. Int J Radiat Oncol Biol Phys 2005;61(5):1337–47.

31. Karlsson P, Cole BF, Price KN, et al. The role of the number of uninvolved lymph nodes in predicting locoregional recurrence in breast cancer. J Clin Oncol 2007; 25(15):2019–26.

32. Kunkler IH, Canney P, van Tienhoven G, et al. Elucidating the role of chest wall irradiation in 'intermediate-risk' breast cancer: the MRC/EORTC SUPREMO trial. Clin Oncol (R Coll Radiol) 2008;20(1):31–4.

33. Paik S, Tang G, Shak S, et al. Gene expression and benefit of chemotherapy in women with node-negative, estrogen receptor-positive breast cancer. J Clin Oncol 2006;24(23):3726–34.

34. Goldstein LJ, Gray R, Badve S, et al. Prognostic utility of the 21-gene assay in hormone receptor-positive operable breast cancer compared with classical clinicopathologic features. J Clin Oncol 2008;26(25):4063–71.

35. Albain KS, Barlow WE, Shak S, et al. Prognostic and predictive value of the 21-gene recurrence score assay in postmenopausal women with node-positive, oestrogen-receptor-positive breast cancer on chemotherapy: a retrospective analysis of a randomised trial. Lancet Oncol 2010;11(1):55–65.

36. van de Vijver MJ, He YD, van't Veer LJ, et al. A gene-expression signature as a predictor of survival in breast cancer. N Engl J Med 2002;347(25):1999–2009.

37. Buyse M, Loi S, van't Veer L, et al. Validation and clinical utility of a 70-gene prognostic signature for women with node-negative breast cancer. J Natl Cancer Inst 2006;98(17):1183–92.

38. Cardoso F, Van't Veer L, Rutgers E, et al. Clinical application of the 70-gene profile: the MINDACT trial. J Clin Oncol 2008;26(5):729–35.

39. Cheng SH, Horng CF, West M, et al. Genomic prediction of locoregional recurrence after mastectomy in breast cancer. J Clin Oncol 2006;24(28):4594–602.

40. Nuyten DS, Kreike B, Hart AA, et al. Predicting a local recurrence after breast-conserving therapy by gene expression profiling. Breast Cancer Res 2006;8(5): R62.

41. Kreike B, Halfwerk H, Armstrong N, et al. Local recurrence after breast-conserving therapy in relation to gene expression patterns in a large series of patients. Clin Cancer Res 2009;15(12):4181–90.

42. Mamounas EP, Tang G, Fisher B, et al. Association between the 21-gene recurrence score assay and risk of locoregional recurrence in node-negative, estrogen receptor-positive breast cancer: results from NSABP B-14 and NSABP B-20. J Clin Oncol 2010;28(10):1677–83.

43. Solin LJ, Gray R, Goldstein LJ, et al. Prognostic value of biologic subtype and the 21-gene recurrence score relative to local recurrence after breast conservation treatment with radiation for early stage breast carcinoma: results from the Eastern Cooperative Oncology Group E2197 study. Breast Cancer Res Treat 2012;134(2): 683–92.

44. Rastogi P, Anderson SJ, Bear HD, et al. Preoperative chemotherapy: updates of National Surgical Adjuvant Breast and Bowel Project Protocols B-18 and B-27. J Clin Oncol 2008;26(5):778–85.

45. Mauriac L, MacGrogan G, Avril A, et al. Neoadjuvant chemotherapy for operable breast carcinoma larger than 3 cm: a unicentre randomized trial with a 124-month median follow-up. Institut Bergonie Bordeaux Groupe Sein (IBBGS). Ann Oncol 1999;10(1):47–52.

46. van der Hage JA, van de Velde CJ, Julien JP, et al. Preoperative chemotherapy in primary operable breast cancer: results from the European Organization for Research and Treatment of Cancer trial 10902. J Clin Oncol 2001;19(22): 4224–37.

47. Untch M, Fasching PA, Konecny GE, et al. Pathologic complete response after neoadjuvant chemotherapy plus trastuzumab predicts favorable survival in human epidermal growth factor receptor 2-overexpressing breast cancer: results from the TECHNO trial of the AGO and GBG study groups. J Clin Oncol 2011; 29(25):3351–7.

48. Mamounas EP, Brown A, Anderson S, et al. Sentinel node biopsy after neoadjuvant chemotherapy in breast cancer: results from National Surgical Adjuvant Breast and Bowel Project Protocol B-27. J Clin Oncol 2005;23(12):2694–702.

49. Nagar H, Mittendorf EA, Strom EA, et al. Local-regional recurrence with and without radiation therapy after neoadjuvant chemotherapy and mastectomy for clinically staged T3N0 breast cancer. Int J Radiat Oncol Biol Phys 2011;81(3): 782–7.

50. McGuire SE, Gonzalez-Angulo AM, Huang EH, et al. Postmastectomy radiation improves the outcome of patients with locally advanced breast cancer who achieve a pathologic complete response to neoadjuvant chemotherapy. Int J Radiat Oncol Biol Phys 2007;68(4):1004–9.

51. Fowble BL, Einck JP, Kim DN, et al. Role of postmastectomy radiation after neoadjuvant chemotherapy in stage II-III breast cancer. Int J Radiat Oncol Biol Phys 2012;83(2):494–503.

52. Le Scodan R, Selz J, Stevens D, et al. Radiotherapy for stage II and stage III breast cancer patients with negative lymph nodes after preoperative chemotherapy and mastectomy. Int J Radiat Oncol Biol Phys 2012;82(1):e1–7.

53. Purushotham A, Pinder S, Cariati M, et al. Neoadjuvant chemotherapy: not the best option in estrogen receptor-positive, HER2-negative, invasive classical lobular carcinoma of the breast? J Clin Oncol 2010;28(22):3552–4.

54. Mamounas E. Pathologic response: implications for local therapy. 2007. Available at: http://ctep.cancer.gov/highlights/docs/mamounas.pdf. Accessed September 4, 2012.

55. Huang EH, Strom EA, Perkins GH, et al. Comparison of risk of local-regional recurrence after mastectomy or breast conservation therapy for patients treated with neoadjuvant chemotherapy and radiation stratified according to a prognostic index score. Int J Radiat Oncol Biol Phys 2006;66(2):352–7.

Contemporary Radiotherapy in Head and Neck Cancer
Balancing Chance for Cure with Risk for Complication

Alvin R. Cabrera, MD[a],*, David S. Yoo, MD, PhD[a],
David M. Brizel, MD[a,b]

KEYWORDS

- Head and neck neoplasms • Radiotherapy • Intensity modulated radiotherapy
- Radiation effects • Adverse effects • Dose fractionation

KEY POINTS

- Altered fractionation strategies improve outcome compared with conventional once-daily treatment of patients with locally advanced disease being treated with radiation therapy alone.
- Technological advances in diagnostic imaging and radiation delivery have improved the therapeutic ratio, with better disease delineation and sparing of normal tissues.
- Concurrent chemoradiation with intensity-modulated radiation therapy constitutes the standard nonsurgical therapy for locally advanced squamous cell head and neck cancer.
- Intensification strategies that add molecularly targeted agents to standard chemoradiation have resulted in increased toxicity but not improved efficacy to date.
- For patients who initially present with lymph node involvement, after chemoradiation PET-CT can distinguish those who do not require adjuvant neck dissection from those who do.

RADIATION THERAPY: BIOLOGIC BASIS AND FRACTIONATION

Approximately 49,000 cases of head and neck squamous cell cancer (HNSCC) are diagnosed in the United States annually; nearly 60% present with locally advanced but nonmetastatic disease.[1] Locoregional recurrence is the predominant pattern of failure from which most fatalities result. As a locoregional therapy, radiotherapy (RT) plays a primary role in treatment.

The authors have nothing to disclose.
Authors ARC and DSY contributed equally to the preparation of this article.
[a] Department of Radiation Oncology, Duke University Medical Center, Box 3085, Durham, NC 27710, USA; [b] Division of Otolaryngology, Department of Surgery, Duke University Medical Center, Box 3085, Durham, NC 27710, USA
* Corresponding author. Duke University Medical Center, Morris Clinic Building, Box 3085, Durham, NC 27710.
E-mail address: alvin.cabrera@duke.edu

Surg Oncol Clin N Am 22 (2013) 579–598
http://dx.doi.org/10.1016/j.soc.2013.02.001
1055-3207/13/$ – see front matter © 2013 Elsevier Inc. All rights reserved.

surgonc.theclinics.com

Ionizing radiation causes cytotoxic effects via free radical–mediated DNA damage. This process precipitates a cascade of physicochemical reactions that lead to single-strand and double-strand DNA breaks, loss of reproductive integrity, and cell death. In the earliest days of RT, treatments often involved single large doses (fractions) of radiation.[2] Unfortunately, clinical responses were often accompanied by significant early and late toxicities. More protracted fractionated courses of RT were subsequently devised, which spread the treatment course out via the delivery of multiple smaller doses, with significantly reduced toxicity.

Four "Rs" underlying the radiobiology of fractionation have been described: repair of sublethal injury, cell repopulation, redistribution into more radiosensitive phases of the cell cycle, and reoxygenation.[3] These concepts have influenced the way RT is delivered for all types of cancer, including HNSCC. Nonmalignant cells more efficiently repair radiation-induced DNA damage than their malignant counterparts. Therefore, multiple radiation fractions give normal tissues time to repair sublethal damage, preferentially killing tumor cells. However, longer overall treatment times promote repopulation of both normal and cancerous cells. Consequently, as fractionated regimens become more protracted, they typically require higher total doses to achieve similar degrees of tumor control. Nonetheless, the delivery of each dose within a fractionated regimen redistributes more cells into the more radiosensitive G2/mitosis phase of the cell cycle, which enhances radiation-induced cell kill. One final advantage of fractionation is that it promotes tumor reoxygenation. Hypoxic cells are 2.5 to 3 times more resistant to a given dose of radiation than their well-oxygenated counterparts. Tumor hypoxia adversely affects the prognosis of head and neck cancer.[4–6]

Strategies to improve tumor control must be balanced against the ability of patients to tolerate the acute side effects of treatment and the potentially irreversible chronic toxicities that may subsequently occur. A conventional fractionation regimen used to treat HNSCC typically consists of once-daily 2 gray (Gy) fractions, five fractions per week, over 7 weeks, to a total dose of 70 Gy. This treatment is relatively well-tolerated with manageable mucositis; roughly one-third of patients experience some degree of grade 3 acute toxicity, and 2-year locoregional control (LRC) and overall survival (OS) rates are around 45%.[7] Altered fractionation regimens, such as hyperfractionation and accelerated fractionation, represent radiobiology-based approaches to improve treatment efficacy.

Hyperfractionation is designed to deliver higher total doses of RT to improve disease control without increasing late toxicity relative to conventional fractionation. Pure hyperfractionation regimens keep the same overall treatment time as conventional therapy but achieve higher doses via delivery of smaller, multiple daily fractions. Smaller individual doses of RT allow for preferential repair of sublethal DNA damage in normal tissues that are responsible for the development of late side effects compared with tumor cells. A commonly used regimen is 1.2 Gy twice daily, ten fractions per week, over 7 weeks, to a total dose of 81.6 Gy.

Pure accelerated regimens deliver the same or slightly reduced total dose of RT in a shorter overall treatment time relative to conventional fractionation. The goal of the condensed timeframe is to overcome tumor repopulation, which accelerates 3 to 4 weeks after RT initiation.[8] A typical regimen developed by the Danish Head and Neck Cancer Group (DAHANCA) uses 2 Gy fractions, six fractions per week, to a total dose of 70 Gy in 6 weeks. Hybrid regimens combine elements of hyperfractionation and acceleration. The concomitant boost regimen of the Radiation Therapy Oncology Group (RTOG) delivers a total dose of 72 Gy over 6 weeks, using 1.8 Gy daily fractions in the morning with the addition of a second 1.5 Gy fraction in the afternoon on the last 12 days of treatment to combat accelerated tumor repopulation.[9]

Multiple trials have compared altered fractionation to conventional fractionation in locally advanced HNSCC. RTOG 9003 randomized 1073 subjects to standard 70 Gy versus pure hyperfractionation 81.6 Gy versus concomitant boost 72 Gy versus a split-course hybrid regimen of 67.2 Gy in 1.6 Gy twice-daily fractions over 6 weeks, with a scheduled 2-week break after 38.4 Gy. All three altered fractionation regimens caused significantly worse acute toxicity than standard RT but no increase in late effects. The hyperfractionated and concomitant boost arms had significantly better LRC than the standard arm with a trend toward improved disease-free survival (DFS). Overall survival was the same among the different arms. Subjects in the split course arm had control rates similar to the standard arm, suggesting that the treatment break had allowed for tumor repopulation.[7] Altered fractionation studies published by the DAHANCA group (70 Gy in 6 weeks) and the European Organization for Research and Treatment of Cancer (EORTC; 1.15 Gy twice-daily to 80.5 Gy in 7 weeks) have shown similar improvements in LRC at the cost of increased but manageable acute toxicity.[10,11]

Other trials have explored very accelerated fractionation regimens, delivering approximately 70 to 72 Gy over 5 weeks. These studies have shown improvements in LRC but at the cost of significantly higher rates of acute and late toxicities.[12] Highly toxic regimens that require scheduled or unanticipated treatments breaks are self-defeating as prolongation to allow for repair and repopulation of normal tissues allows the same for cancer cells. Retrospective analyses have shown that extension of overall treatment time adversely affects local control, perhaps by 1% to 2% per day.[13–15]

Altered fractionation regimens represent the successful translation of fundamental radiobiologic principles into clinical solutions that balance the dual goals of cancer control and treatment toxicity. A meta-analysis of individual patient data from 15 trials with 6515 patients showed an absolute 5-year LRC benefit of 6.4%, which translated into a 3.4% benefit in 5-year OS with altered fractionation strategies.[16] These data provide the foundation for HNSCC management with RT as a single modality. However, treatment of locally advanced disease has evolved with a shift toward intensification with concurrent systemic agents.

TREATMENT TOXICITY

Benefits of treatment intensification, whether through altered fractionation or combined modality therapy, come at the price of increased acute and late toxicities.[17,18] The RTOG toxicity criteria define acute effects as those developing within 90 days from RT commencement and late toxicities after 90 days.[19] The distinction is somewhat arbitrary because some late complications, such as chronic edema or necrosis of soft tissue or bone, may result from severe acute insults. The term consequential late effect is often used to describe this phenomenon.

Common acute toxicities include mucositis, dermatitis, taste alteration, dry mouth, anorexia, and fatigue. Radiation-induced mucositis is the most significant of these and can cause significant pain and distress; it is usually the limiting factor to therapeutic intensification. Decreases in oral fluid and nutritional intake may require treatment breaks for intensive supportive care, including feeding tube placement.

Pathologic examination of inflamed mucosa reveals shallow ulcerations caused by depletion of the epithelial stem cell layer with denudation and subsequent formation of raised pseudomembranes composed of inflammatory cells, interstitial exudate, fibrin, and cell debris.[20] Deep ulceration requiring prolonged healing may lead to consequential late mucosal effects. Some ulcers never heal and may result in soft tissue or bone necrosis.[21] Attempts to mitigate RT-induced oral mucositis have focused on the use of palifermin, a recombinant human keratinocyte growth factor.[22] In two phase III trials, palifermin reduced the incidence of observed grade 3 to 4 mucositis but without differences in subject-reported pain scores, narcotic usage, or duration of treatment breaks.[23,24] Its role in HNSCC management remains investigational.

Potential late effects from HNSCC RT include chronic xerostomia, dysphagia, osteoradionecrosis, fibrosis, trismus, atrophy, hypothyroidism, brachial plexopathy, and carotid artery injury. Development of late complications is multifactorial with contributions from both patient-specific and treatment-related characteristics including age, inherent normal tissue radiosensitivity, primary tumor location and size, RT fraction size, total dose, irradiated volume, and the inclusion of other treatments such as surgery and/or chemotherapy.[17,21,25]

Compared to definitive RT alone, surgery and postoperative RT resulted in significantly higher rates of late subcutaneous fibrosis on retrospective review of two prospective Trans Tasman Radiation Oncology Group (TROG) trials. The study compared 172 patients who received definitive RT (59.4 Gy, 1.8 Gy twice-daily) versus 52 patients who received surgery and postoperative RT (50.4–54 Gy, 1.8 Gy twice-daily). Despite receiving lower radiation doses, postoperative patients had significantly higher rates of subcutaneous fibrosis (34% vs 16%, $P<.01$).[26] Review of three prospective RTOG trials showed a 43% incidence of severe ($\geq$grade 3) late pharyngeal or laryngeal toxicity following concurrent chemoradiation (CRT). Multivariable analysis found that older age, advanced tumor (T) stage, location of disease in the larynx or hypopharynx, and neck dissection after CRT correlated significantly with the development of severe late toxicity.[17] A similar impact of posttherapy neck dissection on late dysphagia was reported by Fox Chase Cancer Center, with relative risk (RR) of feeding tube dependence significantly higher at 18 months (RR 4.7) and 24 months (RR 7.7).[27] These retrospective findings are hypothesis-generating only, but they inform the evolving role of adjuvant neck dissection following definitive RT or CRT.

The most common late complication in HNSCC patients treated with RT is xerostomia. Chronic dry mouth due to permanent damage to salivary glands has significant impact on patient quality of life causing difficulties with chewing and swallowing, disturbances in speech and sleep, and increased susceptibility to oral infections, dental caries, tooth loss, and osteonecrosis. Pharmacologic attempts to reduce the incidence of RT-induced xerostomia have centered on radioprotector compounds such as amifostine. A thiol-containing prodrug, amifostine preferentially accumulates in the kidneys and salivary glands where it is subsequently metabolized into an active free radical scavenger.[28] In a phase III trial, the addition of amifostine to conventional RT alone significantly reduced the incidence of greater than or equal to grade 2 acute xerostomia (78% vs 51%, $P<.001$) and greater than or equal to grade 2 chronic xerostomia 1 year post-RT (57% vs 34%, $P = .002$). The beneficial effects of amifostine on duration and severity of xerostomia persisted 2 years posttreatment without compromising disease control or OS.[29] Side effects of amifostine, including nausea or vomiting and hypotension, developed in nearly two-thirds of subjects, but less than 10% experienced greater than or equal to grade 3 toxicity. Still, 21% discontinued amifostine before the end of RT.[30]

Amifostine was tested in patients treated with conventionally fractionated RT alone using nonconformal techniques that did not spare the parotid glands. Its efficacy in those treated with CRT and/or with modern parotid-sparing RT techniques, such as intensity-modulated RT (IMRT), is unclear. Small phase II-III trials suggest a benefit in the setting of CRT, but level I evidence is lacking.[31,32] Given its side-effect profile, the widespread adoption of IMRT, and the increasing use of CRT, amifostine has not established a significant role in current HNSCC management.

Despite increased late toxicities with multimodality approaches, the worst possible complication remains uncontrolled disease. Therefore, intensive treatment strategies that maximize tumor control should be offered to suitable patients willing and able to tolerate therapy. Honest discussions between providers and patients allow for establishment of reasonable goals and realistic expectations of therapy.

TREATMENT PLANNING AND DELIVERY

Minimizing unnecessary irradiation of adjacent tissues while maximizing dose delivery to tumor represents a fundamental and effective strategy to reduce complications. Advances in imaging technology and treatment delivery have revolutionized the ability to visualize deep structures and design treatments where the regions of high-dose delivery conform closely to target volumes. CT, MRI, and positron-emitting tomography (PET) provide complementary anatomic and functional information for radiation treatment planning.

The typical planning process for external beam RT in HNSCC requires: (1) reproducible immobilization with a thermoplastic mask; (2) simulation CT scan, preferably with intravenous contrast enhancement; (3) export of resulting CT images into a treatment planning software system with registration/fusion of other available imaging datasets (MRI, PET-CT) as clinically indicated; (4) delineation/contouring of all target volumes and normal tissue structures; (5) determination of the optimal number of beams and their respective angles and apertures; (6) generation and optimization of the treatment plan; (7) critical plan evaluation to ensure appropriate target coverage and normal tissue sparing; and (8) plan review and confirmation via quality assurance before treatment delivery.[33]

Target delineation and designation are essential components of RT planning (**Fig. 1**). Gross tumor volume (GTV) corresponds to clinically and/or radiographically apparent disease. The clinical target volume (CTV) encompasses GTV and areas of suspected subclinical, microscopic involvement, including regional nodal basins. Planning target volume (PTV) includes the CTV plus 3 to 5 mm margin to account for anatomic motion and variability in patient or beam setup.[34]

Complex target volumes are common in head and neck cancers, and concave PTVs frequently abut organs such as the parotid glands, pharyngeal constrictor muscles, optic structures, and spinal cord. IMRT has revolutionized the treatment of HNSCC because it is capable of generating very conformal dose distributions around irregularly shaped tumors with steep dose fall-off immediately beyond target boundaries (**Fig. 2**). Unlike conventional radiation techniques, which use static field apertures of uniform beam intensities, IMRT subdivides each beam into thousands of smaller beamlets of varying intensities. The intensity of each beamlet is determined iteratively via computer to generate treatment plans that meet prespecified dose parameters.[35] A typical IMRT treatment plan is designed to ensure that greater than or equal to 95% of the PTV receives the prescribed dose, whereas the maximum dose to the spinal cord with margin is less than 45 to 50 Gy, and the mean dose to at least one parotid gland is less than 26 Gy.

Lower doses to the parotids allow for better recovery of salivary function and less xerostomia.[36] Quantitative scintigraphy studies have found IMRT considerably more effective than amifostine in protection of salivary gland function.[37,38] Two small phase III trials from Hong Kong randomized subjects with nasopharyngeal cancer to IMRT or conventional RT. The use of IMRT was associated with lower

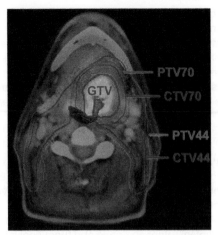

Fig. 1. Target volume definitions. CT simulation and ^{18}F-fluorodeoxyglucose (FDG) PET scan obtained from a patient with a locally advanced squamous cell carcinoma of the base of tongue. The two studies are registered and fused in the treatment planning software system. The radiation oncologist then manually contours the normal tissue structures and target volumes. The gross tumor volume (GTV) represents the clinically apparent and FDG-avid primary tumor in the left base of tongue. The clinical target volume (CTV)70 accounts for microscopic extension around the GTV. The planning target volume (PTV)70 expansion around the CTV70 allows for uncertainties in daily set-up and patient motion. The CTV44 includes the potential microscopic disease in the bilateral regional lymph nodes, with a margin expansion (PTV44) to minimize the risk of missing the intended target volume.

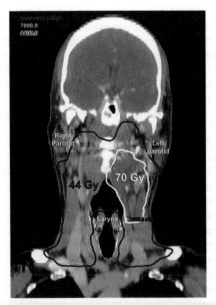

Fig. 2. Target volume coverage and normal tissue sparing with IMRT. Representative coronal slice with overlay of the 44 Gy and 70 Gy isodose lines. The PTV44 (*orange*) and PTV70 (*magenta*) structures are included, as are the parotid glands and larynx. The use of IMRT allows for steep dose gradients that ensure adequate target volume coverage while minimizing irradiation of normal structures.

rates of late xerostomia, greater recovery of salivary flow, and higher quality of life scores.[39,40]

The PARSPORT study, a multicenter phase III trial from the United Kingdom, randomized 94 subects with oropharyngeal or hypopharyngeal squamous cell carcinomas to IMRT or conventional RT. Contralateral mean parotid doses were 22.4 Gy with IMRT versus 60 Gy with conventional RT (P<.0003).[41] Greater than or equal to grade 2 xerostomia, as assessed by the Late Effects of Normal Tissue (LENT SOMA) scale, was significantly lower with IMRT at 12 months (38% vs 74%) and 24 months (29% vs 83%). Subjects treated with IMRT also had greater objective recovery in salivary secretion and clinically significant improvements in dry-mouth–specific and global quality of life scores. No differences were noted in LRC or OS.[42]

One essential tool radiation oncologists use to determine whether a treatment plan achieves the desired dose specifications is the cumulative dose-volume histogram (DVH). The radiation dose to a given target or normal structure is plotted on the X axis and percentage of the volume of that structure is plotted on the Y axis. Each point on the curve represents the percent volume of a particular structure receiving at least the indicated dose. For example, the DVH in **Fig. 3** represents an IMRT plan in which 97% of the mandible is receiving at least 10 Gy, 87% is receiving at least 30 Gy, and 34% is receiving at least 50 Gy. In essence, DVH plots are designed to graphically display entire dose distributions for target volumes and normal tissue structures in a comprehensible format.[35] The responsibility of the radiation oncologist is to recognize the clinically relevant dose-volume relationships for each normal tissue structure and understand their associated complication probabilities.[43,44]

Different normal tissues require different dose and/or volume constraints.[45] For example, radiation beyond tolerance to any segment of the spinal cord may result in permanent damage and myelopathy. Therefore, an acceptable RT plan may restrict the maximum dose to the cord below 45 to 50 Gy to minimize the risk of catastrophic paralysis, even at the expense of target volume coverage. Other organs function in a more parallel fashion and entire sections may be removed or destroyed with the remaining subunits still performing the necessary functions. For these organs, such as the parotid gland, a mean dose constraint more accurately reflects the risk of toxicity development than a maximum dose constraint.

PRINCIPLES OF THERAPY
Radiation Therapy Doses

For head and neck cancers, greater numbers of tumor clonogens require higher RT doses for eradication.[46] Consequently, radiation dose prescriptions are usually made according to the disease burden with higher doses being delivered to regions of gross disease versus subclinical microscopic disease (**Table 1**). Doses of 45 to 50 Gy given with 1.8 to 2 Gy fractions are typically used for areas at risk of harboring microscopic disease, such as elective nodal basins. Regions with larger but still subclinical deposits of disease, such as positive margins or extracapsular extension (ECE), require doses of 60 to 66 Gy. Finally, areas of gross disease receive greater than or equal to 70 Gy. Of note, the dose levels for elective volumes are sufficient to cause permanent xerostomia without careful planning. Also, for patients with nodal disease with clinical and/or radiographic signs of ECE, an upfront neck dissection in lieu of definitive CRT results in only minimal radiation dose reduction from 70 Gy to 66 Gy with concurrent chemotherapy and also exposes the patient to a higher risk of chronic toxicity[17] from trimodality therapy that often is not necessary.[47]

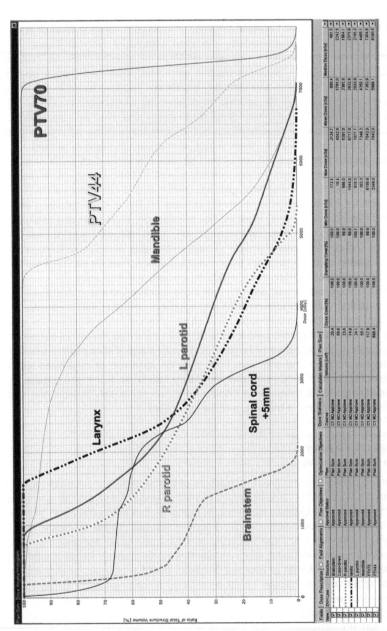

Fig. 3. Dose-volume histogram. Optimal radiation treatment plans balance tumor coverage with sparing of normal structures. The DVH graphically illustrates the dose-volume relationship for any contoured structure.

Table 1 Dose prescriptions in HNSCC		
	Gross Tumor	**Elective Nodal Regions**
Definitive RT	70 Gy	44 Gy with chemo 50 Gy without chemo
	Tumor Bed	**Elective Nodal Regions**
Adjuvant RT	−Margins/ECE: 60 Gy +Margins/ECE: 66 Gy	44 Gy with chemo 50 Gy without chemo

Surgery Versus Radiation Therapy

The fundamental goal of HNSCC management is to deliver therapy that maximizes the probability of cure while minimizing the risks of toxicity that compromise patient function and quality of life. For early stage (I and II) disease, single modality surgery or single modality RT are generally considered to be equivalent with respect to efficacy. The choice of treatment modality, which should be based on which platform will cause less functional impairment, will typically vary according to the anatomic location of the primary tumor.

Curative regimens for more advanced stage disease commonly require a multimodality approach. Both patients and providers must recognize the potential for increased acute and late toxicities requiring significant and sustained supportive care and rehabilitation. Therefore, decisions regarding the roles of surgery, RT, and chemotherapy are best made within a multidisciplinary setting, along with input from colleagues in oral surgery, speech pathology, nutrition, social work, and others.

The choice of whether to use surgery or RT as the primary treatment modality often revolves around the issue of resectability for patients with locally advanced, nonmetastatic disease. The distinction between resectable and unresectable continues to evolve with improvements in resection techniques and reconstruction options. Patients with otherwise technically resectable disease may still not be surgical candidates for several reasons, including medical comorbidities and the inability or refusal to live with the functional deficits potentially resulting from surgery.

Treatment strategies for patients with locally advanced but resectable disease include both primary surgical and nonsurgical options. Nonsurgical organ function preservation became a viable approach following the 1991 publication of the Department of Veterans Affairs (VA) larynx trial, which demonstrated similar survival outcomes in patients randomized to total laryngectomy with adjuvant postoperative RT versus induction chemotherapy followed by RT in responders.[48] The three-arm RTOG 9111 study compared the VA larynx induction regimen versus CRT versus RT alone, and showed that larynx preservation rates could be further improved with the use of CRT.[49] Survival rates were similar because subjects who failed were successfully salvaged surgically.[50] One randomized study from Singapore with 119 subjects directly compared CRT with upfront surgery and RT in resectable HNSCCs (excluding nasopharyngeal and salivary gland primary sites). There was no difference in 3-year DFS and OS between the two arms with a median follow-up of 6 years.[51] These trials suggest that, for properly selected patients, surgical resection may be replaced with an organ function–sparing approach without compromising survival outcomes.

Not all patients are appropriate for organ preservation therapy. For example, a T4 larynx primary that has destroyed the organ with resultant aspiration and dysphagia may have better long-term function with upfront surgery followed by adjuvant RT. RTOG 9111 excluded subjects with large-volume T4 disease and recent consensus guidelines for future larynx preservation studies recommend exclusion of those with evidence of baseline laryngeal dysfunction.[52] Appropriate patient selection and individualized treatment plans tailored to maximize cure and minimize functional deficits remain crucial to the process of multidisciplinary management of locally advanced HNSCC patients.

Surgery and Radiation Therapy

Primary resection followed by postoperative RT or CRT remains a standard treatment option in locally advanced HNSCC patients. Pathologic findings that are associated with increased recurrence risk include high T stage or large tumor size,[53–57] increasing number of positive nodes,[58–60] positive low cervical nodes,[59,61] perineural invasion (PNI),[62–64] bone invasion,[65] vascular invasion,[55,58,66] positive margins,[67–72] and ECE.[60,73] These risk factors are reflected in the suggested indications for adjuvant RT in the National Comprehensive Cancer Network guidelines: pathologic T3-4 and/or N2-3 disease, nodal disease in levels IV-V, PNI, lymphovascular invasion, positive margins, or ECE.[74] In particular, positive margins and ECE seem to carry significantly elevated recurrence risk; concurrent chemotherapy is recommended with postoperative RT when these pathologic features are present.

In one retrospective series, 3-year local control rates with surgery alone were 41% for those with positive margins and 31% with ECE. These rates improved to 49% and 66%, respectively, with postoperative RT. The presence of both risk factors resulted in 0% local control with surgery alone versus 68% with RT.[75] For patients with positive margins or ECE who receive postoperative RT, retrospective analyses have shown higher doses associated with better local control rates, suggesting more intensive therapy may improve outcomes.[76,77]

Two subsequent phase III trials examined the addition of concurrent chemotherapy to postoperative RT in high-risk disease. EORTC 22931 included patients with positive margins, ECE, pT3-4 or N2-3 disease, PNI, vascular invasion, or level IV or V nodal involvement in oral cavity or oropharyngeal tumors. Compared to RT alone, CRT had significantly better 5-year LRC (82% vs 69%), progression-free survival (PFS; 47% vs 36%), and OS (53% vs 40%) but no difference in distant metastases (21% vs 25%). Concurrent chemotherapy increased the risk of greater than or equal to grade 3 acute mucositis but not late toxicity.[78]

RTOG 9501 enrolled subjects with positive margins, ECE, or greater than or equal to 2 positive lymph nodes. In 2004, initial publication showed that CRT significantly improved LRC (82% vs 72%) and DFS (hazard ratio [HR] 0.78) but not distant metastases (20% vs 23%) or OS (HR 0.84, $P = .19$). Chemotherapy increased greater than or equal to grade 3 acute toxicity but not late complications.[79] With longer follow-up, the improvements in LRC and DFS were no longer significant for the entire study population. However, subjects with positive margins or ECE retained the LRC and DFS benefits initially seen with concurrent chemotherapy.[80]

Finally, a pooled analysis of both EORTC and RTOG trials found that only those subjects with positive margins and/or ECE achieved statistically significant benefits from CRT in terms of LRC, DFS, and OS.[81] Taken together, these findings support the use of postoperative CRT in patients with positive margins and/or ECE. For other high-risk indications, the addition of chemotherapy to postoperative RT results in increased acute toxicity without obvious benefits in LRC or survival.

Definitive Radiation Therapy and Chemotherapy

The standard of care for patients with unresectable or inoperable locally advanced disease is CRT. The superiority of CRT over RT alone was established by several landmark trials that completed accrual in the 1990s. The addition of concurrent chemotherapy to either standard once-daily radiation[49,82–84] or altered fractionation regimens[85–88] consistently showed improved outcomes with the combined modality approach for all head and neck primary sites. The most recent meta-analysis of chemotherapy in head and neck cancer (MACH-NC), derived from the individual subject data from 17,346 subjects in 93 randomized trials published through 2000, showed 5-year absolute survival benefits of 8.9% (oral cavity), 8.1% (oropharynx), 5.4% (larynx), and 4% (hypopharynx) for concomitant therapy.[89] The beneficial effects of concurrent therapy were seen with either polychemotherapy combinations or monotherapy with single agent cisplatin alone.[90]

Altered fractionation is superior to standard fractionation when RT alone is used for treatment of locally advanced disease.[91] Whether altered fractionation RT with chemotherapy provided additional benefit beyond standard fractionation RT with chemotherapy was addressed by two recently published phase III trials. The Groupe Oncologie Radiothérapie Tête et Cou (GORTEC) 99-02 study randomized 840 subjects to one of three arms: standard RT (70 Gy in 7 weeks) with three cycles of concurrent carboplatin/5-FU, accelerated RT (70 Gy in 6 weeks) with two cycles of concurrent carboplatin/5-FU, and a regimen of "very accelerated fractionation" (VAF; 64.8 Gy in 3.5 weeks, 1.8 Gy BID) without chemotherapy. With median follow-up of 5.2 years, there was no benefit for the accelerated concurrent regimen compared with standard therapy in terms of LRC, distant metastases, PFS, or OS. Both chemotherapy-containing arms were superior to VAF RT alone.[92]

The RTOG 0129 study randomized 721 subjects to one of two arms: altered frac-tionation (72 Gy in 6 weeks) with two cycles of cisplatin versus standard fractionation (70 Gy in 7 weeks) with three cycles of cisplatin. There were no significant differences in 3-year PFS, OS, grade 3 to 4 acute or late toxicity.[93] Moreover, the 2009 update of MACH-NC reported similar survival benefits from the addition of concurrent chemo-therapy to either standard or altered fractionation RT regimens.[90] These findings in aggregate strongly suggest that further RT dose or fractionation intensification do not improve outcome in the presence of concurrent chemotherapy.

The need to reduce treatment failure and improve survival persists in locally advanced HNSCC despite the use of intensive multimodality therapy. Multiple rational strategies have been used in attempts to further intensify therapy beyond the CRT standard. Overexpression of the epidermal growth factor receptor (EGFR) is associ-ated with worse LRC and survival in HNSCC patients treated with RT alone.[94] The addition of cetuximab, an anti-EGFR antibody, to RT alone improved both LRC and OS in stage III-IV oropharynx, larynx, and hypopharynx patients.[95,96] However, the addition of cetuximab to CRT has been shown to increase toxicity (mucositis and skin reactions) but not improve 2-year PFS or OS compared with CRT alone.[97]

The targeting of hypoxic tumor cells in HNSCC was investigated with the addition of the hypoxia-selective agent tirapazamine to cisplatin-based CRT. Despite promising phase I-II results, the addition of tirapazamine to CRT did not improve OS in a phase III study conducted by the TROG in 861 subjects who were not evaluated for the pres-ence of tumor hypoxia a priori.[98] Moreover, attempts to correct anemia with erythropoiesis-stimulating agents have resulted in worse OS.[99,100]

Sequential strategies with induction chemotherapy and CRT attempted to combine potential improvements in distant metastatic disease control with the LRC benefits already seen with CRT to further improve survival in HNSCC. Taxane-based induction regimens were superior to platinum and 5FU without a taxane delivered before defin-itive CRT or RT alone in the TAX 323 and TAX 324 trials.[101,102] However, the sequential approach of taxane-based induction chemotherapy followed by CRT did not improve

3-year PFS or OS compared with definitive CRT alone in two separate phase III trials.[103,104] Moreover, the addition of induction chemotherapy has been associated with significant toxicity and poor treatment compliance, with approximately one-third of the TAX study subjects failing to complete the regimen. These studies demonstrate that more intensive, aggressive therapy beyond standard CRT is not synonymous with better therapy.

One confounding factor in these trials has been the increasing predominance of oropharynx primary disease and the emergence of human papillomavirus (HPV) status as an independent prognostic factor in this site. There are different outcomes and demographic profiles of patients with HPV-positive and HPV-negative tumors and a growing awareness that these are distinct disease entities that likely require different management strategies.[105] In RTOG 0129, 60% of the study population had oropharyngeal tumors, most of whom were HPV-positive on retrospective analysis. Subjects with HPV-positive tumors had significantly better 3-yr OS compared with HPV-negative patients (82.4% vs 57.1%).[93] Similar differences in survival as a function of HPV status have also been reported on retrospective reviews of the TROG and TAX 324 trials.[106,107]

For HPV-negative tumors, outcomes remain poor, and more effective therapies are still needed. For HPV-positive tumors, studies are underway to determine whether the excellent outcomes currently attained may be maintained with less intensive treatment regimens. For example, RTOG 1016 is a phase III study currently comparing CRT to a putatively less toxic but equally efficacious combination of cetuximab and RT.

One strategy to reduce treatment intensity in all HNSCC patients is to limit the use of adjuvant neck dissections to those patients with clear evidence of persistent or recurrent disease following definitive RT or CRT. Multiple series have reported increased late toxicities in subjects treated with RT or CRT and surgery. Older retrospective series have suggested high rates of residual nodal disease following CRT, poor correlation of clinical response with pathologic findings, and potential DFS and OS benefits from planned neck dissections.[108–110] Recent advances in radiation techniques and functional metabolic imaging have redefined these issues, however, and orchestrated an evolution in management strategy.[111]

For example, when planned neck dissections were institutional policy regardless of treatment response, areas of gross nodal disease often received only 55 to 60 Gy to minimize potential postoperative complication risk.[85] This dose reduction likely contributed to the high observed rates of pathologic residual disease. IMRT markedly improves the ability to deliver 70 Gy to gross nodal disease in the neck without delivering the same high dose to surrounding structures. Furthermore, clinical and/or CT response assessment has been replaced with PET-CT scans obtained 10 to 12 weeks after completion of therapy. A meta-analysis with 51 studies and 2335 subjects reported a negative predictive value for PET-CT in the posttreatment neck of 94.5% (95% CI, 93.1%–95.7%).[112]

A recent prospective study has further examined the utility of PET-CT to direct management of the post-CRT neck.[47] Per institutional protocol, subjects with negative PET scans at 12 weeks, regardless of residual nodal abnormalities on CT, underwent observation. Subjects with positive PET scans had adjuvant neck dissection, whereas those with equivocal scans had a repeat PET-CT at 4 to 6 weeks (**Fig. 4**). In 112 consecutive subjects, 62 had a complete response by both CT and PET criteria, with no isolated nodal failures at a median follow-up of 28 months. Of the 41 subjects with residual CT masses but negative PET scans, there were also no isolated nodal failures after observation. Nine subjects had positive neck disease on PET scans, one with pulmonary metastases as well. Of the eight subjects proceeding to neck

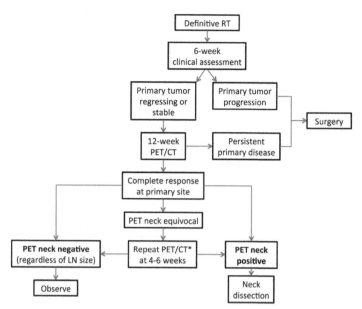

Fig. 4. PET-directed management of the posttreatment neck. This algorithm outlines the use of PET-CT to guide management of the neck after definitive RT or CRT at Duke University Medical Center. If the repeat PET/CT remains equivocal, it is considered a positive study and neck dissection is performed. (*Adapted from* Porceddu SV, Pryor DI, Burmeister E, et al. Results of a prospective study of positron emission tomography-directed management of residual nodal abnormalities in node-positive head and neck cancer after definitive radiotherapy with or without systemic therapy. Head Neck 2011;33(12):1675–82; with permission.)

dissection, two had isolated nodal failures. With this PET-based strategy, 41 subjects who would have otherwise undergone adjuvant neck dissection were spared surgery without subsequent nodal failures.

SUMMARY

Advances in radiobiology and physics have allowed radiation oncologists to maximize radiation's tumoricidal effects and minimize normal tissue toxicity. For many HNSCC patients, RT plays an integral role in their multidisciplinary care. As the population of long-term survivors grows, so does the number of patients able to experience the chronic effects of therapy. Therefore, balancing cure with complication remains the primary challenge, demanding prudent and individualized application of the various treatment modalities in appropriately selected patients to optimize the therapeutic effect.

REFERENCES

1. American Cancer Society. Cancer facts & figures 2010. Atlanta (GA): American Cancer Society; 2010.
2. Bernier J, Hall EJ, Giaccia A. Radiation oncology: a century of achievements. Nat Rev Cancer 2004;4(9):737–47.
3. Withers HR. The four R's of radiotherapy. Adv Radiat Biol 1975;5:241–71.

4. Brizel DM, Dodge RK, Clough RW, et al. Oxygenation of head and neck cancer: changes during radiotherapy and impact on treatment outcome. Radiother Oncol 1999;53(2):113–7.
5. Brizel DM, Sibley GS, Prosnitz LR, et al. Tumor hypoxia adversely affects the prognosis of carcinoma of the head and neck. Int J Radiat Oncol Biol Phys 1997;38(2):285–9.
6. Nordsmark M, Bentzen SM, Rudat V, et al. Prognostic value of tumor oxygenation in 397 head and neck tumors after primary radiation therapy. An international multi-center study. Radiother Oncol 2005;77(1):18–24.
7. Fu KK, Pajak TF, Trotti A, et al. A Radiation Therapy Oncology Group (RTOG) phase III randomized study to compare hyperfractionation and two variants of accelerated fractionation to standard fractionation radiotherapy for head and neck squamous cell carcinomas: first report of RTOG 9003. Int J Radiat Oncol Biol Phys 2000;48(1):7–16.
8. Withers HR, Taylor JM, Maciejewski B. The hazard of accelerated tumor clonogen repopulation during radiotherapy. Acta Oncol 1988;27(2):131–46.
9. Fu KK, Clery M, Ang KK, et al. Randomized phase I/II trial of two variants of accelerated fractionated radiotherapy regimens for advanced head and neck cancer: results of RTOG 88-09. Int J Radiat Oncol Biol Phys 1995;32(3): 589–97.
10. Horiot JC, Le Fur R, N'Guyen T, et al. Hyperfractionation versus conventional fractionation in oropharyngeal carcinoma: final analysis of a randomized trial of the EORTC cooperative group of radiotherapy. Radiother Oncol 1992;25(4): 231–41.
11. Overgaard J, Hansen HS, Specht L, et al. Five compared with six fractions per week of conventional radiotherapy of squamous-cell carcinoma of head and neck: DAHANCA 6 and 7 randomised controlled trial. Lancet 2003;362(9388): 933–40.
12. Skladowski K, Maciejewski B, Golen M, et al. Continuous accelerated 7-days-a-week radiotherapy for head-and-neck cancer: long-term results of phase III clinical trial. Int J Radiat Oncol Biol Phys 2006;66(3):706–13.
13. Barton MB, Keane TJ, Gadalla T, et al. The effect of treatment time and treatment interruption on tumour control following radical radiotherapy of laryngeal cancer. Radiother Oncol 1992;23(3):137–43.
14. Fowler JF, Lindstrom MJ. Loss of local control with prolongation in radiotherapy. Int J Radiat Oncol Biol Phys 1992;23(2):457–67.
15. Maciejewski B, Preuss-Bayer G, Trott KR. The influence of the number of fractions and of overall treatment time on local control and late complication rate in squamous cell carcinoma of the larynx. Int J Radiat Oncol Biol Phys 1983; 9(3):321–8.
16. Baujat B, Bourhis J, Blanchard P, et al. Hyperfractionated or accelerated radiotherapy for head and neck cancer. Cochrane Database Syst Rev 2010;(12). CD002026.
17. Machtay M, Moughan J, Trotti A, et al. Factors associated with severe late toxicity after concurrent chemoradiation for locally advanced head and neck cancer: an RTOG analysis. J Clin Oncol 2008;26(21):3582–9.
18. Trotti A, Bellm LA, Epstein JB, et al. Mucositis incidence, severity and associated outcomes in patients with head and neck cancer receiving radiotherapy with or without chemotherapy: a systematic literature review. Radiother Oncol 2003;66(3):253–62.

19. Cox JD, Stetz J, Pajak TF. Toxicity criteria of the Radiation Therapy Oncology Group (RTOG) and the European Organization for Research and Treatment of Cancer (EORTC). Int J Radiat Oncol Biol Phys 1995;31(5):1341–6.

20. Symonds RP. Treatment-induced mucositis: an old problem with new remedies. Br J Cancer 1998;77(10):1689–95.

21. Trotti A. Toxicity in head and neck cancer: a review of trends and issues. Int J Radiat Oncol Biol Phys 2000;47(1):1–12.

22. Brizel DM, Murphy BA, Rosenthal DI, et al. Phase II study of palifermin and concurrent chemoradiation in head and neck squamous cell carcinoma. J Clin Oncol 2008;26(15):2489–96.

23. Henke M, Alfonsi M, Foa P, et al. Palifermin decreases severe oral mucositis of patients undergoing postoperative radiochemotherapy for head and neck cancer: a randomized, placebo-controlled trial. J Clin Oncol 2011;29(20): 2815–20.

24. Le QT, Kim HE, Schneider CJ, et al. Palifermin reduces severe mucositis in definitive chemoradiotherapy of locally advanced head and neck cancer: a randomized, placebo-controlled study. J Clin Oncol 2011;29(20):2808–14.

25. O'Sullivan B, Levin W. Late radiation-related fibrosis: pathogenesis, manifestations, and current management. Semin Radiat Oncol 2003;13(3):274–89.

26. Wratten CR, Poulsen MG, Williamson S, et al. Effect of surgery on normal tissue toxicity in patients treated with accelerated radiotherapy. Acta Oncol 2002; 41(1):56–62.

27. Lango MN, Egleston B, Ende K, et al. Impact of neck dissection on long-term feeding tube dependence in patients with head and neck cancer treated with primary radiation or chemoradiation. Head Neck 2010;32(3):341–7.

28. Yuhas JM, Spellman JM, Culo F. The role of WR-2721 in radiotherapy and/or chemotherapy. Cancer Clin Trials 1980;3(3):211–6.

29. Wasserman TH, Brizel DM, Henke M, et al. Influence of intravenous amifostine on xerostomia, tumor control, and survival after radiotherapy for head-and-neck cancer: 2-year follow-up of a prospective, randomized, phase III trial. Int J Radiat Oncol Biol Phys 2005;63(4):985–90.

30. Brizel DM, Wasserman TH, Henke M, et al. Phase III randomized trial of amifostine as a radioprotector in head and neck cancer. J Clin Oncol 2000;18(19): 3339–45.

31. Antonadou D, Pepelassi M, Synodinou M, et al. Prophylactic use of amifostine to prevent radiochemotherapy-induced mucositis and xerostomia in head-and-neck cancer. Int J Radiat Oncol Biol Phys 2002;52(3):739–47.

32. Buntzel J, Glatzel M, Kuttner K, et al. Amifostine in simultaneous radiochemotherapy of advanced head and neck cancer. Semin Radiat Oncol 2002; 12(1 Suppl 1):4–13.

33. Kutcher GJ, Coia L, Gillin M, et al. Comprehensive QA for radiation oncology: report of AAPM Radiation Therapy Committee Task Group 40. Med Phys 1994;21(4):581–618.

34. International Commission on Radiation Units and Measurements. Prescribing, recording, and reporting photon beam therapy. Bethesda (MD): International Commission on Radiation Units and Measurements; 1993.

35. Khan FM. The physics of radiation therapy. 4th edition. Philadelphia: Lippincott Williams & Wilkins; 2010.

36. Eisbruch A, Ship JA, Kim HM, et al. Partial irradiation of the parotid gland. Semin Radiat Oncol 2001;11(3):234–9.

37. Munter MW, Hoffner S, Hof H, et al. Changes in salivary gland function after radiotherapy of head and neck tumors measured by quantitative pertechnetate scintigraphy: comparison of intensity-modulated radiotherapy and conventional radiation therapy with and without Amifostine. Int J Radiat Oncol Biol Phys 2007; 67(3):651–9.

38. Rudat V, Munter M, Rades D, et al. The effect of amifostine or IMRT to preserve the parotid function after radiotherapy of the head and neck region measured by quantitative salivary gland scintigraphy. Radiother Oncol 2008;89(1):71–80.

39. Pow EH, Kwong DL, McMillan AS, et al. Xerostomia and quality of life after intensity-modulated radiotherapy vs. conventional radiotherapy for early-stage nasopharyngeal carcinoma: initial report on a randomized controlled clinical trial. Int J Radiat Oncol Biol Phys 2006;66(4):981–91.

40. Kam MK, Leung SF, Zee B, et al. Prospective randomized study of intensity-modulated radiotherapy on salivary gland function in early-stage nasopharyngeal carcinoma patients. J Clin Oncol 2007;25(31):4873–9.

41. Guerrero Urbano MT, Clark CH, Kong C, et al. Target volume definition for head and neck intensity modulated radiotherapy: pre-clinical evaluation of PARSPORT trial guidelines. Clin Oncol 2007;19(8):604–13.

42. Nutting CM, Morden JP, Harrington KJ, et al. Parotid-sparing intensity modulated versus conventional radiotherapy in head and neck cancer (PARSPORT): a phase 3 multicentre randomised controlled trial. Lancet Oncol 2011;12(2):127–36.

43. Emami B, Lyman J, Brown A, et al. Tolerance of normal tissue to therapeutic irradiation. Int J Radiat Oncol Biol Phys 1991;21(1):109–22.

44. Marks LB, Yorke ED, Jackson A, et al. Use of normal tissue complication probability models in the clinic. Int J Radiat Oncol Biol Phys 2010;76(Suppl 3):S10–9.

45. Withers HR, Taylor JM, Maciejewski B. Treatment volume and tissue tolerance. Int J Radiat Oncol Biol Phys 1988;14(4):751–9.

46. Fletcher GH. Lucy Wortham James Lecture. Subclinical disease. Cancer 1984; 53(6):1274–84.

47. Porceddu SV, Pryor DI, Burmeister E, et al. Results of a prospective study of positron emission tomography-directed management of residual nodal abnormalities in node-positive head and neck cancer after definitive radiotherapy with or without systemic therapy. Head Neck 2011;33(12):1675–82.

48. Induction chemotherapy plus radiation compared with surgery plus radiation in patients with advanced laryngeal cancer. The Department of Veterans Affairs Laryngeal Cancer Study Group. N Engl J Med 1991;324(24):1685–90.

49. Forastiere AA, Goepfert H, Maor M, et al. Concurrent chemotherapy and radiotherapy for organ preservation in advanced laryngeal cancer. N Engl J Med 2003;349(22):2091–8.

50. Weber RS, Berkey BA, Forastiere A, et al. Outcome of salvage total laryngectomy following organ preservation therapy: the Radiation Therapy Oncology Group trial 91-11. Arch Otolaryngol Head Neck Surg 2003;129(1):44–9.

51. Soo KC, Tan EH, Wee J, et al. Surgery and adjuvant radiotherapy vs concurrent chemoradiotherapy in stage III/IV nonmetastatic squamous cell head and neck cancer: a randomised comparison. Br J Cancer 2005;93(3):279–86.

52. Lefebvre JL, Ang KK. Larynx preservation clinical trial design: key issues and recommendations-a consensus panel summary. Int J Radiat Oncol Biol Phys 2009;73(5):1293–303.

53. Magnano M, Bongioannini G, Lerda W, et al. Lymphnode metastasis in head and neck squamous cells carcinoma: multivariate analysis of prognostic variables. J Exp Clin Cancer Res 1999;18(1):79–83.

54. de Visscher JG, van den Elsaker K, Grond AJ, et al. Surgical treatment of squamous cell carcinoma of the lower lip: evaluation of long-term results and prognostic factors–a retrospective analysis of 184 patients. J Oral Maxillofac Surg 1998;56(7):814–20 [discussion: 820–1].

55. Close LG, Brown PM, Vuitch MF, et al. Microvascular invasion and survival in cancer of the oral cavity and oropharynx. Arch Otolaryngol Head Neck Surg 1989;115(11):1304–9.

56. Foote RL, Buskirk SJ, Stanley RJ, et al. Patterns of failure after total laryngectomy for glottic carcinoma. Cancer 1989;64(1):143–9.

57. Magnano M, De Stefani A, Lerda W, et al. Prognostic factors of cervical lymph node metastasis in head and neck squamous cell carcinoma. Tumori 1997; 83(6):922–6.

58. Olsen KD, Caruso M, Foote RL, et al. Primary head and neck cancer. Histopathologic predictors of recurrence after neck dissection in patients with lymph node involvement. Arch Otolaryngol Head Neck Surg 1994;120(12):1370–4.

59. Lefebvre JL, Castelain B, De la Torre JC, et al. Lymph node invasion in hypopharynx and lateral epilarynx carcinoma: a prognostic factor. Head Neck Surg 1987;10(1):14–8.

60. Snow GB, Annyas AA, van Slooten EA, et al. Prognostic factors of neck node metastasis. Clin Otolaryngol Allied Sci 1982;7(3):185–92.

61. Cerezo L, Millan I, Torre A, et al. Prognostic factors for survival and tumor control in cervical lymph node metastases from head and neck cancer. A multivariate study of 492 cases. Cancer 1992;69(5):1224–34.

62. Hosal AS, Unal OF, Ayhan A. Possible prognostic value of histopathologic parameters in patients with carcinoma of the oral tongue. Eur Arch Otorhinolaryngol 1998;255(4):216–9.

63. Soo KC, Carter RL, O'Brien CJ, et al. Prognostic implications of perineural spread in squamous carcinomas of the head and neck. Laryngoscope 1986; 96(10):1145–8.

64. Hinerman RW, Mendenhall WM, Morris CG, et al. Postoperative irradiation for squamous cell carcinoma of the oral cavity: 35-year experience. Head Neck 2004;26(11):984–94.

65. Lee WR, Mendenhall WM, Parsons JT, et al. Radical radiotherapy for T4 carcinoma of the skin of the head and neck: a multivariate analysis. Head Neck 1993;15(4):320–4.

66. Yilmaz T, Hosal AS, Gedikoglu G, et al. Prognostic significance of vascular and perineural invasion in cancer of the larynx. Am J Otolaryngol 1998;19(2):83–8.

67. Looser KG, Shah JP, Strong EW. The significance of "positive" margins in surgically resected epidermoid carcinomas. Head Neck Surg 1978;1(2):107–11.

68. Amdur RJ, Parsons JT, Mendenhall WM, et al. Postoperative irradiation for squamous cell carcinoma of the head and neck: an analysis of treatment results and complications. Int J Radiat Oncol Biol Phys 1989;16(1):25–36.

69. Zieske LA, Johnson JT, Myers EN, et al. Squamous cell carcinoma with positive margins. Surgery and postoperative irradiation. Arch Otolaryngol Head Neck Surg 1986;112(8):863–6.

70. Wang ZH, Million RR, Mendenhall WM, et al. Treatment with preoperative irradiation and surgery of squamous cell carcinoma of the head and neck. Cancer 1989;64(1):32–8.

71. Vikram B, Strong EW, Shah JP, et al. Failure at the primary site following multimodality treatment in advanced head and neck cancer. Head Neck Surg 1984;6(3):720–3.

72. Chen TY, Emrich LJ, Driscoll DL. The clinical significance of pathological findings in surgically resected margins of the primary tumor in head and neck carcinoma. Int J Radiat Oncol Biol Phys 1987;13(6):833–7.

73. Gavilan J, Prim MP, De Diego JI, et al. Postoperative radiotherapy in patients with positive nodes after functional neck dissection. Ann Otol Rhinol Laryngol 2000;109(9):844–8.

74. Pfister DG, Ang KK, Brizel DM, et al. Head and neck cancers. J Natl Compr Canc Netw 2011;9(6):596–650.

75. Huang DT, Johnson CR, Schmidt-Ullrich R, et al. Postoperative radiotherapy in head and neck carcinoma with extracapsular lymph node extension and/or positive resection margins: a comparative study. Int J Radiat Oncol Biol Phys 1992;23(4):737–42.

76. Peters LJ, Goepfert H, Ang KK, et al. Evaluation of the dose for postoperative radiation therapy of head and neck cancer: first report of a prospective randomized trial. Int J Radiat Oncol Biol Phys 1993;26(1):3–11.

77. Zelefsky MJ, Harrison LB, Fass DE, et al. Postoperative radiation therapy for squamous cell carcinomas of the oral cavity and oropharynx: impact of therapy on patients with positive surgical margins. Int J Radiat Oncol Biol Phys 1993; 25(1):17–21.

78. Bernier J, Domenge C, Ozsahin M, et al. Postoperative irradiation with or without concomitant chemotherapy for locally advanced head and neck cancer. N Engl J Med 2004;350(19):1945–52.

79. Cooper JS, Pajak TF, Forastiere AA, et al. Postoperative concurrent radiotherapy and chemotherapy for high-risk squamous-cell carcinoma of the head and neck. N Engl J Med 2004;350(19):1937–44.

80. Cooper JS, Zhang Q, Pajak TF, et al. Long-term follow-up of the RTOG 9501/ intergroup phase III trial: postoperative concurrent radiation therapy and chemotherapy in high-risk squamous cell carcinoma of the head and neck. Int J Radiat Oncol Biol Phys 2012;84(5):1198–205.

81. Bernier J, Cooper JS, Pajak TF, et al. Defining risk levels in locally advanced head and neck cancers: a comparative analysis of concurrent postoperative radiation plus chemotherapy trials of the EORTC (#22931) and RTOG (# 9501). Head Neck 2005;27(10):843–50.

82. Adelstein DJ, Li Y, Adams GL, et al. An intergroup phase III comparison of standard radiation therapy and two schedules of concurrent chemoradiotherapy in patients with unresectable squamous cell head and neck cancer. J Clin Oncol 2003;21(1):92–8.

83. Al-Sarraf M, LeBlanc M, Giri PG, et al. Chemoradiotherapy versus radiotherapy in patients with advanced nasopharyngeal cancer: phase III randomized Intergroup study 0099. J Clin Oncol 1998;16(4):1310–7.

84. Calais G, Alfonsi M, Bardet E, et al. Randomized trial of radiation therapy versus concomitant chemotherapy and radiation therapy for advanced-stage oropharynx carcinoma. J Natl Cancer Inst 1999;91(24):2081–6.

85. Brizel DM, Albers ME, Fisher SR, et al. Hyperfractionated irradiation with or without concurrent chemotherapy for locally advanced head and neck cancer. N Engl J Med 1998;338(25):1798–804.

86. Huguenin P, Beer KT, Allal A, et al. Concomitant cisplatin significantly improves locoregional control in advanced head and neck cancers treated with hyperfractionated radiotherapy. J Clin Oncol 2004;22(23):4665–73.

87. Jeremic B, Shibamoto Y, Milicic B, et al. Hyperfractionated radiation therapy with or without concurrent low-dose daily cisplatin in locally advanced squamous cell

carcinoma of the head and neck: a prospective randomized trial. J Clin Oncol 2000;18(7):1458–64.

88. Staar S, Rudat V, Stuetzer H, et al. Intensified hyperfractionated accelerated radiotherapy limits the additional benefit of simultaneous chemotherapy—results of a multicentric randomized German trial in advanced head-and-neck cancer. Int J Radiat Oncol Biol Phys 2001;50(5):1161–71.

89. Blanchard P, Baujat B, Holostenco V, et al. Meta-analysis of chemotherapy in head and neck cancer (MACH-NC): a comprehensive analysis by tumour site. Radiother Oncol 2011;100(1):33–40.

90. Pignon JP, le Maitre A, Maillard E, et al. Meta-analysis of chemotherapy in head and neck cancer (MACH-NC): an update on 93 randomised trials and 17,346 patients. Radiother Oncol 2009;92(1):4–14.

91. Bourhis J, Overgaard J, Audry H, et al. Hyperfractionated or accelerated radiotherapy in head and neck cancer: a meta-analysis. Lancet 2006;368(9538): 843–54.

92. Bourhis J, Sire C, Graff P, et al. Concomitant chemoradiotherapy versus acceleration of radiotherapy with or without concomitant chemotherapy in locally advanced head and neck carcinoma (GORTEC 99-02): an open-label phase 3 randomised trial. Lancet Oncol 2012;13(2):145–53.

93. Ang KK, Harris J, Wheeler R, et al. Human papillomavirus and survival of patients with oropharyngeal cancer. N Engl J Med 2010;363(1):24–35.

94. Ang KK, Berkey BA, Tu X, et al. Impact of epidermal growth factor receptor expression on survival and pattern of relapse in patients with advanced head and neck carcinoma. Cancer Res 2002;62(24):7350–6.

95. Bonner JA, Harari PM, Giralt J, et al. Radiotherapy plus cetuximab for squamous-cell carcinoma of the head and neck. N Engl J Med 2006;354(6): 567–78.

96. Bonner JA, Harari PM, Giralt J, et al. Radiotherapy plus cetuximab for locoregionally advanced head and neck cancer: 5-year survival data from a phase 3 randomised trial, and relation between cetuximab-induced rash and survival. Lancet Oncol 2010;11(1):21–8.

97. Ang KK, Zhang QE, Rosenthal DI, et al. A randomized phase III trial (RTOG 0522) of concurrent accelerated radiation plus cisplatin with or without cetuximab for stage III-IV head and neck squamous cell carcinomas (HNC). ASCO Meeting Abstracts 2011;29(Suppl 15):5500.

98. Rischin D, Peters LJ, O'Sullivan B, et al. Tirapazamine, cisplatin, and radiation versus cisplatin and radiation for advanced squamous cell carcinoma of the head and neck (TROG 02.02, HeadSTART): a phase III trial of the Trans-Tasman Radiation Oncology Group. J Clin Oncol 2010;28(18):2989–95.

99. Henke M, Laszig R, Rube C, et al. Erythropoietin to treat head and neck cancer patients with anaemia undergoing radiotherapy: randomised, double-blind, placebo-controlled trial. Lancet 2003;362(9392):1255–60.

100. Lambin P, Ramaekers BL, van Mastrigt GA, et al. Erythropoietin as an adjuvant treatment with (chemo) radiation therapy for head and neck cancer. Cochrane Database Syst Rev 2009;(3):CD006158.

101. Posner MR, Hershock DM, Blajman CR, et al. Cisplatin and fluorouracil alone or with docetaxel in head and neck cancer. N Engl J Med 2007;357(17): 1705–15.

102. Vermorken JB, Remenar E, van Herpen C, et al. Cisplatin, fluorouracil, and docetaxel in unresectable head and neck cancer. N Engl J Med 2007; 357(17):1695–704.

103. Cohen EE, Karrison T, Kocherginsky M, et al. DeCIDE: a phase III randomized trial of docetaxel (D), cisplatin (P), 5-fluorouracil (F) (TPF) induction chemotherapy (IC) in patients with N2/N3 locally advanced squamous cell carcinoma of the head and neck (SCCHN). ASCO Meeting Abstracts 2012;30(Suppl 15):5500.

104. Haddad RI, Rabinowits G, Tishler RB, et al. The PARADIGM trial: a phase III study comparing sequential therapy (ST) to concurrent chemoradiotherapy (CRT) in locally advanced head and neck cancer (LANHC). ASCO Meeting Abstracts 2012;30(Suppl 15):5501.

105. Gillison ML, D'Souza G, Westra W, et al. Distinct risk factor profiles for human papillomavirus type 16-positive and human papillomavirus type 16-negative head and neck cancers. J Natl Cancer Inst 2008;100(6):407–20.

106. Rischin D, Young RJ, Fisher R, et al. Prognostic significance of p16INK4A and human papillomavirus in patients with oropharyngeal cancer treated on TROG 02.02 phase III trial. J Clin Oncol 2010;28(27):4142–8.

107. Settle K, Posner MR, Schumaker LM, et al. Racial survival disparity in head and neck cancer results from low prevalence of human papillomavirus infection in black oropharyngeal cancer patients. Canc Prev Res 2009;2(9):776–81.

108. Brizel DM, Prosnitz RG, Hunter S, et al. Necessity for adjuvant neck dissection in setting of concurrent chemoradiation for advanced head-and-neck cancer. Int J Radiat Oncol Biol Phys 2004;58(5):1418–23.

109. McHam SA, Adelstein DJ, Rybicki LA, et al. Who merits a neck dissection after definitive chemoradiotherapy for N2-N3 squamous cell head and neck cancer? Head Neck 2003;25(10):791–8.

110. Stenson KM, Haraf DJ, Pelzer H, et al. The role of cervical lymphadenectomy after aggressive concomitant chemoradiotherapy: the feasibility of selective neck dissection. Arch Otolaryngol Head Neck Surg 2000;126(8):950–6.

111. Ferlito A, Corry J, Silver CE, et al. Planned neck dissection for patients with complete response to chemoradiotherapy: a concept approaching obsolescence. Head Neck 2010;32(2):253–61.

112. Gupta T, Master Z, Kannan S, et al. Diagnostic performance of post-treatment FDG PET or FDG PET/CT imaging in head and neck cancer: a systematic review and meta-analysis. Eur J Nucl Med Mol Imaging 2011;38(11):2083–95.

Present and Future Innovations in Radiation Oncology

Lewis Rosenberg, MD, PhD*, Joel Tepper, MD*

KEYWORDS

- Image guidance • Proton • Radiosensitizer • Dose painting • Radiosurgery

KEY POINTS

- Innovations in image guidance have made radiation delivery more accurate and reproducible and may reduce side effects and improve effectiveness.
- Charged particle therapy, such as proton radiation, can overcome the physical limitations of X rays but has some practical limitations.
- Sensitizers are commonly used during radiation to improve tumor control, and protectors are being developed to reduce radiation's adverse effects.
- Functional imaging, such as positron emission tomography, is already used to define targets of radiation and may eventually be used to design more intelligent and complex treatments.
- Altered fractionation is becoming less alternative because many fractionation schemes such as those used in radiosurgery are being studied and adopted.

INTRODUCTION

The practice of radiation oncology has changed greatly in the past few decades and continues to change at a brisk pace. These changes are fed by innovations in engineering, computing, physics, and biology.

An example will help to illustrate the changes that have taken place in radiation oncology. Let us compare a sample patient with rectal cancer treated today with one treated several decades ago. A few decades ago, radiation oncology was practiced in 2 dimensions (ie, with radiographs instead of computed tomography [CT]). A radiation oncologist would have obtained plain radiographs of this patient's pelvis and would have drawn fields by hand with crayon on the radiographs similar to the one shown in **Fig. 1**. The design of these fields would have been based on an understanding of soft tissue anatomy and the natural spread of disease, but bony anatomy

Department of Radiation Oncology, University of North Carolina, 101 Manning Drive, Chapel Hill, NC 27514, USA
* Corresponding author.
E-mail addresses: lewisar3@yahoo.com; joel_tepper@med.unc.edu

Surg Oncol Clin N Am 22 (2013) 599–618
http://dx.doi.org/10.1016/j.soc.2013.02.007
1055-3207/13/$ – see front matter © 2013 Elsevier Inc. All rights reserved.

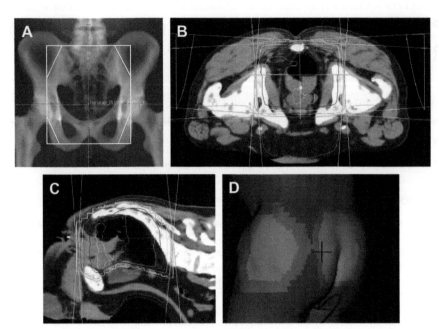

Fig. 1. Examples of treatment planning interfaces in a patient with rectal cancer. (*A*) Representation of a traditional radiation field for the treatment of rectal cancer. (*B, C*) Axial and sagittal images of a modern treatment plan. Four perpendicular radiation fields are best visualized in the axial view. The colored lines represent radiation doses. (*D*) Surface rendering of the treatment plan showing the entrance and exit of the beams on the surface of the body. Because of beam divergence, beams are larger when exiting the body. The jagged lines are a result of the rectangular shape of the multicollimator leaves, which shape the beam.

would have served as the only direct guide. A technician would have cut blocks comprised of a lead-based alloy to match these drawings, and these heavy blocks would have been placed in the machine head daily by radiation therapists at the time of treatment. Radiation doses would have been calculated by hand to a few points of interest.

Today, nearly all patients undergoing radiotherapy are planned using 3-dimensional information from a CT. The radiation oncologist sits in front of a computer and draws fields with a mouse that can be viewed in any dimension. **Fig. 1**B–D provides examples of some of the information available to radiation oncologists when planning a treatment. Inclusion of a target or exclusion of normal tissues is achieved with more confidence. Doses to targets and normal structures (in this case femoral heads, bladder, small bowel, and so forth) can be accurately and quickly determined to any point in 3 dimensions. What ensues is an iterative process whereby the radiation oncologist fine-tunes a plan in an environment in which the consequences of field changes are immediately calculated and known. Furthermore, treatment-planning software itself is capable of some decision making in a process known as *inverse planning*.

The delivery of radiotherapy has also changed. Field-shaping blocks are rarely cut by hand because treatment machines are now equipped with small movable leaves that are able to shape fields quickly and easily. Checking the patients' position during radiation has also improved substantially. Once limited to the use of plain radiographs, radiation oncologists may now choose from a wide variety of image-guidance techniques that provide 3-dimensional information and can, in some situations, even monitor patients' position while the beam is on. Finally, patients today commonly undergo treatment with chemotherapy concurrent with a course of radiotherapy.

This review describes innovations in radiation oncology as well as exciting, potentially field-changing technologies still in development. The authors describe the practical implications as well as the limitations of these innovations. The authors have attempted to include the most influential and recent innovations, but this report is in no way exhaustive; because of space constraints, the authors have excluded concepts that some would deem quite important.

IMAGE GUIDANCE
Introduction

A typical daily radiation treatment lasts at least several minutes. If a patient's position deviates from what is expected even by a small amount, the tumor may be underdosed or normal tissue may be inappropriately exposed to radiation. Dealing with patients' position and motion is one of the fundamental issues of radiotherapy. If there is no mechanism in place to check the patients' position, a treatment machine has no knowledge of the patients' location and the linear accelerator will continue ignorantly streaming X rays regardless of where the patients may be. To reduce the chance of motion error, almost all modern radiotherapy is guided by imaging obtained in the treatment room with patients in the treatment position.[1]

The simplest, and most frequently used, form of image guidance involves acquiring plain radiographs while patients are in the treatment position. These portal films are simple to acquire and are adequate for many situations, but there are significant limitations. First, soft tissues (which are often the most relevant for localizing tumors) are poorly visualized. Second, image quality in general is often poor because of the use of a very high-energy photon beam optimized for treatment rather than imaging (**Fig. 2**). Third, portal films acquired before treatment yield no information about motion while the radiation beam is on.

The limitations of using portal films for image guidance are well demonstrated with the example of prostate cancer treatment. Although the bony pelvis may seem to be positioned properly, the prostate may move substantially between or even during radiation treatments. For example, a rectal air bubble may displace the prostate anteriorly over 1 cm.[2,3] A treatment plan using portal imaging alone for image guidance would be ignorant of this motion. Faced with this knowledge, the treating radiation oncologist is faced with either expanding the margins of the radiation fields, which will place more normal tissue in the field, or using narrow fields but risk missing the target. In modern radiation oncology, more advanced forms of image-guided radiotherapy (IGRT) are commonly used for situations in which portal films are inadequate. Most of these technologies have become common only in the past decade. (It is important to note that IGRT typically refers to technologies more advanced than portal films, although literally, radiographs are a form of image guidance.)

IGRT for Interfraction Motion

Interfraction motion refers to changes in patient position from one treatment to the next. A course of radiation typically consists of many individual treatments (or fractions) of radiation delivered daily. There are many methods to account and correct for interfraction motion that are superior to portal films. One solution is to obtain 3-dimensional imaging with the use of CT. A CT scan may be acquired in the treatment

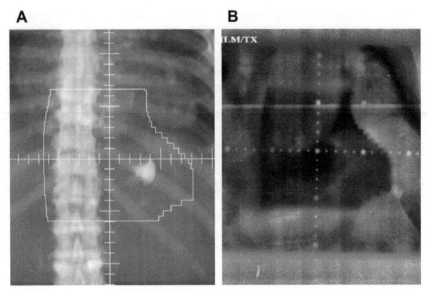

Fig. 2. Digitally reconstructed radiograph (DRR) versus portal. (*A*) This DRR is an image reconstructed from a CT intended to emulate a plain radiograph. (*B*) A portal image obtained with megavoltage photons. Commonly, radiation oncologists compare these images to check patients' position. The poor image quality of the megavoltage radiograph is readily apparent in this example.

vault in several manners. First, a treatment vault may contain a CT scanner that is literally built on rails and is able to roll over the treatment table and the stationary patient (**Fig. 3**). Second, some treatment machines have the capability of generating a CT by rotating the gantry 360° around patients while acquiring an image; the result of this technique is termed a *cone beam CT*.[1] There are many other ways of accounting for interfraction motion, such as through the use of ultrasound or by implantation of radiopaque markers in soft tissues that can be visualized easily with films. Although very useful for many situations, the main limitation to all of these methods is that they do not account for motion during treatment or intrafraction motion. If patients move during treatment, radiation continues unperturbed.

IGRT for Intrafraction Motion

There are many systems that can account for intrafraction motion. These systems can automatically stop treatment or sound a warning if movement is detected and will resume once adjustments are made. Let us again use the example of prostate cancer. One solution to intrafraction motion for prostate cancer uses radiofrequency transponders that are implanted into the prostate before the start of radiation. During radiation, sensors track the position of these transponders, which act as a surrogate for prostate position. If one of the transponders moves outside of its expected range, treatment stops, and the radiation therapists reposition the patient. This radiofrequency transponder method can localize the prostate to within a few millimeters.[4]

Intrafraction motion is particularly relevant in cases when tumors are in or adjacent to the lung and move with respiration. The traditional and simple method of compensating for respiratory motion is to expand the borders of the radiation fields to achieve adequate margins throughout respiration, with the obvious drawback being larger

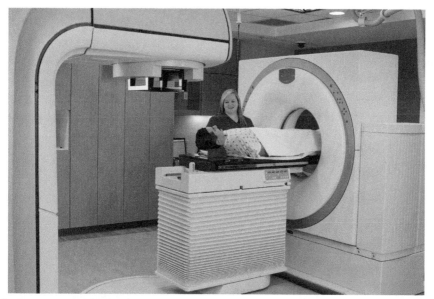

Fig. 3. CT on rails. This technology is one example of an advanced form of image guidance. The CT unit shown in the picture can roll back and forth and obtain images of patients while lying still on the treatment couch. These images can be compared with the treatment-planning CT and the position is verified. (*Courtesy of* Mark Kostich, Chapel Hill, NC; with permission.)

fields with increased dose to normal tissues. More advanced solutions to respiratory motion management include systems that predict the position of the target and turn the beam on and off as the target moves into and out of position in a process known as *respiratory gating*. Respiratory gating systems do not directly see the tumor. Instead, these respiratory gating systems track an easily detectable surrogate marker on the skin or implanted near the tumor and predict the position of the target based on these surrogates.[5,6]

For example, the authors' institution uses a stereoscopic system, which is a collection of cameras that can recognize body position. This system essentially watches the rise and fall of the abdomen and from this information can predict where the target is throughout the breathing cycle.[6] Respiratory gating is often used in the treatment of breast cancer, for which radiation fields may include significant cardiac tissue at full expiration, but greatly exclude the heart during inspiration. For the treatment of breast cancer, patients are often instructed to inhale and hold their breath to increase the distance between the chest wall and heart.[7,8]

A drawback of respiratory gating systems is that the radiation beam is turned on and off with each breath and the total duration of treatment is increased. There is at least one commercially available system, the CyberKnife (Accuray, Sunnyvale, CA), that actually moves with the target throughout respiration. The CyberKnife is a compact linear accelerator that is mounted on a powerful robotic arm that is capable of very fine and fast movements (**Fig. 4**). The x-ray beam remains on as the robotic arm moves back and forth with respiration, keeping the beam on target.[9] There are other respiratory tracking systems in development that use a robotic couch that moves patients with each breath instead of moving the beam.[10]

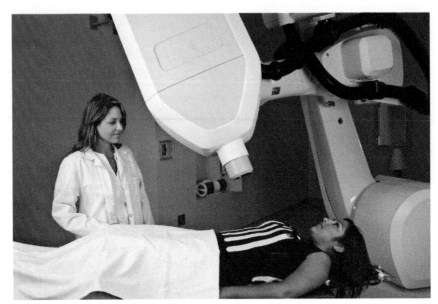

Fig. 4. CyberKnife. This machine is comprised of a compact linear accelerator mounted on a robotic arm. See text for more details. (*Courtesy of* Mark Kostich, Chapel Hill, NC; with permission.)

The Future of Image Guidance

The ideal image-guidance system would track real anatomy instead of surrogate markers, continuously track during treatment, and make automatic adjustments to compensate for movement. To this end, radiotherapy machines coupled with magnetic resonance imaging (MRI) are in development by at least 2 organizations, one based in Germany and another in Ohio.[11,12] These machines are being designed to continuously and quickly acquire MRI images during radiotherapy and to automatically interpret images within small fractions of a second. Automatic and fast interpretation of images is a substantial computational challenge. Successful development of MRI-coupled linear accelerators, therefore, would represent both an engineering and computing achievement. If and when these devices are used in patient care, they have the potential to be a very important tool for IGRT.

PARTICLE BEAM THERAPY (PROTONS AND SO FORTH)
The Problem with X Rays

Despite all of the innovative gadgets adopted by radiation oncologists in the past decades, they are still limited by the physical laws of high-energy X rays, which are used to deliver most radiotherapy. An x-ray beam loses a constant percentage of its energy per distance traveled through a patient. A typical x-ray beam used for treatment loses about 3% of its dose per centimeter traveled. The x-ray beam's remaining energy decreases exponentially through a patient and the beam exits on the other side of the patient, destined toward the wall of the vault with substantial remaining energy.[13] The usual solution is to aim multiple x-rays beams from many angles at the target, so that only at the convergence of the beams is the dose high (as a rough approximation of this procedure, think of 4 flashlights aimed at a single spot). Even with these efforts, there is substantial dose deposited in tissues where it is unwanted.

Charged Particle Radiation, in Theory

High-energy protons and other charged particles behave in a fundamentally different way. They deposit little dose through much of their path, then deposit more dose at the end of their paths, resulting in a pattern termed a *Bragg peak* (**Fig. 5**). Furthermore, the depth of the Bragg peak can be adjusted either by changing the energy of the proton or by adding material between the proton source and the body. With these methods, a tumor may be treated to a high dose while sparing shallower normal tissues.[14] Because protons save much of their dose deposition for the end of their paths, a treatment with protons will typically deliver less dose to normal tissues than will a photon treatment.

Studies have evaluated the theoretical advantage of protons over X rays. Studies comparing protons with X rays for prostate cancer show that protons reduce mean rectal dose 25% to 59% and mean bladder dose 19% to 50%.[15–17] Similarly, proton therapy for lung cancer reduces the dose to the lung, spinal cord, esophagus, and heart.[18] Perhaps the largest theoretical benefit in using proton therapy is in the treatment of pediatric patients requiring radiotherapy to the brain or the craniospinal axis. Normal tissues of children and adolescents likely have higher inherent radiosensitivity, and children also have a lifetime to experience late effects of treatment. Proton therapy for craniospinal irradiation for pediatric medulloblastoma has been explored and demonstrates an impressive reduction in the radiation dose to normal tissues. An illustration of this concept is in **Fig. 6**.[19]

Carbon ions offer further theoretical advantages over protons. Carbon ions, like protons, deposit more energy at the end of their paths in the form of a Bragg peak. Unlike X rays or protons, carbon ions have a characteristic termed high *relative biologic effectiveness* (RBE). RBE is a measure of how effective radiation is per unit of energy deposited. Simply put, particles with a high RBE, such as carbon ions, kill more cells for a given amount of energy deposited.[20] Furthermore, for carbon ions, the RBE increases only at the end of the path, whereas in the earlier portions of the path, the RBE is the same as X rays or protons. Practically, this property of carbon ions means that not only is the dose delivered where it is wanted but the dose also has more effect than that of X rays or protons. Carbon ions have another potential advantage. As they deposit dose in tissue, carbon ions generate positron-emitting isotopes. If a patient is placed in a positron emission tomography (PET) scanner immediately following treatment, the dose deposited may be directly evaluated. Although this application may seem obscure, the ability to directly visualize and confirm dose deposition is quite exciting to the radiation oncologist.[21]

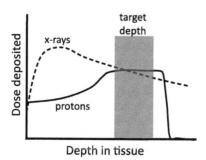

Fig. 5. Depth dose profiles of a proton field versus a photon field. To dose the target as indicated, the integral dose (area under the curve) of the photon field will be greater than the proton field.

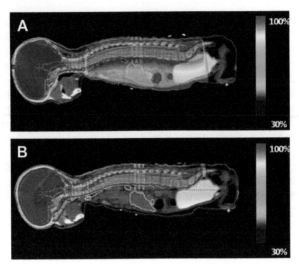

Fig. 6. Craniospinal irradiation treatment planned with photons (*A*) versus protons (*B*). The color keys at the right of the images show the percentage of prescribed dose delivered. Note that the proton plan spares the anterior thorax and abdomen. (*From* Yoon M, Shin DH, Kim J, et al. Craniospinal irradiation techniques: a dosimetric comparison of proton beams with standard and advanced photon radiotherapy. Int J Radiat Oncol Biol Phys 2011;81(3):637–46; with permission.)

Charged Particle Radiation, in Practice

Radiation oncologists are drawn toward particle therapy because of these theoretical advantages and the attractive plans generated by their treatment planning systems, but the actual clinical benefits of particle therapy are not so easily known, and the literature lacks good randomized evidence in its favor. Furthermore, there are potential disadvantages to proton therapy when compared with x-ray therapy. First, because of the exquisite sensitivity of the path of protons to the patients' position and tissue type, they are less forgiving than X rays and there is more uncertainty as to where radiation is actually being delivered.[22] To compensate for this uncertainty, the region targeted with radiation is typically slightly larger, which might place normal tissues at a higher risk of adverse effects.[22] Second, image-guidance and field-shaping technology lags behind x-ray radiotherapy, although this problem may be overcome given more time and engineering advancements.

The decision to treat with particle therapy is often based on a predicted reduction in normal tissue toxicity, but this improvement is often predicted to be small. For example, for the treatment of prostate cancer with intensity modulated radiation therapy (IMRT), the modern rate of grade 3 late genitourinary and gastrointestinal toxicities may be as low as 5% and 1%, respectively.[23] These data suggest little room for improvement for these parameters beyond current x-ray–based therapy. In addition, the irradiated volumes that result in toxicity are often in the target so that they will always receive a high dose of radiation regardless of the modality. A recent retrospective study has shown no detectable reduction in morbidity with protons for prostate cancer, possibly because of the limitations described in the previous paragraph.[24]

Cost is certainly one of the single most significant limitations to the widespread adoption of particle therapy. Individual proton facilities cost between $100 million and $225 million.[25] Even with some very favorable assumptions, some individuals have argued that the cost is not worth the potential small gains for many cancers.[26] Despite these astronomic costs and the practical limitations of protons, there is a proton boom in the United States. Based on the Particle Therapy Co-operative Group's Web site, which tracks all facilities treating with particle therapy, there are currently 34 proton and 6 carbon ion operating facilities in the world. The United States has 10 operating proton facilities, with 6 more under construction.[27] When the dust settles, proton and carbon ion therapy will likely have an important place in the treatment of certain cancers, but particle therapy seems unlikely to replace X rays as the standard modality for most treatments any time soon.

RADIATION MODULATORS
Radiosensitizers

Chemical radiosensitization has become the standard of care for many solid tumors over the past several decades. Starting with some gastrointestinal tumors in the 1950s and then becoming standard for anal cancer in the 1970s,[28] concurrent chemotherapy grew in favor and has become standard for many situations after proving itself through randomized trials throughout the 1990s and 2000s.[29] At present, the most agents used as radiosensitizers are common chemotherapies, such as cisplatin or 5-fluorouracil (5FU). The functions of these chemotherapeutic agents are in no way limited to radiosensitization and result in significant side effects.

The optimal radiation sensitizer is an agent that increases the effectiveness of radiation without increasing side effects (**Fig. 7**). Current radiation sensitizers are far from this ideal and also increase side effects. Targeted biologic compounds with mechanisms of action more specific to radiation sensitization are under study with the hope that they may be more efficacious with fewer systemic effects. Epithelial growth factor receptor (EGFR) and its associated pathways are often activated in tumor cells. EGFR inhibitors act as radiosensitizers, perhaps partially because of their ability to slow tumor repopulation.[30] One EGFR inhibitor has been well studied as a radiosensitizer: A randomized controlled study of head and neck cancers published in 2006 showed that the addition of cetuximab to radiotherapy improved median survival from 29 to 49 months.[31] Clinical trials with standard chemotherapy agents had shown similar improvements, but this was a landmark study because it was the first randomized trial to show a benefit with the use of a targeted biologic compound.

Other novel pharmaceuticals show promise as radiosensitizers. For example, the use of poly (ADP-ribose) polymerase (PARP) inhibitors as radiosensitizers has

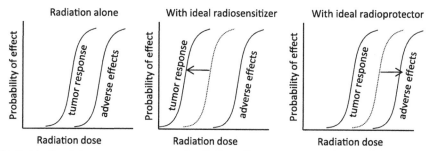

Fig. 7. Idealized dose response curves of radiation effects on tumor and normal tissues. With ideal radiosensitization, the tumor response curve is shifted to the left, so that a lower dose of radiation will shrink or kill the tumor. With ideal radioprotection, the normal tissue response curve is shifted to the right, so that a higher dose of radiation is needed to damage normal tissues.

generated much interest and enthusiasm. PARP is an enzyme that is important in DNA damage repair pathways. In response to DNA damage, it catalyzes the production of the polymer poly (ADP-ribose), which recruits many proteins involved in DNA repair.[32] Because the effects of radiation are ultimately dependent on DNA damage, it stands to reason that an inhibitor of DNA repair would sensitize cells to radiation. Several companies have recently synthesized a new generation of potent and selective PARP inhibitors, and early clinical trials combining these with radiation are underway.[33]

Another strategy to radiosensitize tumors is to promote apoptosis when exposed to radiation. One of the hallmarks of malignant transformation is resistance to apoptosis.[34] Great efforts have been put forth in an attempt to counteract this behavior from a variety of approaches. Laboratory studies have shown that promoters of apoptosis do have radiosensitizing properties. For example, drugs that activate the so-called death-receptors, such as those that mimic tumor necrosis factor –related apoptosis-inducing ligand, act as radiosensitizers in vitro.[35] Another drug shown to induce apoptosis, AT-101 (or gossypol), is being evaluated as a radiosensitizer in ongoing clinical trials for the treatment of glioblastoma multiforme and esophageal cancer. These results are not yet published.[30]

Normal Tissue Protectors

Another strategy to modulate the effects of radiotherapy is to protect normal tissues from adverse sequelae. An ideal radioprotector would protect normal tissues from the effects of radiation while leaving tumor sensitive to radiation (see **Fig. 7**).

Although much research has been devoted to the development of radioprotectors, there are only a handful of agents in clinical use. The free-radical scavenger amifostine is approved as an agent to reduce the incidence of xerostomia with radiation to the salivary glands.[36] Amifostine tends to accumulate preferentially in normal tissues and does not seem to affect tumor control or cure. Because of the significant side effects, amifostine is not widely used. Another radioprotector used clinically is palifermin, which is a recombinant human keratinocyte growth factor. It is used to prevent mucositis in patients undergoing total body irradiation to reduce the incidence of severe mucositis. Palifermin is undergoing further evaluation as a radioprotector in other contexts, but results have been mixed; there remains concern about inadvertent tumor protection.[37]

Many other radioprotectors are being evaluated in the laboratory and in clinical trials, many of which have antioxidant properties. One such antioxidant radioprotector worth mentioning is tempol. A phase I clinical trial demonstrated the ability of tempol, when applied topically to the scalp, to prevent alopecia in patients undergoing whole brain radiotherapy. This result is striking because it demonstrates the potential of radioprotectors to prevent what is typically thought to be an unavoidable side effect of radiotherapy.[38] Many other compounds are at various levels of investigation, including growth factors, protease inhibitors, angiotensin-converting enzyme inhibitors, nonsteroidal antiinflammatory drugs, and transforming growth factor –beta inhibitors.[37] Radioprotectors have not become a standard part of radiotherapy as have sensitizing agents, but there are exciting radioprotectors in development with the potential to substantially improve the treatment of patients undergoing radiation.

FUNCTIONAL IMAGING

The use of imaging to identify targets and normal structures is an essential component of modern radiation oncology. Most imaging modalities in use today, such as MRI or

CT, provide structural information about tissues but do not give any functional information.[39] Functional imaging, which may provide information about the behavior of tissues rather than only anatomic information, may be extremely useful to radiation oncologists. For example, such information may help physicians direct the radiation dose at regions of tumor that are resistant to radiation or reduce radiation to normal tissues that are more functional.[40]

PET is by far the most frequently used functional imaging modality in oncology. PET uses a tracer that includes a positron emitting radionuclide incorporated into a metabolite (**Fig. 8**). Tracers are designed to localize to a region or regions of interest, a property that is typically based on the normal function of the metabolite. For example, the most common tracer used for PET imaging is ^{18}F-2-fluoro-2-deoxy-D-glucose (FDG), which is useful to detect anatomic regions that have accelerated glucose metabolism, a common characteristic of neoplasms.[39] Positrons emitted from the tracer travel a short distance and are annihilated when they come into contact with an electron, a process that generates 2 photons that travel 180° from one another. These 2 photons are ultimately detected by the PET scanner.[41] Because the photons always travel exactly away from each other, when they hit the detector at about the same moment, their origin can be determined. Single-photon emission computed tomography (SPECT) is another functional imaging modality that is conceptually similar to PET; however, PET uses positron emitting radionuclides, whereas SPECT uses single-photon emitting tracers that are directly detected.[42]

Improved Delineation of Tumors with Functional Imaging

Radiation oncologists frequently use PET as a component of treatment planning, and studies have shown that the use of FDG-PET can have significant influence on the

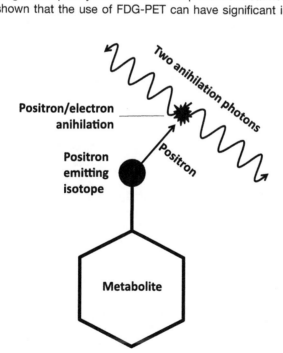

Fig. 8. PET tracer. A PET tracer is composed of a metabolite that incorporates an isotope that emits a positron. The emitted positron is annihilated when it contacts an electron, an interaction that emits 2 photons that are ultimately detected by the scanner.

definition of target volume and improves the consistency of target definition between physicians (**Fig. 9**).[43,44] Although FDG is the most commonly used tracer, PET is by no means limited to a glucose-based tracer. Any metabolite that incorporates a positron-emitting radionuclide can be used for various purposes, some that may be quite useful for radiation targeting. For example, amino acid–based tracers, such as 11C-methionine, may be used to better delineate gliomas, an approach that is undergoing study.[45]

Dose Painting with Functional Imaging

As it is used in practice today by radiation oncologists, PET and other functional imaging modalities yield essentially binary information: tumor is present or it is not. In the future, functional imaging modalities may be developed (or existing technologies might be refined) that yield valuable information about various parts of tumors. In theory, such imaging modalities could differentiate regions of tumor that are radioresistant from those that are radiosensitive. Higher doses could be prescribed to the resistant regions and lower doses to the more sensitive regions, whereas today, the entire tumor is prescribed a uniform dose. This concept is known as *dose painting*.

Several PET tracers are being evaluated that may eventually be used in dose painting. For example, regions of a tumor undergoing accelerated proliferation may be radioresistant, simply because tumor growth outpaces cell killing. The PET tracer 3'-deoxy-3'-[^{18}F] fluorothymidine (FLT) accumulates in proliferating cells[46] and has been proven to correlate well with other markers of cell proliferation.[47] Very early studies have suggested that FLT-PET may be useful to identify regions of tumors requiring more dose for eradication.[48] Similarly, because oxygen is a potent radiation sensitizer, hypoxic regions of tumor may be radioresistant. PET tracers, such as [18F] fluoromisonidazole, indicate hypoxic areas, and additional radiation may be directed to these regions.[49] Before dose painting within tumors is incorporated into practice, several questions must be addressed including the following: (1) Does functional imaging accurately identify regions of tumor with the predicted characteristics, such as hypoxia or accelerated growth? (2) Do these regions correspond with differences in radiosensitivity? (3) What doses of radiation is required to adequately treat the radioresistant or radiosensitive regions?

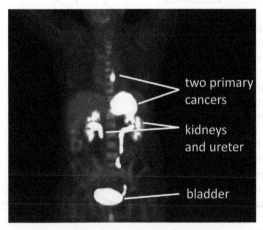

Fig. 9. FDG-18 PET of a patient with a large gastric adenocarcinoma and a second primary cancer of the esophagus. The boundaries of this patient's tumor were difficult to see with CT alone, so a PET was used to better plan radiotherapy to these tumors.

Sparing Normal Tissues with Functional Imaging

Functional imaging might also be used to better avoid critical normal tissues. When planning a course of radiation therapy, normal tissues are typically thought of as functionally homogenous, meaning one part is as functional as any other. This philosophy is often not true. A simple example of functional heterogeneity of normal tissues can be illustrated by renal function, whereby one kidney may contribute much more to total glomerular filtration than the other. With knowledge of this differential function, a radiation oncologist may design beams to spare a more functional kidney at the cost of sacrificing a defunct kidney. There is a functional imaging scan that uses dimercaptosuccinic acid (a photon-emitting radionuclide) that is able to show differential function of kidneys.[50] In the authors' department, in fact, they frequently order this scan and adjust their beams accordingly.

It is also known that there is functional heterogeneity in other organs, such as lung, liver, and bone marrow. Several groups are studying the possibility of selectively avoiding areas of these organs that are more active.[51] For example, lung SPECT (using the tracer [^{99m}Tc] macroaggregated albumin) can differentiate highly functional regions of lung from those that are less active. Several groups have performed theoretical studies showing potential benefits to using this information in radiation-treatment planning. In theory, those parts of the lung that are better perfused and aerated may be preferentially spared from radiation.[51] Sparing highly functional regions of liver and bone marrow may also reduce adverse effects of radiation; but these studies are in the early stages, and these techniques have not yet been adopted.[51,52]

NONSTANDARD FRACTIONATION
Introduction

A simple experiment involving the sterilization of rams' testicles was one of the seminal experiments that ushered in the modern era of radiation therapy. Regaud, in the 1920s, demonstrated that rams could be sterilized by exposing their testicles to a single dose of radiation but that this procedure consistently resulted in significant skin toxicity. By administering the dose of radiation in multiple smaller increments, or fractions, he was able to still sterilize the rams but spare the skin from severe toxicity.[20] This experiment demonstrated that simply by modifying the fractionation scheme of radiation, one could modify its effects in a tissue-dependent manner. Since that time, the science of radiobiology has confirmed that there are 3 main factors that determine the effects of radiation: total dose, dose per fraction, and total duration of treatment. These concepts have led to much experimentation on various fractionation schemes, usually in an attempt to treat tumors more effectively while sparing normal tissues. Ninety years after the discovery of fractionated radiation, we are still trying to determine the optimal fractionation schemes for many diseases.

It is important here to define several terms. *Standard fractionation* refers to treatment with daily fractions of 1.8 Gy to 2 Gy daily. *Hypofractionation* refers to radiation delivered at a dose more than 2 Gy daily, and *hyperfractionation* is radiation delivered at a dose less than 1.8 Gy daily (*hyper* refers to more fractions to achieve the same dose, and *hypo* refers to fewer fractions to achieve the same dose). This topic may seem a bit esoteric, but altered fractionation is poised to change much of the practice of radiation oncology and in some ways it already has. This review focuses on hypofractionation, or high dose per fraction, because this subject represents most of the recent innovations concerning altered fractionation.

Moderate Hypofractionation

Hypofractionation ranges from doses slightly more than 2 Gy daily to very high doses administered in a single or few fractions (for example 20 Gy in a single fraction for a brain metastasis). There are 2 main rationales for hypofractionation. First, it may be more effective for certain cancers; second, it typically reduces total treatment time, which improves patient convenience and often cost.[53] Radiation for breast conservation therapy is one of the best-studied areas of hypofractionation. Multiple randomized trials have evaluated hypofractionation for breast conservation and essentially demonstrated equivalency with standard fractionation.[54–56] For example, a Canadian study randomized patients with early stage breast cancer undergoing postlumpectomy radiation to 50.0 Gy in 25 fractions versus 42.5 Gy in 16 fractions. In a publication in 2010, it was demonstrated that after a median follow-up of 12 years, there was no difference in oncologic outcomes or cosmesis.[56] Hypofractionation in this context does not improve outcomes; it is intended to be an equivalent treatment that is faster and cheaper. The publication of this and other similar trials is changing the standard of care for a very common radiotherapy treatment.

Hypofractionation is theorized to be more effective in certain types of cancer, such as prostate cancer; but the reasons for this advantage are complex and are beyond the scope of this review.[57] A handful of smaller randomized controlled trials have been published that compare standard fractionation for prostate cancer with hypofractionation, and several large randomized trials are ongoing.[58–60] In one study based in Italy, men with high-risk prostate cancer were randomized to a standard course of 8 weeks of radiation (80 Gy in 2 Gy fractions, 5 days each week) versus a hypofractionated course of 5 weeks of radiation (62 Gy in 3.1 Gy fractions, 4 days each week). Early results with about 3 years of follow-up showed a lower biochemical failure rate in the hypofractionated group without higher toxicity.[58] It will be many years before this and other trials are sufficiently mature to change the standard of care for radiation therapy to the prostate, but preliminary results support the radiobiologic theory that prostate cancer may be better controlled with hypofractionation. These data on breast, prostate, and other cancers are beginning to shake radiation oncologists' unwavering faith in standard fractionation.

Extreme Hypofractionation: Radiosurgery

Radiosurgery represents the extreme of hypofractionation. Radiosurgery refers to radiation treatment whereby high doses of radiotherapy are delivered in 5 or fewer fractions. It is certainly not a true surgery, although it bears some resemblance to surgery in that it is typically completed in a single (or very few) settings; it typically renders tissue in the high-dose region nonfunctional while sparing surrounding tissues. The idea that radiosurgery burns or ablates may be useful from a functional or radiographic point of view but it is simply not correct histologically. Under the microscope, changes to normal tissues after radiosurgery may actually be subtle and delayed and typically involve vascular changes several months following treatment.[61]

As described earlier, the effects of radiation depend on total dose and dose per fraction. These factors are related in the following manner: With a higher dose per fraction, a lower total dose is needed to achieve the same effect on a tumor. For example, a single dose of 15 or 20 Gy delivered during radiosurgery is likely biologically equivalent to delivering 50 or 70 Gy with standard fractionation (1.8–2.0 Gy per fraction). It is not uncommon for multiple fractions of very high doses to be delivered during radiosurgery, such as 45 Gy or 60 Gy in 3 fractions. When such doses are delivered, the biologic equivalent dose is much higher than what is ever delivered with standard fractionation.[62,63]

Why is radiosurgery not used for all tumors? Radiosurgery has a devastating effect on tissues in the high-dose region and in tissues immediately surrounding this region. It is most useful for small, well-delineated tumors because a rim of surrounding tissue will also receive a high dose of radiation. The larger and more irregularly shaped a tumor is, the more normal tissue will receive a high dose of radiation. For example, if a physician attempted to treat a large non–small cell lung cancer (NSCLC) with lymph nodes in the mediastinum using radiosurgical doses, damage to normal tissues, including the lung and esophagus, would likely be severe and the treatment would at least result in significant morbidity and possibly the death of the patient. In cases whereby large volumes of normal tissues are infield, the axiom *fractionation is your friend* still holds true.

In the clinic, radiosurgery is now coming of age, but the concept is more than 50 years old. Lars Leksell first used the word *radiosurgery* in 1951 and developed the first machine dedicated to radiosurgery in 1968, the GammaKnife, which was (and still is) used to treat intracranial targets.[64] With advances in imaging and engineering, along with a better clinical understanding of its function in cancer therapy, radiosurgery is becoming a standard offering in radiation oncology departments. There several machines that have been specifically engineered to treat patients with radiosurgery, including the Gammaknife (Elekta, Stockholm, Sweden) and CyberKnife (Accuray, Sunnyvale, CA), and other machines that look more like standard treatment machines with radiosurgery capabilities. The one common element that all machines capable of delivering radiosurgery have in common is accuracy to within millimeters. Various methods are used to achieve such accuracy, which typically involves careful tracking of patients' movement during the actual treatment. It is worthwhile noting that it is advances in engineering that have improved accuracy that have allowed radiosurgery to blossom.

Radiosurgery in practice

Radiosurgery for brain metastases is one of the best examples of an innovation that has recently changed the practice of oncology. Radiosurgery for brain metastases is one of the most common uses of the technology and typically yields a control rate of 60% to 90% for the treated lesions.[65] Many randomized clinical trials have evaluated the efficacies and side effects of surgery, radiosurgery, and whole brain radiation for brain metastases.[66–71] The results of most of these trials have looked favorable for radiosurgery and have led many to suggest that treatment with radiosurgery alone without whole brain radiation is the preferred approach for brain metastases.[68] This practice represents a dramatic shift from the past approach, which was essentially whole brain radiation therapy for all patients.

Another situation whereby the use of radiosurgery has grown quickly in recent years is in the treatment of early primary NSCLC. This approach has been validated in several prospective trials and retrospective studies and seems to yield control rates similar to surgery.[63,72,73] An ongoing randomized clinical trial is comparing radiosurgery with resection for early NSCLC.[74] The results of this study combined with other data may make radiosurgery a standard option for the treatment of patients with early stage NSCLC.

Radiosurgery is also used at times for primary brain tumors, base of skull tumors, prostate cancer, renal cell carcinoma, and primary and secondary liver cancers. The radiosurgical data for these sites is less mature than it is for brain and lung metastases.[75,76] Radiosurgery is quickly becoming a component of standard practice for radiation oncologists and promises to continue growing at a brisk pace.

SUMMARY

Radiation oncology has changed rapidly in recent decades and it continues to change at a daunting pace. The radiation oncology innovations that typically come to mind and are commonly discussed include engineering advances, such image guidance and charged particle therapy. Ultimately, advances in radiobiology, such as concurrent therapy with targeted biologic agents and treatment planning with functional imaging, may prove to be equally if not more revolutionary. It is difficult to predict what the practice of radiation oncology will look like in 20 years, but it is easy to predict that it will differ substantially from current practice.

REFERENCES

1. Chen GT, Sharp GC, Mori S. A review of image-guided radiotherapy. Radiol Phys Technol 2009;2(1):1–12.
2. Perez-Romasanta LA, Lozano-Martin E, Velasco-Jimenez J, et al. CTV to PTV margins for prostate irradiation. Three-dimensional quantitative assessment of interfraction uncertainties using portal imaging and serial CT scans. Clin Transl Oncol 2009;11(9):615–21.
3. Stephans KL, Xia P, Tendulkar RD, et al. The current status of image-guided external beam radiotherapy for prostate cancer. Curr Opin Urol 2010;20(3):223–8.
4. Button MR, Staffurth JN. Clinical application of image-guided radiotherapy in bladder and prostate cancer. Clin Oncol (R Coll Radiol) 2010;22(8):698–706.
5. Willoughby TR, Forbes AR, Buchholz D, et al. Evaluation of an infrared camera and X-ray system using implanted fiducials in patients with lung tumors for gated radiation therapy. Int J Radiat Oncol Biol Phys 2006;66(2):568–75.
6. Hughes S, McClelland J, Tarte S, et al. Assessment of two novel ventilatory surrogates for use in the delivery of gated/tracked radiotherapy for non-small cell lung cancer. Radiother Oncol 2009;91(3):336–41.
7. Vikstrom J, Hjelstuen MH, Mjaaland I, et al. Cardiac and pulmonary dose reduction for tangentially irradiated breast cancer, utilizing deep inspiration breath-hold with audio-visual guidance, without compromising target coverage. Acta Oncol 2011;50(1):42–50.
8. Giraud P, Yorke E, Jiang S, et al. Reduction of organ motion effects in IMRT and conformal 3D radiation delivery by using gating and tracking techniques. Cancer Radiother 2006;10(5):269–82.
9. Gibbs IC, Loo BW Jr. CyberKnife stereotactic ablative radiotherapy for lung tumors. Technol Cancer Res Treat 2010;9(6):589–96.
10. Buzurovic I, Yu Y, Podder TK. Active tracking and dynamic dose delivery for robotic couch in radiation therapy. Conf Proc IEEE Eng Med Biol Soc 2011; 2011:2156–9.
11. Raaymakers BW, Lagendijk JJ, Overweg J, et al. Integrating a 1.5 T MRI scanner with a 6 MV accelerator: proof of concept. Phys Med Biol 2009;54(12):N229–37.
12. Verellen D, De Ridder M, Linthout N, et al. Innovations in image-guided radiotherapy. Nat Rev Cancer 2007;7(12):949–60.
13. Khan FM. The physics of radiation therapy. 4th edition. Philadelphia: Lippincott Williams & Wilkins; 2010.
14. Durante M, Loeffler JS. Charged particles in radiation oncology. Nat Rev Clin Oncol 2010;7(1):37–43.
15. Chera BS, Vargas C, Morris CG, et al. Dosimetric study of pelvic proton radiotherapy for high-risk prostate cancer. Int J Radiat Oncol Biol Phys 2009;75(4): 994–1002.

16. Mock U, Bogner J, Georg D, et al. Comparative treatment planning on localized prostate carcinoma conformal photon- versus proton-based radiotherapy. Strahlenther Onkol 2005;181(7):448–55.

17. Trofimov A, Nguyen PL, Coen JJ, et al. Radiotherapy treatment of early-stage prostate cancer with IMRT and protons: a treatment planning comparison. Int J Radiat Oncol Biol Phys 2007;69(2):444–53.

18. Zhang X, Li Y, Pan X, et al. Intensity-modulated proton therapy reduces the dose to normal tissue compared with intensity-modulated radiation therapy or passive scattering proton therapy and enables individualized radical radiotherapy for extensive stage IIIB non-small-cell lung cancer: a virtual clinical study. Int J Radiat Oncol Biol Phys 2010;77(2):357–66.

19. Fossati P, Ricardi U, Orecchia R. Pediatric medulloblastoma: toxicity of current treatment and potential role of proton therapy. Cancer Treat Rev 2009;35(1):79–96.

20. Hall EJ, Giaccia AJ. Radiobiology for the radiologist. 6th edition. Philadelphia: Lippincott Williams & Wilkins; 2006.

21. Weber U, Kraft G. Comparison of carbon ions versus protons. Cancer J 2009; 15(4):325–32.

22. Kagan AR, Schulz RJ. Proton-beam therapy for prostate cancer. Cancer J 2010; 16(5):405–9.

23. Alicikus ZA, Yamada Y, Zhang Z, et al. Ten-year outcomes of high-dose, intensity-modulated radiotherapy for localized prostate cancer. Cancer 2011;117: 1429–37.

24. Sheets NC, Goldin GH, Meyer AM, et al. Intensity-modulated radiation therapy, proton therapy, or conformal radiation therapy and morbidity and disease control in localized prostate cancer. JAMA 2012;307(15):1611–20.

25. Trikalinos TA, Terasawa T, Ip S, et al. Systematic review: charged-particle radiation therapy for cancer. Ann Intern Med 2009;151(8):556.

26. Konski A, Speier W, Hanlon A, et al. Is proton beam therapy cost effective in the treatment of adenocarcinoma of the prostate? J Clin Oncol 2007;25(24): 3603–8.

27. PTCOG. 2011. Available at: http://ptcog.web.psi.ch/ptcentres.html. Accessed March 28, 2012.

28. Nigro ND, Vaitkevicius VK, Buroker T, et al. Combined therapy for cancer of the anal canal. Dis Colon Rectum 1981;24(2):73–5.

29. Kimple RJ. Strategizing the clone wars: pharmacological control of cellular sensitivity to radiation. Mol Interv 2010;10(6):341–53.

30. Verheij M, Vens C, van Triest B. Novel therapeutics in combination with radiotherapy to improve cancer treatment: rationale, mechanisms of action and clinical perspective. Drug Resist Updat 2010;13(1–2):29–43.

31. Bonner JA, Harari PM, Giralt J, et al. Radiotherapy plus cetuximab for locoregionally advanced head and neck cancer: 5-year survival data from a phase 3 randomised trial, and relation between cetuximab-induced rash and survival. Lancet Oncol 2010;11(1):21–8.

32. Rouleau M, Patel A, Hendzel MJ, et al. PARP inhibition: PARP1 and beyond. Nat Rev Cancer 2010;10(4):293–301.

33. Chalmers AJ, Lakshman M, Chan N, et al. Poly(ADP-ribose) polymerase inhibition as a model for synthetic lethality in developing radiation oncology targets. Semin Radiat Oncol 2010;20(4):274–81.

34. Hanahan D, Weinberg RA. The hallmarks of cancer. Cell 2000;100(1):57–70.

35. Verbrugge I, Wissink EH, Rooswinkel RW, et al. Combining radiotherapy with APO010 in cancer treatment. Clin Cancer Res 2009;15(6):2031–8.

36. Hensley ML, Hagerty KL, Kewalramani T, et al. American Society of Clinical Oncology 2008 clinical practice guideline update: use of chemotherapy and radiation therapy protectants. J Clin Oncol 2009;27(1):127–45.

37. Citrin D, Cotrim AP, Hyodo F, et al. Radioprotectors and mitigators of radiation-induced normal tissue injury. Oncologist 2010;15(4):360–71.

38. Metz JM, Smith D, Mick R, et al. A phase I study of topical Tempol for the prevention of alopecia induced by whole brain radiotherapy. Clin Cancer Res 2004; 10(19):6411–7.

39. Torigian DA, Huang SS, Houseni M, et al. Functional imaging of cancer with emphasis on molecular techniques. CA Cancer J Clin 2007;57(4):206–24.

40. Das SK, Ten Haken RK. Functional and molecular image guidance in radiotherapy treatment planning optimization. Semin Radiat Oncol 2011;21(2):111–8.

41. Levin CS. Primer on molecular imaging technology. Eur J Nucl Med Mol Imaging 2005;32(Suppl 2):S325–45.

42. Wahl RL, Herman JM, Ford E. The promise and pitfalls of positron emission tomography and single-photon emission computed tomography molecular imaging-guided radiation therapy. Semin Radiat Oncol 2011;21(2):88–100.

43. Ciernik IF, Dizendorf E, Baumert BG, et al. Radiation treatment planning with an integrated positron emission and computer tomography (PET/CT): a feasibility study. Int J Radiat Oncol Biol Phys 2003;57(3):853–63.

44. van Baardwijk A, Baumert BG, Bosmans G, et al. The current status of FDG-PET in tumour volume definition in radiotherapy treatment planning. Cancer Treat Rev 2006;32(4):245–60.

45. Grosu AL, Weber WA. PET for radiation treatment planning of brain tumours. Radiother Oncol 2010;96(3):325–7.

46. Rasey JS, Grierson JR, Wiens LW, et al. Validation of FLT uptake as a measure of thymidine kinase-1 activity in A549 carcinoma cells. J Nucl Med 2002;43(9): 1210–7.

47. Vesselle H, Grierson J, Muzi M, et al. In vivo validation of 3'deoxy-3'-[(18)F]fluorothymidine ([(18)F]FLT) as a proliferation imaging tracer in humans: correlation of [(18)F]FLT uptake by positron emission tomography with Ki-67 immunohistochemistry and flow cytometry in human lung tumors. Clin Cancer Res 2002; 8(11):3315–23.

48. Troost EG, Bussink J, Hoffmann AL, et al. 18F-FLT PET/CT for early response monitoring and dose escalation in oropharyngeal tumors. J Nucl Med 2010; 51(6):866–74.

49. Bentzen SM, Gregoire V. Molecular imaging-based dose painting: a novel paradigm for radiation therapy prescription. Semin Radiat Oncol 2011;21(2):101–10.

50. Durand E, Prigent A. The basics of renal imaging and function studies. Q J Nucl Med 2002;46(4):249–67.

51. Partridge M, Yamamoto T, Grau C, et al. Imaging of normal lung, liver and parotid gland function for radiotherapy. Acta Oncol 2010;49(7):997–1011.

52. McGuire SM, Menda Y, Ponto LL, et al. A methodology for incorporating functional bone marrow sparing in IMRT planning for pelvic radiation therapy. Radiother Oncol 2011;99(1):49–54.

53. Kavanagh BD, Miften M, Rabinovitch RA. Advances in treatment techniques: stereotactic body radiation therapy and the spread of hypofractionation. Cancer J 2011;17(3):177–81.

54. Bentzen SM, Agrawal RK, Aird EG, et al. The UK Standardisation of Breast Radiotherapy (START) Trial A of radiotherapy hypofractionation for treatment of early breast cancer: a randomised trial. Lancet Oncol 2008;9(4):331–41.

55. Bentzen SM, Agrawal RK, Aird EG, et al. The UK Standardisation of Breast Radiotherapy (START) Trial B of radiotherapy hypofractionation for treatment of early breast cancer: a randomised trial. Lancet 2008;371(9618):1098–107.
56. Whelan TJ, Pignol JP, Levine MN, et al. Long-term results of hypofractionated radiation therapy for breast cancer. N Engl J Med 2010;362(6):513–20.
57. Ko EC, Forsythe K, Buckstein M, et al. Radiobiological rationale and clinical implications of hypofractionated radiation therapy. Cancer Radiother 2011;15(3): 221–9.
58. Arcangeli G, Saracino B, Gomellini S, et al. A prospective phase III randomized trial of hypofractionation versus conventional fractionation in patients with high-risk prostate cancer. Int J Radiat Oncol Biol Phys 2010;78(1):11–8.
59. Norkus D, Miller A, Plieskiene A, et al. A randomized trial comparing hypofractionated and conventionally fractionated three-dimensional conformal external-beam radiotherapy for localized prostate adenocarcinoma: a report on the first-year biochemical response. Medicina (Kaunas) 2009;45(6):469–75.
60. Pollack A, Hanlon AL, Horwitz EM, et al. Dosimetry and preliminary acute toxicity in the first 100 men treated for prostate cancer on a randomized hypofractionation dose escalation trial. Int J Radiat Oncol Biol Phys 2006;64(2):518–26.
61. Oh BC, Pagnini PG, Wang MY, et al. Stereotactic radiosurgery: adjacent tissue injury and response after high-dose single fraction radiation: part I–histology, imaging, and molecular events. Neurosurgery 2007;60(1):31–44 [discussion: 44–5].
62. Anker CJ, Shrieve DC. Basic principles of radiobiology applied to radiosurgery and radiotherapy of benign skull base tumors. Otolaryngol Clin North Am 2009; 42(4):601–21.
63. Nguyen NP, Garland L, Welsh J, et al. Can stereotactic fractionated radiation therapy become the standard of care for early stage non-small cell lung carcinoma. Cancer Treat Rev 2008;34(8):719–27.
64. Ganz JC. Gamma knife neurosurgery. New York: Springer; 2010.
65. Elaimy AL, Mackay AR, Lamoreaux WT, et al. Clinical outcomes of stereotactic radiosurgery in the treatment of patients with metastatic brain tumors. World Neurosurg 2011;75(5–6):673–83.
66. Andrews DW, Scott CB, Sperduto PW, et al. Whole brain radiation therapy with or without stereotactic radiosurgery boost for patients with one to three brain metastases: phase III results of the RTOG 9508 randomised trial. Lancet 2004; 363(9422):1665–72.
67. Aoyama H, Shirato H, Tago M, et al. Stereotactic radiosurgery plus whole-brain radiation therapy vs stereotactic radiosurgery alone for treatment of brain metastases: a randomized controlled trial. JAMA 2006;295(21):2483–91.
68. Chang EL, Wefel JS, Hess KR, et al. Neurocognition in patients with brain metastases treated with radiosurgery or radiosurgery plus whole-brain irradiation: a randomised controlled trial. Lancet Oncol 2009;10(11):1037–44.
69. Kondziolka D, Patel A, Lunsford LD, et al. Stereotactic radiosurgery plus whole brain radiotherapy versus radiotherapy alone for patients with multiple brain metastases. Int J Radiat Oncol Biol Phys 1999;45(2):427–34.
70. Patchell RA, Tibbs PA, Regine WF, et al. Postoperative radiotherapy in the treatment of single metastases to the brain: a randomized trial. JAMA 1998;280(17):1485–9.
71. Patchell RA, Tibbs PA, Walsh JW, et al. A randomized trial of surgery in the treatment of single metastases to the brain. N Engl J Med 1990;322(8):494–500.
72. McGarry RC, Papiez L, Williams M, et al. Stereotactic body radiation therapy of early-stage non-small-cell lung carcinoma: phase I study. Int J Radiat Oncol Biol Phys 2005;63(4):1010–5.

73. Timmerman R, Paulus R, Galvin J, et al. Stereotactic body radiation therapy for inoperable early stage lung cancer. JAMA 2010;303(11):1070–6.
74. RTOG website. Available at: http://www.rtog.org/ClinicalTrials/ProtocolTable/ StudyDetails.aspx?study=1021. Accessed March 14, 2012.
75. Chan MD, Tatter SB, Lesser G, et al. Radiation oncology in brain tumors: current approaches and clinical trials in progress. Neuroimaging Clin N Am 2010;20(3): 401–8.
76. Martin A, Gaya A. Stereotactic body radiotherapy: a review. Clin Oncol (R Coll Radiol) 2010;22(3):157–72.

Index

Note: Page numbers of article titles are in **boldface** type.

A

Ablation, thermal. *See* Thermal ablation.
Anal canal squamous cell carcinoma, 525–532
    contemporary therapy, 526–528
    historical perspective, 525–526
    ongoing areas of investigation in, 528–532
        chemotherapy, 529–530
        imaging, 528–529
        radiation therapy, 530–532
Androgen deprivation therapy, external beam radiation therapy combined with, 487–488

B

Biopsy, role in surgery for extremity sarcomas, 435
Bone fracture, after radiotherapy for extremity sarcomas, 440
Brachytherapy, for definitive management of prostate cancer, 484–486
    for extremity sarcomas, 439
    image-guided, for gynecologic surgeons, **495–509**
        cautions and caveats, 507
        clinical results for, 502–504
        defining T2-weighted MRI targets, 501–502
        film-based treatment planning, 495
        high dose rate applications, 504–505
        interstitial, 505–507
        modern imaging of cervical cancer, 496–501
            computed tomography, 496–497
            magnetic resonance imaging, 497–498
            metabolic and functional imaging, 498–501
Brain tumors, radiotherapy and radiosurgery for, 446–461
    brain metastases, 448–451
        decision making, 450–451
        stereotactic radiosurgery with and without whole-brain, 450
        stereotactic radiosurgery with surgery, 450
        surgery with and without whole-brain, 449
        whole-brain with and without stereotactic radiosurgery, 449–450
        whole-brain with and without surgery, 448–449
    primary tumors, 451–453
        malignant gliomas, 451
        normal tissue toxicity, 453
        radiotherapy, 451–452
        surgery, 451
        surgery, radiotherapy, and chemotherapy, 452–453

Surg Oncol Clin N Am 22 (2013) 619–628
http://dx.doi.org/10.1016/S1055-3207(13)00039-2
1055-3207/13/$ – see front matter © 2013 Elsevier Inc. All rights reserved.

surgonc.theclinics.com

Brain (*continued*)
    radiotherapy techniques, 446–448
      intracranial stereotactic radiosurgery, 446–448
      whole-brain, 446
Breast cancer, radiotherapy after mastectomy, **563–577**
    changing paradigm, 565–566
    impact of neoadjuvant chemotherapy, 571–573
      preoperative nodal evaluation, 571–572
    risk stratification in node-negative cancer, 566–569
    role of genomic prediction tools, 569–571

C

Central nervous system, radiotherapy and radiosurgery for tumors of, **445–461**
    brain tumors, 446–453
    spine and spinal cord tumors, 453–456
Cervical cancer. *See* Gynecologic oncology.
Chemoradiation, for localized gastrointestinal cancers, **511–524**
    esophageal and gastroesophageal cancers, 512–515
    gastric cancer, 515–517
    pancreatic cancer, 517–530
Chemoradiotherapy, in rectal adenocarcinoma, 533–536
    new and investigational regimens, 536–538
Chemotherapy, for head and neck cancer, definitive radiation therapy and, 588–591
    in anal canal squamous cell carcinoma, 529–530
    neoadjuvant, post-mastectomy radiotherapy in setting of, 572–573
    with surgery and radiotherapy for malignant gliomas, 452–453
Colorectal cancer, combined modality therapy for, 414–425
    patient selection and evaluation, 414–417
    sequencing of, 417–418
      external beam radiation, 418
      future possibilities, 424
      intraoperative radiation, 420–424
      surgery for primary and recurrent cancers, 418–420
Combined modality treatment, integration of radiation oncology with surgery, **405–432**
    general patient selection, evaluation, and treatment factors, 406–408
      dose-limiting structures/treatment-related morbidity, 408
      EBRT doses and technique, 407–408
      IORT doses and technique, 408
      patient evaluation, 406–407
      patient selection criteria, 406
      sequencing of, 407
    patient selection and treatment factors by disease site, 408–429
      colorectal, 414–425
      pancreatic cancer, 408–414
      retroperitoneal sarcomas, 425–429
Computed tomography, of cervical cancer, 496–497

D

Doxorubicin, thermosensitive liposome formulations in treatment of hepatocellular carcinoma and hepatic metastases, **545–561**

E

Edema, after radiotherapy for extremity sarcomas, 440–441
Esophageal cancer, chemoradiation for localized, 512–515
    inoperable, 513–515
        current state, 513–514
        future directions, 514–515
    locally advanced resectable, 512–513
        chemotherapy or, 513
        neoadjuvant, 512–513
External beam radiation therapy (EBRT), for definitive management of prostate cancer, 486–488
    for extremity sarcomas, 437–439
    for palliation of metastatic disease in prostate cancer, 489
    for salvage therapy of prostate cancer after prostatectomy, 488–489
    for spine and spinal cord tumors, 453–454
    integration with surgery as combined modality treatment, **405–432**
        doses and technique, 407–408
Extremities, radiation oncology for sarcomas of, **433–443**
    complications of, 438–441
        bone fracture, 439
        edema, 439–441
        wound complications, 438–439
        wound reconstruction, 439
    evidence for use of radiotherapy, 436
    for unresected sarcomas, 436–437
    multidisciplinary evaluation of, 434
    staging workup, 434–435
    surgical considerations, 435–436
        role of biopsy, 435
        surgical margins, 435–436
    technical details of planning for, 437–439
        brachytherapy, 439
        EBRT, 437–439
        IORT, 439
        x-rays, electrons, and particle therapy, 439

F

Fractionation, nonstandard, in radiation oncology, 611–614
    extreme hypofractionation (radiosurgery), 612–614
    moderate hypofractionation, 612
Functional imaging, in radiation oncology, 608–611
    dose painting with, 610
    improved delineation of tumors with, 609–610
    sparing normal tissues with, 611
  of cervical cancer, 498–501

G

Gastric cancer, chemoradiation for localized, 515–517
Gastroesophageal cancer, chemoradiation for localized, 512–515

Gastrointestinal cancers, chemoradiation for localized, **511–524**
    esophageal and gastroesophageal cancers, 512–515
    gastric cancer, 515–517
    pancreatic cancer, 517–530
Genomic prediction tools, role in post-mastectomy radiotherapy, 549–571
Gliomas, malignant, radiotherapy and radiosurgery for, 451–453
Gynecologic oncology, image-guided brachytherapy in, **495–509**
    cautions and caveats, 507
    clinical results for, 502–504
    defining T2-weighted MRI targets, 501–502
    film-based treatment planning, 495
    high dose rate applications, 504–505
    interstitial, 505–507
    modern imaging of cervical cancer, 496–501
        computed tomography, 496–497
        magnetic resonance imaging, 497–498
        metabolic and functional imaging, 498–501

H

Head and neck cancer, contemporary radiotherapy in, **579–598**
    biologic basis and fractionation, 579–581
    principles of therapy, 585–591
        definitive, and chemotherapy, 588–591
        doses, 585–587
        surgery and radiation, 588
        surgery *vs.* radiation, 587–588
    treatment planning and delivery, 583–585
    treatment toxicity, 581–583
Hepatic metastases, treatment with thermal ablation and thermosensitive liposomes,
    545–561
Hepatocellular carcinoma, novel approach to treatment of hepatic metastases and,
    545–561
    chemotherapeutics and thermal ablation, 546–547
    doxorubicin liposome formulation, 547
    future directions, 554–556
    low-temperature-sensitive liposomal doxorubicin (LTSL-Dox), 549–554
        canine studies, 553–554
        human clinical studies, 554
        preclinical studies with, 551–553
    second-generation thermosensitive liposome formulations, 548
    thermal ablation, 546
    thermal ablation and liposomal doxorubicin, 547–548
High dose rate (HDR) brachytherapy, in gynecologic oncology, 504–505

I

Image guidance, in radiation oncology, 601–604
    for interfraction motion, 601–602
    for intrafraction motion, 602–603
    future of, 604

Image-guided brachytherapy. *See* Brachytherapy.

Imaging, in anal canal squamous cell carcinoma, 528–529

Integration, of radiation oncology with surgery as combined modality therapy, **405–432**

Intensity-modulated radiation therapy (IMRT), for definitive management of prostate cancer, 487

    for head and neck cancer, 582–586

    for rectal cancer, 538

Interstitial brachytherapy, image-guided, in gynecologic oncology, 507505

Intraoperative radiation therapy (IORT), for extremity sarcomas, 439

    integration with surgery as combined modality treatment, **405–432**

        doses and technique, 408

L

Liposomes, thermosensitive. *See* Thermosensitive liposomes.

Lung cancer, stereotactic body radiation therapy for primary and metastatic pulmonary malignancies, **463–481**

    complications and risks, 468

        brachial plexopathy, 468

        chest wall/skin toxicity, 468

        pulmonary toxicity, 468

    for pulmonary metastases, 470–476

        differences between treatment of, 475–476

        integrating with systemic therapy, 474–475

        rationale for treatment of limited, 470–474

    for stage I NSCLC, 464–467

    future directions in lung cancer, 469

        optimal dose-fractionation scheme, 469

        surgery *vs.*, 469

        systemic therapy, 469

M

Magnetic resonance imaging (MRI), defining T2-weighted targets in gynecologic oncology, 501–502

    T2-weighted, of cervical cancer, 497–498

Malignant glioma. *See* Gliomas, malignant.

Margins, surgical, role in extremity sarcoma treatment, 435–436

Mastectomy, radiotherapy after, **563–577**

        changing paradigm, 565–566

        impact of neoadjuvant chemotherapy, 571–573

            preoperative nodal evaluation, 571–572

        risk stratification in node-negative cancer, 566–569

        role of genomic prediction tools, 569–571

Metabolic imaging, of cervical cancer, 498–501

Metastatic disease, brain, radiotherapy and radiosurgery for, 448–451

    hepatic, treatment with thermal ablation and thermosensitive liposomes, **545–561**

    in prostate cancer, 488–490

        brachytherapy after definitive radiation, 488

        external beam radiotherapy after prostatectomy, 488–489

        external beam radiotherapy for palliation of, 489

        radiopharmaceuticals for palliation of, 489–490

Metastatic (*continued*)
    pulmonary, stereotactic body radiation therapy for, **463–481**
    to osseous spine, 455–456
Modulators, radiation, in radiation oncology, 607–608
        normal tissue protectors, 608
        radiation sensitizers, 607–608

   N

Neck cancer. *See* Head and neck cancer.
Neoadjuvant therapy, impact on post-mastectomy radiotherapy, 571–573
        in setting of neoadjuvant chemotherapy, 572–573
        preoperative nodal evaluation, 571–572
    short-course radiation therapy in rectal adenocarcinoma, 533–536
Non-small cell lung cancer (NSCLC). *See* Lung cancer.

   P

Pancreatic cancer, chemoradiation for localized, 517–520
        current state, 517–519
            future directions, 519–520
            locally advanced, 517–519
            resectable, 517
    combined modality therapy for, 408–414
        external beam radiation, 409–411
        future possibilities in, 414
        intraoperative radiation, 411
        outcomes in borderline resectable and unresectable, 412–414
        patient evaluation and selection, 408–409
        surgical technique, 411–412
Pancreaticoduodenectomy, technique in combined modality therapy, 411–412
Particle beam therapy, in radiation oncology, 604–607
        charged particle radiation, 605–607
            in practice, 606–607
            in theory, 605–606
        problem with x-rays, 604
Particle therapy, for extremity sarcomas, 439
Patient evaluation, pretreatment, for combined modality treatment with radiation and surgery, 406–407
Patient selection, for combined modality treatment with radiation and surgery, 406
Post-mastectomy radiotherapy. *See* Breast cancer.
Prostate cancer, radiation therapy for, **483–494**
        as definitive management, 484–488
            brachytherapy, 484–486
            external beam, 486–488
        palliation of metastatic disease, 489–490
            external beam, 489
            radiopharmaceuticals, 489–490
        salvage therapy with, 488–489
            brachytherapy after definitive radiation, 488
            external beam after prostatectomy, 488–489

Prostatectomy, external beam radiotherapy after, for prostate cancer salvage therapy, 489–490

Pulmonary malignancies, primary. *See* Lung cancer.

Pulmonary metastases. *See* Lung cancer.

R

Radiation modulators. *See* Modulators, radiation.

Radiation oncology, practical, for surgeons, 405–618

    after mastectomy, **563–577**

       changing paradigm, 565–566

       impact of nepoadjuvant chemotherapy, 571–573

       risk stratification in node-negative cancer, 566–569

       role of genomic prediction tools, 569–571

    chemoradiation for localized gastrointestinal cancers, **511–524**

       esophageal and gastroesophageal cancers, 512–515

       gastric cancer, 515–517

       pancreatic cancer, 517–530

    for anal and rectal cancer, **525–542**

       anal canal squamous cell carcinoma, 525–532

       rectal adenocarcinoma, 532–538

    for extremity sarcomas, **433–443**

       complications of, 438–441

       evidence for use of radiotherapy, 436

       for unresected sarcomas, 436–437

       multidisciplinary evaluation of, 434

       staging workup, 434–435

       surgical considerations, 435–436

       technical details of planning for, 437–438

    for head and neck cancer, **579–598**

       biologic basis and fractionation, 579–581

       principles of therapy, 585–591

       treatment planning and delivery, 583–585

       treatment toxicity, 581–583

    for hepatocellular carcinoma and hepatic metastases, **545–561**

       canine studies with low-temperature sensitive liposomal doxorubicin, 553–554

       chemotherapeutics and thermal ablation, 546–547

       doxorubicin liposome formulation, 547

       future directions, 554–556

       human clinical studies with LTSL-Dox, 554

       preclinical studies with LTSL-Dox, 551–553

       second-generation thermosensitive liposome formulations, 548

       thermal ablation, 546

       thermal ablation and liposomal doxorubicin, 547–548

    for prostate cancer, **483–494**

       as definitive management, 484–488

       palliation of metastatic disease, 489–490

       salvage therapy with, 488–489

    for tumors of central nervous system, **445–461**

       brain tumors, 446–453

       spine and spinal cord tumors, 453–456

Radiation (*continued*)

image-guided brachytherapy for gynecologic surgeons, **495–509**

cautions and caveats, 507

clinical results for, 502–504

defining T2-weighted MRI targets, 501–502

film-based treatment planning, 495

high dose rate applications, 504–505

interstitial, 505–507

modern imaging of cervical cancer, 496–501

integration with surgery as combined modality treatment, **405–432**

general patient selection, evaluation, and treatment factors, 406–408

patient selection and treatment factors by disease site, 408–429

novel approaches with, for hepatocellular carcinoma and hepatic metastases, **545–561**

present and future innovations in, **599–618**

functional imaging, 608–611

image guidance, 601–604

nonstandard fractionation, 611–614

particle beam therapy, 604–607

radiation modulators, 607–608

stereotactic body, for primary and metastatic pulmonary malignancies, **463–481**

complications and risks, 468

for NSCLC, 464–467

for pulmonary metastases, 470–476

future directions in lung cancer, 469

Radiopharmaceuticals, for palliation of metastatic disease in prostate cancer, 489–490

Radiosurgery, extreme hypofractionation, 612–614

stereotactic. *See* Stereotactic radiosurgery.

Rectal adenocarcinoma, 532–538

contemporary radiation therapy, 533–536

long-course chemoradiotherapy, 533–536

neoadjuvant short-course, 533–536

historical perspective on therapy, 532–533

intensity-modulated radiation therapy for, 538

new and investigational chemoradiotherapy regimens, 536–538

Retroperitoneal sarcomas, combined modality therapy for, 425–429

clinical trials, 427–428

EBRT and IORT factors, 425

outcomes of, 426

surgical factors, 425–426

surgical techniques, 426

S

Sarcomas, extremity, radiation therapy for, **433–443**

complications of, 438–441

bone fracture, 439

edema, 439–441

wound complications, 438–439

wound reconstruction, 439

evidence for use of radiotherapy, 436

for unresected sarcomas, 436–437
multidisciplinary evaluation of, 434
staging workup, 434–435
surgical considerations, 435–436
role of biopsy, 435
surgical margins, 435–436
technical details of planning for, 437–439
brachytherapy, 439
EBRT, 437–439
IORT, 439
x-rays, electrons, and particle therapy, 439
retroperitoneal, combined modality therapy for, 425–429
clinical trials, 427–428
EBRT and IORT factors, 425
outcomes of, 426
surgical factors, 425–426
surgical techniques, 426
Selection, patient, for combined modality treatment with radiation and surgery, 406
Sequencing, of radiation and surgery in combined modality therapy, 407
Soft tissue sarcomas. See Sarcomas.
Spinal cord, radiotherapy and radiosurgery for tumors of, 453–461
radiotherapy techniques, 453–454
EBRT, 453–454
metastatic disease to osseous spine, 455–456
primary spine tumors, 454
spinal stereotactic radiosurgery, 454
Spine, radiotherapy and radiosurgery for tumors of, 453–461
radiotherapy techniques, 453–454
EBRT, 453–454
metastatic disease to osseous, 455–456
primary, 454
spinal stereotactic radiosurgery, 454
Stereotactic body radiation therapy, for primary and metastatic pulmonary malignancies, **463–481**
complications and risks, 468
brachial plexopathy, 468
chest wall/skin toxicity, 468
pulmonary toxicity, 468
for pulmonary metastases, 470–476
differences between treatment of, 475–476
integrating with systemic therapy, 474–475
rationale for treatment of limited, 470–474
for stage I NSCLC, 464–467
future directions in lung cancer, 469
optimal dose-fractionation scheme, 469
surgery vs., 469
systemic therapy, 469
Stereotactic radiosurgery, for brain metastases, 449–451
whole-brain radiotherapy with and without, 449–450
with and without whole-brain radiotherapy, 450
with surgery, 450

Stereotactic (*continued*)
  intracranial, for brain tumors, 446–448
  spinal, 454
Surgery, for extremity sarcomas, 435–436
    as sole treatment for, 437
    role of biopsy, 435
    surgical margins, 435–436
  for head and neck cancer, 587–588
    and radiation therapy, 588
    vs. radiation therapy, 587–588
  for malignant gliomas, 451
    with radiotherapy and chemotherapy, 452–453
  integration with radiation oncology as combined modality therapy, **405–432**
    general patient selection, evaluation, and treatment factors, 406–408
      dose-limiting structures/treatment-related morbidity, 408
      EBRT doses and technique, 407–408
      IORT doses and technique, 408
      patient evaluation, 406–407
      patient selection criteria, 406
      sequencing of, 407
    patient selection and treatment factors by disease site, 408–429
      colorectal, 414–425
      pancreatic cancer, 408–414
      retroperitoneal sarcomas, 425–429
  vs. stereotactic body radiation therapy for primary and metastatic pulmonary
    malignancies, 469

T

Thermal ablation, and thermosensitive liposomes in treatment of hepatocellular carcinoma
  and hepatic metastases, **545–561**
Thermosensitive liposomes, wit thermal ablation for hepatocellular carcinoma and hepatic
  metastases, **545–561**
    chemotherapeutics and thermal ablation, 546–547
    doxorubicin liposome formulation, 547
    future directions, 554–556
    low-temperature-sensitive liposomal doxorubicin (LTSL-Dox), 549–554
      canine studies, 553–554
      human clinical studies, 554
      preclinical studies with, 551–553
    second-generation formulations, 548
    thermal ablation and liposomal doxorubicin, 547–548

W

Whole-brain radiotherapy, for brain metastases, 448–450
    surgery with and without, 449
    with and without stereotactic radiosurgery, 449–450
    with and without surgery, 448–449
  for brain tumors, 446
Wound complications, of radiotherapy for extremity sarcomas, 439–440

Printed and bound by CPI Group (UK) Ltd, Croydon, CR0 4YY

03/10/2024

01040442-0003